Pediatric Anesthesiology Revie

MÄNGELEXEMPLAR

37,-
41,-
Med /Täd.

Robert S. Holzman · Thomas J. Mancuso
Navil F. Sethna · James A. DiNardo

Pediatric Anesthesiology Review

Clinical Cases for Self-Assessment

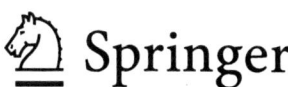 Springer

Robert S. Holzman, MD, FAAP
Senior Associate in Perioperative
Anesthesia
Children's Hospital Boston
Associate Professor of Anaesthesia
Harvard Medical School
Boston, MA
robert.holzman@childrens.harvard.edu

Navil F. Sethna, MB, ChB
Senior Associate in Perioperative
Anesthesia and Pain Medicine
Children's Hospital Boston
Associate Professor of Anaesthesia
Harvard Medical School
Boston, MA
navil.sethna@childrens.harvard.edu

Thomas J. Mancuso, MD, FAAP
Senior Associate in Perioperative
Anesthesia, Critical Care Medicine and
Pain Medicine
Department of Anesthesiology,
Perioperative and Pain Medicine
Children's Hospital Boston
Assistant Professor of Anaesthesia
Harvard Medical School
Boston, MA
thomas.mancuso@childrens.harvard.edu

James A. DiNardo, MD
Senior Associate in Cardiac Anesthesia
Children's Hospital Boston
Associate Professor of Anaesthesia
Harvard Medical School
Boston, MA
james.dinardo@childrens.harvard.edu

Additional material to this book can be download from http://extra.springer.com

ISBN 978-1-4419-1616-7   e-ISBN 978-1-4419-1617-4
DOI 10.1007/978-1-4419-1617-4
Springer New York Dordrecht Heidelberg London

Library of Congress Control Number: 2010925116

Printed on acid-free paper

Springer is part of Springer Science+Business Media (www.springer.com)

Preface

This text is designed for those who would become consultants in pediatric anesthesia. It is based on a curriculum developed over 15 years in our department to illustrate the breadth and depth of the practice of pediatric anesthesia, consisting of weekly meetings between our fellows and many of our faculty who are or who have been associate examiners of the American Board of Anesthesiology. The program is an integral part of the didactic series in the Department of Anesthesiology, Perioperative and Pain Medicine at Children's Hospital Boston.

An ability to explain *why* various data are required before or during the care of a patient or *why* a certain anesthesia care plan was chosen was critical to us in our philosophy of the course, and we have tried to preserve that ideal during the crafting of this text. Although the interactive aspect of a dialog between examiner and examinee cannot be effectively recreated through a textbook, the reader is encouraged – strongly so – to use this book in creative ways to try to mimic the spontaneity achievable through conversation. First of all, a "buddy" system is advisable. Secondly, a small hand-held tape recorder is extremely useful when using the questions as prompts; the contemplative reader will listen critically to the responses he or she has offered into the tape and then hopefully improve as the taping continues. Using materiality as the best endpoint for adequate answers, the discerning reader should attempt to answer the question to the satisfaction of an imaginary partner – whether a parent, a surgeon, a pediatrician, or another anesthesiology colleague calling for help. With practice and introspection, it is amazing how similar, rather than different, the answers are to these diverse audiences.

The written examinations, seen at the beginning of the text as a baseline in pediatric medicine, are primarily knowledge-based, reflecting factual medical information necessary for the subspecialty practice of pediatric anesthesiology.

With this basic guidance, the reader is encouraged to be creative throughout this book to use imagination as well as a fund of knowledge in bringing yourself "into the operating room" and managing the patient in an expert fashion, one that would, in the eyes of peers as well as patients and their families, merit the awarding of "consultant in pediatric anesthesiology."

Boston, MA   Robert S. Holzman
                                                                                Thomas J. Mancuso
                                                                                 Navil F. Sethna
                                                                                James A. DiNardo

Contents

Supplementary materials including interactive quiz available at
extras.springer.com

Part I
Pediatric Medicine for Pediatric Anesthesiologists

Chapter 1
Newborn Medicine

R.S. Holzman et al., *Pediatric Anesthesiology Review: Clinical Cases for Self-Assessment,*
DOI 10.1007/978-1-4419-1617-4_1, © Springer Science+Business Media, LLC 2010

1. In the neonatal period (day 0–28 of life), mortality is higher than any other period in infancy and childhood. Regarding neonatal mortality the following are true:

   1. It is inversely correlated with birth weight with most deaths occurring in neonates with birth weights <1.5 kg.
   2. It is most commonly due to prematurity and its complications.
   3. Most neonatal deaths occur in the first week of life.
   4. The high neonatal mortality in African-American babies is due to the higher rate of premature births in this group.

      A. 1, 2, 3
      B. 1, 3
      C. 2, 4
      D. 4 only
      E. All of the above

2. Regarding apnea of prematurity:

   1. It occurs in nearly all infants born weighing <1,000 gm.
   2. It usually resolves by 36–37 weeks postconceptual age (PCA).
   3. It is treated with theophylline or caffeine.
   4. Infants with this problem require home monitoring until 60 weeks PCA.

      A. 1, 2, 3
      B. 1, 3
      C. 2, 4
      D. 4 only
      E. All of the above

3. Which of the following are associated with poor fetal growth and therefore SGA births?

   1. Reduced uteroplacental blood flow
   2. Intrauterine infection
   3. Chromosomal abnormalities
   4. Poor maternal nutrition

      A. 1, 2, 3
      B. 1, 3
      C. 2, 4
      D. 4 only
      E. All of the above

1. E. All of the above

Low birth weight, which is distinct from preterm birth (see definitions), occurs in approximately 7% of live births in the USA. Mortality of low birth weight infants is higher than mortality of normal birth weight infants by approximately the following:

- MLBW(moderately low birth weight 1,501–2,500 gm) 40 times increased
- VLBW (very low birth weight 1,000–1,500 gm) 200 times increased
- ELBW (extremely low birth weight <1,000 gm) 600 times increased

Mortality for low birth weight infants has decreased with improvements in newborn care. Common causes for mortality in the newborn are different for term and preterm newborns.

Term: congenital anomalies, birth asphyxia, infection, meconium aspiration syndrome.
Preterm: respiratory distress syndrome (RDS), intraventricular hemorrhage (IVH), infection, necrotizing enterocolitis (NEC)

The LBW (<2,500 gm) rate in the USA has increased from 6.6 to 7.5% from 1981 to 1997. The US still lags behind many industrialized countries in neonatal mortality while the rate of teen pregnancy exceeds that of many industrialized countries.

2. A. 1, 2, 3

Apnea is defined as cessation of air flow into the lungs for a specified period of time, usually 1–20 s. Once the known potential causes for apnea have been ruled out, the diagnosis of apnea of prematurity can be made. Infants with apnea of prematurity may be discharged home without monitoring provided they have had 7–10 days free of apneac spells. The incidence of SIDS does increase with decreasing birth weight but apnea of prematurity is not an independent risk factor for SIDS.

3. E. All of the above

Intrauterine growth restriction can be considered a final common pathway for a myriad of influences on the fetus including genetic factors and environmental influences. The intrauterine environment is determined by uterine blood flow, placental function, and placental and umbilical circulation. Maternal factors which affect birth weight include maternal weight gain, maternal age, and medical conditions such as hypertension or diabetes mellitus.

4. What maintenance fluid would you order for a 2 kg, 2 week old who will be NPO for 6 h?

  A. D_5 0.2 NS at 8 mL/h
  B. D_{10} 0.45 NS at 10 mL/h
  C. D_5 LR at 10 mL/h
  D. D_5 0.45 NS at 12 mL/h

5. Which of the following is (are) true regarding maintenance fluids electrolytes and glucose administration to the newborn after the first week of life?

  1. Approximately 100–125 mL/kg/day of water will replace urine output and insensible losses.
  2. Glucose utilization, 6–10 mg/kg/min, can be supplied with D10 given at 100 mL/kg/day.
  3. Excessive sodium losses, due to renal tubular immaturity, must be replaced with 0.9% NS.
  4. Preterm newborns require less fluid than term infants because of their decreased urine output.

  A. 1, 2, 3
  B. 1, 3
  C. 2, 4
  D. 4 only
  E. All of the above

6. Newborns have a difficulty maintaining temperature because:

  1. They have a large surface area relative to their weight.
  2. Their increased tone leads to excessive heat loss.
  3. Shivering thermogenesis is limited.
  4. Brown fat is a poor insulator.

  A. 1, 2, 3
  B. 1, 3
  C. 2, 4
  D. 4 only
  E. All of the above

4. D. D_5 0.2 NS at 8 mL/h

Water administration to term older infants and children is related to caloric expenditure in the following manner on a 1 mL/cal basis.

- 0–10 kg; 100 cal/kg/day divided by 24 h/day = 4 mL/kg/h
- 10–20 kg: 50 cal/kg/day divided by 24 h/day = 2/mL/kg/h
- >20 kg: 20 cal/kg/day divided by 24 h/day = 1 mL/kg/h

Sodium requirements are in the neighborhood of 2–3 mEq/kg/day. 0.2–0.45% NS is adequate for sodium replenishment for children up to 45 kg.

Fluid requirements for the newborn change dramatically in the first few days of life. For DOL #1 the fluid needed by the newborn is 60–80 mL/kg/day, gradually increasing to 100–140 mL/kg/day over the subsequent several days. D_{10} provides sufficient glucose to the newborn.

5. A. 1, 2, 3

The newborn has higher insensible fluid losses than older children. Transdermal evaporative losses are affected by the ambient temperature while respiratory evaporative losses are affected by the humidity. Maintenance glucose requirements can be met with the administration of 6–8 mg/kg/min. D_5 at 100 mL/kg/day provides 5 g/kg/day or 5,000 mg/kg/day of glucose or 3.5 mg/kg/min (5,000 mg/kg/day × 1 day/1440 min/day = 3.5 mg/kg/min). D_{10} given at 100 mL/kg/day will provide 6.7 mg/kg/min of glucose. Normal newborns lose little sodium in the first few days of life, often receiving only D_{10}W during the first 24 h of life. Preterm newborns require more fluid because of increased transdermal losses.

6. B. 1, 3

Surface area/weight in a newborn is 3 times that of an adult. Newborns lose heat at a rate approximately 4 times that of adults. Nonshivering thermogenesis, which occurs in the brown fat, is a neonatal response to cold. In nonshivering thermogenesis, fat is oxidized and oxygen consumption is increased.

7. The neutral thermal environment for a 10-day-old 1.5 kg infant lying on a warm
   mattress in a draft free room of moderate humidity:

   1. Is a room temperature of 34–35°C
   2. Is the environment at which the baby will be actively warmed
   3. Is the environment at which 02 consumption is lowest
   4. Includes warming lights

   A. 1, 2, 3
   B. 1, 3
   C. 2, 4
   D. 4 only
   E. All of the above

8. The Apgar score:

   1. Has a 0–10 scale
   2. Is a useful guide to interventions needed in neonatal resuscitation
   3. Can be used to estimate the likelihood of neonatal acidosis
   4. Was developed in the 1950s by Virginia Apgar, an anesthesiologist

   A. 1, 2, 3
   B. 1, 3
   C. 2, 4
   D. 4 only
   E. All of the above

9. The Apgar score includes all of the following, which are scored 0–2, except:

   1. Heart rate
   2. Presence of gag reflex
   3. Respiratory effort
   4. Tone
   5. Reflex irritability
   6. Color

   A. 1
   B. 2
   C. 3
   D. 4
   E. 5
   F. 6

7. B. 1, 3

The neutral thermal environment is one with the ambient temperature in which the newborn loses the least amount of heat while maintaining normal body temperature. A neutral thermal environment is one in which the infants neither gain nor lose heat. The newborn loses heat by four means:

Convection to the cooler surrounding air
Conduction to the cooler surfaces which contact the newborn's skin
Radiation to nearby solid objects and
Evaporation from moist skin and lungs

Newborns respond to ambient temperature below the neutral thermal environment with increased oxygen consumption to produce heat. The increased oxygen consumption response is limited, however, and once this occurs the temperature of the newborn begins to fall.

8. E. All of the above

This score is of value in assessment of the newborn at birth and the effectiveness of any resuscitation efforts. Apgar scores at 1 and 5 min correlate poorly with longer-term neurologic outcome. The American Academy of Pediatrics and American College of Obstetrics and Gynecology emphasize using the Apgar score only as a tool in evaluating the condition of the newborn at the time of birth.

9. B.

The Apgar score range is 0–10. Term newborns without congenital anomalies with a normal cardiopulmonary adaptation to extrauterine life should have a score of 8–9. Newborns with a score of 0–3 require resuscitation. Most cases of low Apgar scores are due to inadequate ventilation, not to cardiac causes.

In her original work (Apgar, V. Current Research in Anesthesia and Analgesia 1953:32;260), Dr Virginia Apgar demonstrated that the score could differentiate between infants born to mothers who had general vs. spinal anesthesia.

10. A newborn whose Apgar score was 2 at 1 min has been intubated and is being adequately and appropriately ventilated. The heart rate is now 70/min. The next intervention should be:

1. Volume expansion with 10 cc/kg isotonic fluid
2. Correction of acidosis with NaHCO3, 1 Meq/kg slowly
3. Observation and active warming in the special care nursery
4. Closed cardiac massage

    A. 1, 2, 3
    B. 1, 3
    C. 2, 4
    D. 4 only
    E. All of the above

11. Intraventricular hemorrhage in preterm infants has been associated with:

1. Acidosis
2. Hypoxemia
3. Cerebral blood flow alterations
4. Germinal matrix hyperplasia

    A. 1, 2, 3
    B. 1, 3
    C. 2, 4
    D. 4 only
    E. All of the above

12. Possible consequences of germinal matrix (GMH)/intraventricular hemorrhage (IVH) include:

1. A normal neurologic exam after grade I IVH
2. Posthemorrhagic hydrocephalus (PHH)
3. Motor and cognitive deficits in 50% of infants with grade IV IVH
4. Hydrocephalus in virtually all infants with grade III–IV IVH

    A. 1, 2, 3
    B. 1, 3
    C. 2, 4
    D. 4 only
    E. All of the above

10. D.

The goals of neonatal resuscitation are to prevent morbidity and mortality of hypoxic-ischemic damage and to reestablish spontaneous respiratory effort and cardiac output. Although the 1-min Apgar score is useful in evaluation of the newborn, there are occasions when intervention should be immediate. Please review resuscitation of the newborn in one of the references.

11. A. 1, 2, 3

Immature vessels in the gelatinous subependymal germinal matrix of preterm newborns are subject to various forces predisposing the preterm to intraventricular hemorrhage (IVH). Contributory factors include: prematurity, respiratory distress syndrome (RDS), pneumothorax, hypotension, hypertension, and increased venous pressure. Most IVH occurs within the first week of life and can present with seizures, apnea, cardiovascular instability, and acidosis. The risk for IVH decreases with increasing gestational age. In many surveys, approximately one-half of infants with birth weights <1,500 gm have imaging evidence of IVH.

12. E. All of the above

The incidence of IVH increases with decreasing birth weight: 60–70% of 500–750 gm infants and 10–20% of 1,000–1,500 gm infants have IVH. There are four grades defined by ultrasound (done through the anterior fontanelle):

Grade I.   Bleeding in germinal matrix
Grade II.   Blood in ventricle filling <50% of the ventricle
Grade III.   >50% of ventricle filled with blood
Grade IV.   Grade III+intraparenchymal blood

Marked clinical deterioration (apnea, seizures, metabolic acidosis, decreased tone) accompanies the occurrence of the IVH, usually within the first week of life. Neurological sequelae are more severe in newborns with the more severe grades of IVH.

13. The initial laboratory evaluation of a healthy neonate with normal perinatal history who has a brief seizure should include:

    1. Measurement of electrolytes, Ca, glucose
    2. Neuro imaging
    3. An EEG
    4. A lumbar puncture

        A. 1, 2, 3
        B. 1, 3
        C. 2, 4
        D. 4 only
        E. All of the above

14. Regarding neonatal respiratory distress syndrome (RDS):

    1. It is rare in infants born after 30 weeks gestation.
    2. It is due to surfactant deficiency.
    3. Lung compliance is decreased in infants with RDS.
    4. It is associated with the premature closure of the PDA (patent ductus arteriosus).

        A. 1, 2, 3
        B. 1, 3
        C. 2, 4
        D. 4 only
        E. All of the above

15. Which of the following are features of RDS?

    1. Grunting
    2. Nasal flaring
    3. Air bronchograms on CXR
    4. Central cyanosis with peripheral plethora

        A. 1, 2, 3
        B. 1, 3
        C. 2, 4
        D. 4 only
        E. All of the above

13. E. All of the above

The most common cause of seizures in the newborn is hypoxic-ischemic encephal-opathy. Other causes include: infectious, metabolic, hemorrhagic (see above), and structural abnormalities. Seizure types in the newborn include:

Myoclonic, involving the extremities
Focal, often involving the facial muscles
Subtle, involving chewing, blinking, respiratory alterations including apnea and
Multifocal clonic seizures

14. A. 1, 2, 3

RDS occurs in approximately 75% of infants born at <28 weeks gestation and in about 5% of those born after 37 weeks. Increased incidence (controlling for gestational age) is seen in infants of diabetic mothers, multifetal pregnancies, and cesarean delivery. Preterm white males have the highest incidence. Surfactant deficiency leads to higher surface tension within alveoli, the development of atelectaisis, and a decreased FRC leading to hypoxemia.

15. A. 1, 2, 3

Rapid, shallow breathing, indicative of poor compliance, is seen within minutes of birth in RDS. The natural course is one of progressive cyanosis and dyspnea. Newborns with RDS exhibit nasal flaring, grunting (in an effort to develop end-expiratory distending airway pressure), and tachypnea. Affected, untreated infants may develop mixed acidosis, hypotension, temperature instability, and apnea.

16. Therapies for RDS include:

    1. Distending airway pressure
    2. Administrative of sodium bicarbonates
    3. Surfactant administration
    4. Hypertonic fluid administration

       A. 1, 2, 3
       B. 1, 3
       C. 2, 4
       D. 4 only
       E. All of the above

17. Transient tachypnea of the newborn (TTN):

    A. Is primarily seen in prematures born between 30 and 34 weeks of gestation
    B. Can progress to chronic lung disease if untreated
    C. Resolves within 24–48 h
    D. Has a CXR identical to that seen with RDS

18. The ductus arteriosus:

    1. Has right to left blood flow in the normal fetus
    2. Closes in the postnatal period as a result of higher oxygen tension in the blood
    3. If open in the preterm, may lead to congestive heart failure
    4. If open in the newborn, causes a characteristic harsh diastolic murmur

       A. 1, 2, 3
       B. 1, 3
       C. 2, 4
       D. 4 only
       E. All of the above

19. The diagnosis of PDA is supported by:

    A. The presence of a shadow at the aortic knob on CXR
    B. The presence of diminished peripheral pulses due to excessive pulmonary blood flow
    C. The presence of pulses paradoxicus
    D. The findings of bounding pulses, tachypnea, and a systolic murmur

16. B. 1, 3

Impaired gas exchange in the lung is the basic pathophysiology requiring treatment. Warm humidified oxygen should be given to maintain $SpO_2 > 90\%$. If this is not accomplished with an F_iO_2 of 60%, CPAP via nasal prongs should be started. At this point administration of exogenous surfactant via endotracheal tube should also be considered and assisted mechanical ventilation may be needed. Surfactant administration should be started within the first 24 h of life and may be repeated every 6–12 h for up to 2–4 doses depending upon the clinical situation.

17. C. Resolves within 24–48 h

TTN is seen in newborns following an uneventful term vaginal or cesarean delivery. The infants may have a minimal oxygen requirement. TTN resolves within 2–3 days. It is thought to be due to delayed absorption of fetal lung fluid. CXR will show prominent pulmonary vascular markings, fluid lines in the fissures, and overaeration.

18. A. 1, 2, 3

In the fetus, RV output is 66% of the combined ventricular output and the ductus arteriosus carries 90% of that RV output to the descending aorta, with 10% going to the lungs. In the normal newborn, the patent ductus arteriosus (PDA) may have a continuous murmur, often described as machine-like. In newborns, a large PDA may present with bounding pulses, cardiomegaly, and other signs of CHF. Bounding peripheral pulses are the result of increased LV stroke volume due to the increased LV volume load and diastolic runoff due to the low diastolic pressure. A small PDA may be asymptomatic.

19. D. The findings of bounding pulses, tachypnea, and a systolic murmur

The CXR in a newborn with a large PDA will show increased pulmonary vascular markings and possibly cardiomegaly. The ECHO will show an enlarged left atrium, picked up by an abnormal LA/Ao ratio and flow through the PDA itself can be detected by Doppler. The ductus can often be seen with 2D ECHO. The LA is enlarged due to the R to L shunt through the PDA. Spontaneous closure of the PDA beyond infancy is rare. The risk of endarteritis is such that all PDAs should be closed either surgically or via catheter closure.

20. Which of the following maternal/perinatal factors is (are) often associated with congenital heart disease?

    1. The presence of a chromosomal abnormality
    2. Maternal rubella infection
    3. Maternal alcohol abuse during pregnancy
    4. Maternal cocaine use during pregnancy

        A. 1, 2, 3
        B. 1, 3
        C. 2, 4
        D. 4 only
        E. All of the above

21. In persistent pulmonary hypertension of the newborn (PPHN):

    1. Pulmonary blood flow is decreased.
    2. There is systemic hypoxemia.
    3. Blood flow through the PDA is right to left.
    4. The systemic vascular resistance is much lower than it was during fetal life.

        A. 1, 2, 3
        B. 1, 3
        C. 2, 4
        D. 4 only
        E. All of the above

22. At birth, the right ventricle:

    A. Is hypoplastic
    B. Is approximately as thick walled as the left ventricle
    C. Has much thicker walls than the left ventricle
    D. Has poor contractility until PVR decreases

23. Which of the following congenital heart defects is the most common in full-term newborns?

    A. Coarctation of the aorta
    B. Tetralogy of fallot
    C. Patent ductus arteriosus
    D. Ventricular septal defect
    E. Hypoplastic left heart syndrome

20. A. 1, 2, 3

Infants born to mothers who abused cocaine have many problems but an increased incidence of congenital heart disease is not one of them. Problems these children *do* have as a result of intrapartum cocaine exposure include spontaneous abortion, preterm birth, IUGR, microcephalus, abnormal EEG, poor expressive language and verbal comprehension and later behavioral problems.

21. A. 1, 2, 3

PPHN may occur in term and postterm infants after birth asphyxia, meconium aspiration, group B streptococal sepsis, or polycythemia. The normal decline in pulmonary vascular resistance (PVR) which usually occurs after birth does not occur. Excessively high PVR leads to a return to a fetal pattern of circulation, with increased right to left flow through the PDA from the RV and markedly diminished pulmonary blood flow. Labile hypoxemia, out of proportion to CXR findings, is seen. Hypoxemia, hypercarbia, and acidosis worsen the degree of pulmonary vaso-constriction. A transthoracic echocardiogram can confirm the diagnosis and rule out other causes of profound hypoxemia such as congenital heart disease.

22. B. Is approximately as thick walled as the left ventricle

During fetal life the RV delivers approximately 90% of its output to the systemic circulation via the open ductus arteriosus and 10% to the very high resistance pulmonary circulation. The ECG of a newborn shows prominent right-sided forces with right axis deviation and large R waves. The upright T waves in the precordial leads seen at birth often revert to negative within a few days of birth.

23. D. Ventricular septal defect

Ventricular septal defects (VSD) comprise approximately 25% of all congenital cardiac lesions, exclusive of PDA's in preterms, bicuspid aortic valves, and peripheral pulmonic stenosis. The majority are of the membranous type, located posteroinferi-orly, anterior to the septal leaflet of the tricuspid valve. The severity of the VSD can be characterized by the ratio of pulmonary to systemic flow (Qp:Qs). An infant with a ventricular septal defect with a Qp:Qs>2:1 will exhibit clinical signs and symp-toms of congestive heart failure (CHF) such as effortless tachypnea, diaphoresis, and poor feeding (the equivalent of "exercise intolerance" in the newborn).

24. Hypoglycemia is seen in the following neonates:

    1. SGA newborns
    2. Infants with polycythemia/hyperviscosity
    3. Preterm newborns
    4. Infants with Beckwith–Wiedeman Syndrome (macroglossia, visceromegaly, omphalocele)

       A. 1, 2, 3
       B. 1, 3
       C. 2, 4
       D. 4 only
       E. All of the above

25. Hypoglycemia in the term neonate:

    1. Is diagnosed only by the presence of signs and symptoms not a specific number
    2. Should only be treated if it occurs after the first 3–4 h of life
    3. Is very rarely seen in large, term infants
    4. Can be defined as a glucose of <40 gm%

       A. 1, 2, 3
       B. 1, 3
       C. 2, 4
       D. 4 only
       E. All of the above

26. Symptoms and signs of hypoglycemia in the neonates include:

    1. Tremors or seizures
    2. Apnea
    3. Lethargy
    4. Poor feeding

       A. 1, 2, 3
       B. 1, 3
       C. 2, 4
       D. 4 only
       E. All of the above

24. E. All of the above

There are four groups of newborns at risk for hypoglycemia: infants of diabetic mothers, IUGR newborns, very immature and/or ill newborns, and newborns with metabolic/genetic disorders such as galactosemia, glycogen storage diseases, etc.

25. D. 4

The incidence of hypoglycemia varies with the definition used, the population studied, and the method of measurement. In term infants, a glucose of less than 35 mg% requires intervention, while symptomatic infants with glucose measurements >40 mg% also may be treated. Preterm newborns are *not* more tolerant of low glucose than full-term newborns. Term infants and preterm newborns are equally at risk for severe neurodevelopmental sequelae if left with a low serum glucose.

26. E. All of the above

In the newborn, hypoglycemia may present with neurologic (apnea, seizures, lethargy, coma) or sympathomimetic (pallor, palpitations, diaphoresis) symptoms. The brain in a newborn uses glucose at a rate of approximately 20 mg/min or 4–5 mg/100 gm brain/min. The rate of glucose utilization of 5–7 mg/kg/min for a 3.5 kg newborn leads to an overall rate of glucose utilization of 17–24 mg/min.

27. In the treatment of glucose of <25 mg% in a newborn, an IV bolus of 200–300 mg/kg glucose (2–3 mL/kg of D_{10}) is given, followed by:

1. 4 mL/kg/h of D_{10} (6.7 mg/kg/min glucose)
2. D_5.2 NS at maintenance
3. 6–8 mg/kg/min glucose
4. Glucagon 0.3 mg/kg IM up a maximum of 1.0 mg

   A. 1, 2, 3
   B. 1, 3
   C. 2, 4
   D. 4 only
   E. All of the above

28. Regarding hemoglobin in the newborn:

1. The mean venous hemoglobin in term infants is 18 gm/dL.
2. Preterm infants' physiologic anemia lasts longer and is lower than that of full-term infants.
3. Hemoglobin concentration increases during the first few days of life as plasma volume decreases.
4. RBC survival is normal (120 days) in term infants.

   A. 1, 2, 3
   B. 1, 3
   C. 2, 4
   D. 4 only
   E. All of the above

29. The physiologic anemia (expected drop in hemoglobin) of infancy:

1. Is due to decreased erythtopoiesis in the oxygen rich postnatal environment
2. Occurs more rapidly and has a lower nadir in preterm infants compared with term infants
3. Occurs at 10–12 weeks of age in term infants
4. Has its nadir at 9–10 gm/dL in term infants

   A. 1, 2, 3
   B. 1, 3
   C. 2, 4
   D. 4 only
   E. All of the above

27. B. 1, 3

Treating hypoglycemia with larger amounts of glucose than 200–300 mg/kg results in rebound hypoglycemia. If the hypoglycemic newborn is seizing, 400 mg/kg may be given. The infusion is begun following the bolus and the glucose level is closely followed afterward. The prognosis of asymptomatic hypoglycemia is generally quite good. If hypoglycemia is accompanied by seizures it is associated with abnormal intellectual development.

28. A. 1, 2, 3

Hemoglobin levels in very low birth weight (VLBW) infants are 1–2 gm lower than those of term infants.

29. E. All of the above

The anemia of prematurity occurs at 1–3 months and may present with pallor, apnea, poor weight gain, tachypnea, and tachycardia. As the total hemoglobin concentration drops, the concentration of fetal hemoglobin decreases; the newborn makes more Hb A, a hemoglobin that releases oxygen more readily than fetal Hb. The P_{50} of fetal hemoglobin is a PaO_2 of 19 mmHg while that in the adult, with no fetal Hb, is a PaO_2 of 32 mmHg.

30. Neonatal Polycythemia:

    1. Is seen in infants of diabetic mothers
    2. Is diagnosed with a venous Hct > 65%
    3. Is treated with partial exchange transfusion in symptomatic infants
    4. Can lead to development of seizures, CNS damage, or necrotizing entero-
       colitis (NEC)

    A. 1, 2, 3
    B. 1, 3
    C. 2, 4
    D. 4 only
    E. All of the above

31. Polycythemia in the neonate (a venous Hct > 65% on two separate specimens):

    1. Is commonly idiopathic
    2. Occurs in infants of diabetic mothers
    3. Is associated with prolonged labor and fetal distress
    4. Occurs in newborns with intrauterine growth restriction

    A. 1, 2, 3
    B. 1, 3
    C. 2, 4
    D. 4 only
    E. All of the above

32. Polycythemia in the neonate should be treated:

    1. In all infants whose venous Hct is >65%
    2. With simple phlebotomy to reduce the Hct to <60%
    3. With exchange transfusion to reduce the Hct to <45%
    4. With partial exchange transfusion in all symptomatic infants whose venous
       Hct is >65% on two separate specimens

    A. 1, 2, 3
    B. 1, 3
    C. 2, 4
    D. 4 only
    E. All of the above

30. E. All of the above

With increases in hematocrit from 40 to 60%, blood viscosity changes very little. With increases above 65%, blood viscosity increases rapidly. The incidence of polycythemia is increased in

- Babies born at altitude
- Postmature vs. term infants
- SGA babies
- Infants after delayed clamping of the umbilical cord
- Infants of diabetic mothers

31. A. 1, 2, 3

Clinical manifestations of polycythemia include: lethargy, tachypnea, respiratory distress, hypoglycemia, and thrombocytopenia. Infants may appear ruddy or plethoric. Severe complications also may occur such as seizures, necrotizing enterocolitis (NEC), and pulmonary hypertension (PPHN). Although studies are not conclusive, it appears that long-term sequelae such as neurodevelopmental abnormalities can be prevented by treatment of affected infants with partial exchange transfusion.

32. D. 4

The goal of the partial exchange transfusion is to reduce the hematocrit to <50%. The long-term prognosis of polycythemia is unclear. Some adverse outcomes reported include problems with speech, fine motor control, and perhaps lower IQ scores. Partial exchange transfusion, when performed through an umbilical vein, is associated with an increased incidence of NEC.

33. "Physiologic" hyperbilirubinemia in the healthy term newborn:

   1. Usually does not exceed 8–9 mg/dL of unconjugated (indirect) bilirubin
   2. Is seen only in breast fed infants
   3. Can be partly accounted for by the low levels of glucuronyl transferase in the newborn
   4. Is diagnosed with a bilirubin level >15 mg/dL within the first week of life

       A. 1, 2, 3
       B. 1, 3
       C. 2, 4
       D. 4 only
       E. All of the above

34. Factors which weight in the decision to institute phototherapy treatment for unconjugated hyperbilirubinemia include:

   1. The neonate's gestational age
   2. The neonate's chronological age
   3. The presence of other illnesses such as sepsis or respiratory distress
   4. The neonate's Hgb concentration

       A. 1, 2, 3
       B. 1, 3
       C. 2, 4
       D. 4 only
       E. All of the above

35. Bilirubin results from hemolysis. Causes of hemolysis in the newborn associated with hyperbilirubinemia include:

   1. Cephaolhematoma
   2. Rh or ABO incompatibility
   3. Circulating bacterial endotoxin from group B Streptococcus
   4. Sickle-cell trait

       A. 1, 2, 3
       B. 1, 3
       C. 2, 4
       D. 4 only
       E. All of the above

33. B. 1, 3

Jaundice is observed in approximately 60% of term and 80% of preterm infants during the first week of life. The color results from accumulation of unconjugated (indirect-reacting) bilirubin in the skin. "Physiologic jaundice" appears on day 2 or 3 of life but jaundice appearing at this time may also represent a more severe form. Clinical jaundice and indirect hyperbilirubinemia are reduced upon exposure of the skin to visible light in the blue (420–470 nm) range. Conventional phototherapy is applied continuously and the baby should be turned to expose the maximum amount of skin. The eyes should be covered. Complications of phototherapy include loose stools, rashes, and dehydration. Exchange transfusion is another more definitive but also more invasive procedure to lower bilirubin.

34. A. 1, 2, 3

There are many algorithms for the use of phototherapy. In general, phototherapy for unconjugated hyperbilirubinemia is begun at lower bilirubin concentrations in younger, smaller, and sicker infants and infants in whom the rate of rise of unconjugated bilirubin is more rapid.

35. A. 1, 2, 3

The causes include factors which increase the amount of bilirubin presented to the liver for conjugation (hemolysis, infection, shortened red blood cell lifespan) or factors which decrease the liver's ability to conjugate the bilirubin (liver immaturity, enzyme deficiency, prematurity, hypothyroidism).

36. Bilirubin toxicity:

    1. May be seen in term neonates whose bilirubin level exceeds 25 mg/dL
    2. Need not be seen in term infants whose bilirubin exceeds 30 mg/dL
    3. May be seen in preterm infants weighing <1,500 gm whose bilirubin level exceeds 15 mg/mg/dL
    4. Results from damage to the basal ganglia and cranial nerve nuclei

      A. 1, 2, 3
      B. 1, 3
      C. 2, 4
      D. 4 only
      E. All of the above

37. The clinical signs of bilirubin toxicity include:

    1. Lethargy
    2. High-pitched cry
    3. Rigidity
    4. Choreathetosis

      A. 1, 2, 3
      B. 1, 3
      C. 2, 4
      D. 4 only
      E. All of the above

38. A mother with type O^+ blood delivers a 35-week, 2,600 gm infant with type A^+ blood. She is breast feeding. On day 2 of life the infant's indirect bilirubin is 12 mg/dL. Management includes:

    1. Cessation of breast feeding for 2–3 days
    2. Coombs test, Hb, RBC morphology and indices
    3. Partial exchange transfusion
    4. Observation with daily bilirubin measurements

      A. 1, 2, 3
      B. 1, 3
      C. 2, 4
      D. 4 only
      E. All of the above

36. E. All of the above

Kernicterus is the neurologic syndrome resulting from deposition of unconjugated bilirubin in brain cells. The relationship between serum bilirubin levels and kernicterus in healthy term infants is uncertain. The less mature the infant, the greater the susceptibility to kernicterus. Suggested maximum unconjugated bilirubin levels (in mg/dL) in relatively healthy preterms are:

- <1,000 gm: 12–13
- 1,000–1,250: 12–14
- 1,250–1,500: 14–16
- 1,500–2,000: 16–20

37. E. All of the above

More long-term neurologic problems associated with kernicterus include mental retardation, choreoathetosis, spastic diplegia, and deafness. The incidence of kernicterus at autopsy in hyperbilirubinemic preterm newborns ranges from 2 to 16%.

38. C. 2, 4

Evaluation of a well newborn with clinical jaundice involves a search for the etiology before deciding that the cause is "physiologic." While it is true that breast fed infants have higher bilirubin measurements than comparable formula fed infants, breast feeding is rarely held. Overall approximately 7% of term infants have bilirubin levels >13 mg% while less than 3% have levels >15 mg.

39. Group B Streptococcal sepsis in the newborn:

    1. May occur early, within the first 72 h after birth, primarily with bacteremia
    2. May occur later, between 10 and 30 days of age often including meningitis
    3. Is fatal in 10–15% of cases
    4. Will be less likely by treatment of women colonized with the bacteria with appropriate antibiotics during labor

       A. 1, 2, 3
       B. 1, 3
       C. 2, 4
       D. 4 only
       E. All of the above

40. Congenital Rubella infections are characterized by:

    1. Various congenital cardiac defects
    2. Cataracts
    3. Intrauterine growth retardation
    4. Brain calcifications

       A. 1, 2, 3
       B. 1, 3
       C. 2, 4
       D. 4 only
       E. All of the above

41. A newborn with a vesicular rash, retinopathy, and meningoencephalitis likely has:

    A. Group B Streptococcal infection
    B. Congenital rubella infection
    C. Congenital Herpes Simplex Virus infection
    D. Chlamydia infection

42. Which of the following are risk factors for the development of BPD or Chronic Lung Disease (CLD) of infancy?

    1. Lower gestational age
    2. Prolonged mechanical ventilation and oxygen therapy
    3. Male gender
    4. Exchange transfusion

       A. 1, 2, 3
       B. 1, 3
       C. 2, 4
       D. 4 only
       E. All of the above

39. E. All of the above

Sepsis in the newborn may present with a variety of signs and symptoms including apnea, tachypnea, temperature instability, metabolic acidosis, hypoxemia, or DIC. Initial empirical treatment of infants suspected of having systemic bacterial infection usually consists of an aminoglycoside and ampicillin.

40. A. 1, 2, 3

Congenital rubella affects virtually all organ systems. IUGR is the most common manifestation. Other findings include developmental delay, anemia, blueberry muffin skin lesions, structural cardiac defects (PDA, PA stenosis), hearing loss, microphthalmia, cataracts, and meningoencephalitis. Brain calcifications are seen in children with congenital toxoplasmosis or congenital cytomegalovirus infection, two other parts of the TORCH (Toxoplasmosis, Others, Rubella, Cytomegalovirus, Herpes) acronym of congenital infections.

41. C. Congenital Herpes Simplex Virus infection

Most cases of neonatal herpes occur due to infection during delivery with most cases manifesting themselves in the first month of life. One-third of infected infants will never have a skin lesion while symptoms of encephalitis (lethargy, seizures, poor tone) occur in 50–80%. Newborns with postnatal infection also often have keratoconjunctivitis. Acyclovir is the mainstay of treatment for HSV. Newborns with intrauterine infection may also present with microcephaly.

42. A. 1, 2, 3

Chronic lung disease results from injury to the newborn lungs from mechanical ventilation and oxygen therapy. It is defined as an oxygen requirement in an infant beyond 36 weeks postconceptual age. Uncomplicated RDS begins to improve in the third or fourth day while infants developing CLD show X-ray and clinical worsening. Most affected infants recover by 6–12 months but some may have respiratory symptoms throughout childhood. Right-sided heart failure may be seen in severely affected infants.

43. Bronchopulmonary dysplasia (BPD) or chronic lung disease (CLD) of infancy:

    1. Is only seen in infants who suffered severe RDS
    2. Is caused by oxygen toxicity
    3. Is characterized by hypoxia and hypercarbia
    4. Is seen as often in ex-full-term infants as in ex-preterm newborns

    A. 1, 2, 3
    B. 1, 3
    C. 2, 4
    D. 4 only
    E. All of the above

44. IM Vitamin K is given to newborns:

    1. To make up for the relative deficiency of vitamin K in breast milk
    2. Because newborns have inadequate stores of vitamin K
    3. Because the newborn lacks sufficient bacterial flora to produce Vitamin K
    4. To prevent hemorrhagic disease of the newborn due to lack of Vitamin K-dependent coagulation factors

    A. 1, 2, 3
    B. 1, 3
    C. 2, 4
    D. 4 only
    E. All of the above

45. Which of the following are characteristics of human milk?

    1. It has a casein/whey ratio = 1/4.
    2. It meets all the nutritional needs of infants for only the first 1–2 months of life.
    3. It contains lactose.
    4. Its iron content is adequate for the first year of life.

    A. 1, 2, 3
    B. 1, 3
    C. 2, 4
    D. 4 only
    E. All of the above

43. B. 1, 3

Treatment of CLD includes: nutritional support, fluid restriction, maintenance of adequate oxygenation, and vigorous treatment of infection. Recovery is dependent on growth of healthy new lung tissue. Medications often used to treat these children are diuretics, bronchodilators, and dexamethasone. Infants with CLD often exhibit growth failure, psychomotor retardation, nephrolithiaisis (from long-term diuretic therapy and TPN), osteopenia, and subglottic stenosis (form long-term/multiple intubations).

44. E. All of the above

A moderate decrease in some coagulation factors (II, VII, IX, X) occurs in all newborns between the second and third day of life. These gradually return to normal by the 10th day of life. Hemorrhagic disease of the newborn is characterized by GI, nasal, intracranial, or postcircumcision bleeding. Vitamin K administration prevents the fall in Vitamin K-dependent factors in term infants but is not effective in all preterm newborns.

45. B. 1, 3

There are several advantages to breast feeding: allergy to cow's milk is avoided, human milk contains antibodies, is free of contaminating bacteria, contains macrophages, lactoferrin, and it supplies many important nutrients to the infant. Supplements of iron and Vitamin D should be started at 4–6 months. If the water supply is not adequately fluoridated, the infant should receive this as a supplement as well.

46. Instillation of 1% Silver Nitrate into the conjunctival sac of newborns shortly after birth:

    1. Is an effective strategy for preventing gonoccal ophthalmia neonatorum
    2. Will not prevent Chlamydia conjunctivitis
    3. Can be replaced by instillation of 1% tetracycline ophthalmic ointment
    4. Should not be considered adequate treatment of ophthalmia neonatorum

        A. 1, 2, 3
        B. 1, 3
        C. 2, 4
        D. 4 only
        E. All of the above

46. E. All of the above

Other routines of newborn care include warming and drying to help conserve heat, treatment of the umbilical cord with triple dye, bacitracin or another bactericidal agent, and screening for various diseases (these are state specific).

Chapter 2
Respiratory System

R.S. Holzman et al., *Pediatric Anesthesiology Review: Clinical Cases for Self-Assessment*, DOI 10.1007/978-1-4419-1617-4_2, © Springer Science+Business Media, LLC 2010

1. Respiratory syncytial virus (RSV):

    1. Is the second most important lower respiratory tract pathogen in early childhood
    2. Causes infected cells to form characteristic syncytia
    3. Confers lifelong immunity after one infection
    4. Infects well over 1 million children annually

        A. 1, 2, 3
        B. 1, 3
        C. 2, 4
        D. 4 only
        E. All of the above

2. Which of the following are part of the clinical presentation of RSV bronchiolitis?

    1. It is commonly seen in children less than 2 years of age.
    2. Young infants with the illness may have lethargy and apnea.
    3. Respiratory distress (caused by small airways obstruction).
    4. Wheezes, rales, and ronchi all may be heard on auscultation of the lungs.

        A. 1, 2, 3
        B. 1, 3
        C. 2, 4
        D. 4 only
        E. All of the above

3. Respiratory syncytial virus (RSV) can cause:

    1. An upper respiratory illness
    2. Bronchiolitis
    3. Otitis media
    4. Pneumonia

        A. 1, 2, 3
        B. 1, 3
        C. 2, 4
        D. 4 only
        E. All of the above

1. C. 2, 4

RSV is the most important respiratory tract pathogen in childhood. It is the major cause of bronchiolitis and pneumonia in children less than 1 year of age, although placentally transmitted antibody may offer protection for the first 4–6 weeks of life. RSV is a medium-sized RNA virus which produces characteristic syncytial cytopathology. The occurrence of outbreaks each fall and winter and the very high incidence in the first year of life are characteristics not seen with other respiratory viruses.

2. E. All of the above

Infants and children infected with RSV first present with the rhinorrhea, then cough accompanied by audible and auscultatory wheezing. There is intermittent fever and the clear rhinorrhea persists throughout the illness. Hospitalized infants with RSV have normal CXRs only about 10% of the time.

3. E. All of the above

RSV most often causes coryza and pharyngitis, often with fever. In 10–40% of infected children, there is lower respiratory tract involvement (pneumonia, bronchiolitis). RSV infection is usually an outpatient illness. Generally, 1–3% of infected infants are hospitalized.

4. Infection with RSV:

  1. Is very common among infants
  2. Often leads to more serious respiratory distress in infants aged 2–6 months
  3. Occurs in epidemics annually during the months of November through April
  4. Confers lifelong immunity to the RSV virus

  A. 1, 2, 3
  B. 1, 3
  C. 2, 4
  D. 4 only
  E. All of the above

5. The pathologic changes brought about by RSV infection include:

  1. Necrosis of the respiratory epithelium
  2. Edema of the submucosa
  3. Destruction of cilia
  4. Small airway obstruction by edema and necrotic cells

  A. 1, 2, 3
  B. 1, 3
  C. 2, 4
  D. 4 only
  E. All of the above

6. Infection with RSV leads to more severe respiratory distress in:

  1. Ex-preterm newborns
  2. Infants with seizure disorders
  3. Children with congenital heart disease
  4. Infants with sickle cell trait

  A. 1, 2, 3
  B. 1, 3
  C. 2, 4
  D. 4 only
  E. All of the above

4. A. 1, 2, 3

Annual epidemics of RSV occur during the 4–5 months of the winter. It is estimated that up to 50% of susceptible infants undergo infection during each epidemic. Infection is almost universal by the second birthday. Reinfection occurs at a rate of 10–20% per epidemic throughout childhood with higher rates in day care settings.

5. E. All of the above

The pathology seen in the lung includes: necrosis of the respiratory epithelium, mucus secretion, and edema of the submucosa. These changes lead to mucus plugging of the small airways with distal hyperinflation or atelectaisis.

6. B. 1, 3

Infection of immunocompromised infants with RSV often results in more severe disease. RSV infection in the first few weeks following bone marrow or solid organ transplant can be as high as 50%. Children for whom immunoprophylaxis is considered useful are ex-preterm newborns with BPD or CLD and ex-preterm newborns discharged from hospital during RSV season.

7. Treatments for RSV bronchiolitis include:

1. Amoxicillin
2. Ribavirin
3. Racemic epinephrine
4. Oxygen

    A. 1, 2, 3
    B. 1, 3
    C. 2, 4
    D. 4 only
    E. All of the above

8. True statements regarding the prognosis for infants with RSV bronchiolitis include:

1. Infants who develop the illness are more likely to have recurrent wheezing later in life.
2. Approximately 1–2% of infants hospitalized with this illness die.
3. 2–5% of hospitalized infants with this illness develop respiratory failure.
4. Anti-RSV antibody administration will dramatically decrease the severity of the illness.

    A. 1, 2, 3
    B. 1, 3
    C. 2, 4
    D. 4 only
    E. All of the above

9. The differential diagnosis of wheezing in children during the first year of life includes:

1. Bronchiolitis (RSV)
2. Ataxia-telangiectasia with pulmonary involvement
3. Gastroesophageal reflux (GER)
4. Cystic fibrosis

    A. 1, 2, 3
    B. 1, 3
    C. 2, 4
    D. 4 only
    E. All of the above

7. C. 2, 4

Most hospitalized infants are hypoxemic, requiring humidified oxygen therapy. A trial of inhaled bronchodilators is often undertaken and continued if the clinical status of the child improves. Antibiotics are *not* useful in *uncomplicated* RSV bronchiolitis. They may be indicated if a consolidated pneumonia develops, however. Ribavirin has been shown to have a modest effect on the course of RSV pneumonia but hospital stay and mortality have not been reduced. Long-term effects are unknown. It is currently recommended only for high-risk infants with RSV such as those with CLD, congenital heart disease, or immunodeficiency.

8. A. 1, 2, 3

Administration of Palivizumab (Synagis), a monoclonal antibody against RSV or RSV-IVIG, high titer antibody against RSV, is recommended for protecting high-risk infants from serious complications of RSV. It has been shown to reduce total hospital days in this population.

9. E. All of the above

Wheezing is a manifestation of obstruction in the lower respiratory tract in children. There are many etiologies:

Acute wheezing. Asthma (intrinsic, exercise, anxiety, or cold induced), infection, airway foreign body, aspiration of GI, oral secretions

Chronic. Asthma (as above), tracheo- or bronchomalacia, airway compression (various vascular compressions, enlarged lymph nodes, tumors), bronchitis, cystic fibrosis, sequelae of RDS (chronic lung disease or bronchopulmonary dysplasia)

10. Asthma, a chronic disease of reversible airways obstruction,

    1. Is characterized by episodes of recurrent wheezing and coughing
    2. Only rarely has an allergic basis in children
    3. Often begins before the 6th birthday
    4. Is decreasing in prevalence and severity

       A. 1, 2, 3
       B. 1, 3
       C. 2, 4
       D. 4 only
       E. All of the above

11. Airway narrowing in asthma is due to:

    1. Thickened basement membranes
    2. Edema of the small airways
    3. Mucus secretion
    4. Increased airway smooth muscle tone

       A. 1, 2, 3
       B. 1, 3
       C. 2, 4
       D. 4 only
       E. All of the above

12. Causes of wheezing in asthmatic children include:

    1. Viral respiratory infections such as RSV infection
    2. Tobacco smoke
    3. Aspirin
    4. Animal dander

       A. 1, 2, 3
       B. 1, 3
       C. 2, 4
       D. 4 only
       E. All of the above

10. A. 1, 2, 3

Asthma is the most frequent admitting diagnosis in children's hospitals. Before puberty, males are affected twice as often as females. Thereafter the incidence is equal. Thirty percent of children who will later be diagnosed as asthmatics are symptomatic by 1 year of age and 80% present by the 4th birthday. Although up to 50% of asthmatic children are nearly symptom-free by 20 years of age, resolution is rare in children with steroid-dependent disease.

11. E. All of the above

The airways obstruction in asthma is due to bronchoconstriction, mucus hypersecretion, mucosal edema, cellular infiltration, and also desquamation of epithelial and inflammatory cells within the airways.

12. E. All of the above

Wheezing is a complex process involving autonomic, immunologic, infectious, endocrine, and psychologic factors. In children with extrinsic or allergic asthma, wheezing results from exposure to environmental factors and these patients have increased IgE against the implicated allergens. Children with intrinsic asthma do not have such antibodies. Viral infections are the most important infectious triggers of asthma (see RSV). Emotional factors may trigger wheezing and children with this chronic disease may suffer emotional consequences from the illness.

13. The changes in the small and large airways that occur in asthma lead to:

1. Increased airways resistance, especially noticeable during exhalation
2. Hypercarbia resulting from decreased respiratory drive
3. Ventilation-perfusion (V/Q) mismatch due to nonuniform airway involvement
4. Increased specific compliance due to much lower resting lung volumes

    A. 1, 2, 3
    B. 1, 3
    C. 2, 4
    D. 4 only
    E. All of the above

14. Pathophysiologic alterations seen in asthmatic children include:

1. Nonuniform small airways obstruction
2. V/Q mismatch
3. Decreased lung compliance as a result of hyperinflation
4. Atelectaisis

    A. 1, 2, 3
    B. 1, 3
    C. 2, 4
    D. 4 only
    E. All of the above

15. Treatment of acute exacerbations of asthma includes:

1. CPAP
2. Steroids
3. Cromolyn
4. Beta agonists

    A. 1, 2, 3
    B. 1, 3
    C. 2, 4
    D. 4 only
    E. All of the above

13. B. 1, 3

PaCO$_2$ is generally low early in asthma attacks, rising as the obstruction worsens. PaO$_2$ is often low during an acute exacerbation and may remain so for several days after the worst of the attack is over. Reversible airway obstruction is a hallmark of asthma, with PEFR and FEV$_1$ increasing at least 10% following bronchodilator administration.

14. E. All of the above

CXR abnormalities often seen in children during acute exacerbations of asthma include hyperinflation, atelectasis, infiltrates, and pneumomediastinum. PEFR and FEV$_1$ are decreased, often by more than 15%. ABG abnormalities are described above.

15. C. 2, 4

Therapy of acute asthma is aimed at lessening bronchoconstriction and reducing inflammation. Oxygen is administered by mask or nasal prongs. Bronchodilation is achieved with various inhaled medications such as beta-2 agonists (albuterol) and/ or cholinergic antagonists (ipratropium bromide). Systemic corticosteroids are often given for a short course. CPAP will likely worsen air trapping and is avoided. Cromolyn is useful for prophylaxis, especially with exercise-induced asthma. Cromolyn is a maintenance medication with little use during acute exacerbations.

16. Regarding the use of theophylline as a treatment for asthma:
    1. The medication has a narrow therapeutic range.
    2. It inhibits phosphodiesterase and is an adenosine receptor antagonist.
    3. It is effective orally and intravenously.
    4. Side effects include sleep disturbances, nausea, vomiting, and headaches.

    A. 1, 2, 3
    B. 1, 3
    C. 2, 4
    D. 4 only
    E. All of the above

17. Which of the following are common side effects of nebulized albuterol?
    1. Nausea and vomiting
    2. Jitteriness, sleep disturbances
    3. Suppression of adrenal secretion
    4. Tachycardia

    A. 1, 2, 3
    B. 1, 3
    C. 2, 4
    D. 4 only
    E. All of the above

18. Complications of asthma seen in children with asthma include:
    1. Pneumothorax
    2. Pneumonia
    3. Pneumomediastinum
    4. Sudden death

    A. 1, 2, 3
    B. 1, 3
    C. 2, 4
    D. 4 only
    E. All of the above

16. E. All of the above

Theophylline may be given orally as a sustained release preparation for children with moderately severe asthma as an alternative to inhaled steroids or cromolyn. It also may be used IV in the treatment of acute severe asthma. The therapeutic range is 10–20 mg%. Toxicity may be seen with serum levels of 25–30 mg%.

17. C. 2, 4

Other treatments for asthma include:

Ipratropium. A cholinergic antagonist, which may cause tachycardia and abdominal pain.
Cromolyn. An inhaled powder, which may cause coughing especially when first used. It is used as a preventive measure in asthma, not a treatment of acute exacerbations.
Albuterol. The jitteriness from albuterol usually occurs with excessive use of either the PO or inhaled forms.

18. E. All of the above

Death from childhood asthma is rare, but mortality rates have been increasing. Mortality rates are several times higher in African-American children than in white children.

19. Clinical manifestations of cystic fibrosis include:

    1. Productive cough and recurrent respiratory infections
    2. Hemoptysis, pneumothorax, and atelectaisis
    3. Maldigestion due to exocrine pancreatic insufficiency
    4. Diabetes insipidus

       A. 1, 2, 3
       B. 1, 3
       C. 2, 4
       D. 4 only
       E. All of the above

20. Cystic fibrosis, the major cause of severe chronic lung disease in children,

    1. Occurs in 1:3,000 white and 1:17,000 black live births
    2. Is characterized by thickened secretions
    3. Primarily involves the pulmonary and gastrointestinal systems
    4. Is inherited as an autosomal dominant trait

       A. 1, 2, 3
       B. 1, 3
       C. 2, 4
       D. 4 only
       E. All of the above

21. Treatments which patients with cystic fibrosis (CF) might receive include:

    1. Pancreatic enzyme replacement, high calorie diets, and fat-soluble vitamin supplements
    2. Antibiotics to control progression of pulmonary infections
    3. Bronchodilator and anti-inflammatory agents
    4. Oxygen

       A. 1, 2, 3
       B. 1, 3
       C. 2, 4
       D. 4 only
       E. All of the above

19. A. 1, 2, 3

CF is characterized by obstruction and infection of the airways and malabsorbtion of many important nutrients. After 10 years of age, 85% of children with cystic fibrosis will develop diabetes mellitus. People with CF have varying degrees of the following respiratory tract problems: failure to clear mucus secretions, dehydrated mucus secretions, and chronic infection in the respiratory tract. The rate of progression of lung disease is the chief determinant of morbidity and mortality. The first lung pathology is bronchiolitis, followed later by bronchiectaisis. Interstitial disease is not a regular feature although eventually fibrosis does develop. The paranasal sinuses are filled with secretions and the epithelial lining is hyperplastic and hypertrophic. The nasal mucosa is edematous and develops polyps.

20. A. 1, 2, 3

The CF gene is most common in Northern and Central Europeans. It codes for a protein called the transmembrane conductance regulator (CFTR) which is expressed largely in epithelial cells of the airways, GI tract, sweat glands, and GU system.

21. E. All of the above

Antibiotics, given PO, IV, and via inhalation, are used to control the progression of lung infection. Steroids are used to treat allergic pulmonary aspergillosis. Antiinflammatory agents may slow the progression of lung disease.

22. Croup, a clinical syndrome of barking cough, hoarseness, and inspiratory stridor, has several causes, including respiratory viruses. Characteristics of croup include:

    1. The illness lasts for 4–6 days.
    2. There is a characteristic CXR finding called the pencil (or steeple) sign indicative of subglottic tracheal narrowing.
    3. Treatment with inhaled racemic epinephrine (0.5 cc of a 2.25% solution) temporarily improves the stridor.
    4. Dexamethasone, 0.3–0.5 mg/kg, is a treatment for the illness.

       A. 1, 2, 3
       B. 1, 3
       C. 2, 4
       D. 4 only
       E. All of the above

23. Clinical characteristics of croup (laryngotracheobronchitis) include:

    1. Mild temperature elevation, rarely reaching 39°C
    2. The presence of a URI (upper respiratory infection) for 1–3 days prior to the onset of stridor
    3. A peak incidence during the ages of 18 months to 3 years
    4. A typical barking cough

       A. 1, 2, 3
       B. 1, 3
       C. 2, 4
       D. 4 only
       E. All of the above

24. Acute epiglottitis presents differently than viral croup in the following was(s):

    1. The course of epiglottitis is much more rapid and fulminating.
    2. The temperature elevation in epiglottitis is greater.
    3. The ages range of children with epiglottitis is older.
    4. Very often other family members of children with epiglottitis have been ill with URI symptoms.

       A. 1, 2, 3
       B. 1, 3
       C. 2, 4
       D. 4 only
       E. All of the above

22. E. All of the above

Croup is the most common form of acute upper airway obstruction and is most commonly caused by a virus. Symptoms are characteristically worse at night. Most children with croup progress to stridor and slight dyspnea and then begin to recover. Agitation and crying, with associated more rapid respiratory rate and turbulent airflow, worsen the situation. Children with croup prefer to sit upright.

23. E. All of the above

Older children are generally not seriously ill. Other family members may have a mild respiratory illness. The nighttime worsening may recur for several consecutive days before the illness resolves.

24. A. 1, 2, 3

Epiglottitis is usually seen in children aged 2–7 years while croup is more often seen in younger children. Epiglottitis is caused by bacteria, croup a virus. Other family members are not acutely ill with respiratory viruses as is the case with croup. Epiglottitis is a severe bacterial infection associated with high fever, rapidly progressing airway obstruction, and dyspnea.

25. Aspirated airway foreign bodies:

    1. Can usually be seen on either a PA or lateral CXR
    2. Most often occur in 2–4-year-old children
    3. Are usually first noted during an acute URI when the child has more severe symptoms than usual
    4. May not be noted until sometime after the aspiration episode

       A. 1, 2, 3
       B. 1, 3
       C. 2, 4
       D. 4 only
       E. All of the above

26. Bacterial tracheitis, a cause of upper airway obstruction which occurs as a super infection of viral laryngotracheitis:

    1. Is often caused by coagulase + Staph or Haemophilus Influenzae
    2. Is diagnosed with airway endoscopy
    3. Is regularly treated with endotracheal intubation and IV antibiotics
    4. Is seen only in the teen age years

       A. 1, 2, 3
       B. 1, 3
       C. 2, 4
       D. 4 only
       E. All of the above

27. Regarding acute otitis media (AOM) in children:

    1. Both bacteria and viruses are known causative agents.
    2. Meningitis is a possible complication of untreated bacterial AOM.
    3. It is generally treated with PO antibiotics.
    4. Infants less than 1 month of age with AOM should be thoroughly evaluated for systemic infection.

       A. 1, 2, 3
       B. 1, 3
       C. 2, 4
       D. 4 only
       E. All of the above

25. C. 2, 4

Most airway foreign bodies are not radio-opaque and many are actually food, often peanuts. Although up to 50% of cases of airway foreign body aspiration come to medical attention soon after the aspiration event and the parents give a history of a specific choking episode, a substantial minority of cases are discovered in the evaluation of a child with recurrent wheezing for several months.

26. A. 1, 2, 3

Bacterial tracheitis is one of the laryngotracheal respiratory tract infections affecting children. The other is croup, viral laryngotracheobronchitis, and epiglottitis. Bacterial tracheitis is acute in onset, affects children 4–5 years of age, and is associated with a cough and harsh stridor. Treatment of affected children often involves IV antibiotics, hospitalization, and intubation.

27. E. All of the above

AOM is a very common childhood infection. Management strategies vary. The etiologic agent in a particular case is rarely identified. The tympanic membrane in AOM is red, often bulging, immobile, and the normal landmarks are not seen. With repeated episodes of AOM or with chronic serous OM, pediatricians often refer their patients to an ORL specialist for myringotomy and tube placement. Untreated AOM can develop into acute mastoiditis which can destroy the mastoid air cells.

28. Children with acute sinusitis:

    1. Have URI symptoms (nasal discharge and cough) which persist for more than 10 days
    2. May have persistent daytime cough
    3. May have facial pain and swelling in association with their URI
    4. May complain of headache

        A. 1, 2, 3
        B. 1, 3
        C. 2, 4
        D. 4 only
        E. All of the above

29. Regarding URIs in children:

    1. Mucociliary dysfunction can persist for weeks after recovery from the URI.
    2. Viral URI's predispose children to bacterial infections such as pneumonia, sinusitis, or otitis media.
    3. Nasal discharge, initially watery, becomes mucopurulent after 5–7 days.
    4. Young infants may develop fever to 38C or 39C with uncomplicated URIs.

        A. 1, 2, 3
        B. 1, 3
        C. 2, 4
        D. 4 only
        E. All of the above

30. Children with allergic rhinitis:

    1. Often also have conjunctivitis
    2. Have pale edematous nasal membranes
    3. May have fewer and lessened symptoms during exercise
    4. Often have nasal polyps

        A. 1, 2, 3
        B. 1, 3
        C. 2, 4
        D. 4 only
        E. All of the above

28. E. All of the above

Sinusitis often accompanies the common cold or even allergic rhinitis. The maxillary, ethmoid, and sphenoid sinuses are present at birth and the frontal sinuses develop at around the first birthday. These sinuses gradually become air filled over the first several years of life. Affected children have persistent purulent nasal drainage, nighttime cough, and facial tenderness and pain. Treatment is with PO antibiotics unless extension from the sinuses is considered a possibility.

29. E. All of the above

The common cold or viral URI is a frequent problem in children. These occur most often in the winter months, from early fall through late springs. Toddlers and young school-aged children can have up to 6–9 colds/year. The number/year decreases, with most adults reporting 1–3/URI's year.

30. A. 1, 2, 3

The differential diagnosis of rhinitis in children includes sinusitis, viral URI, nasal foreign body, and allergic rhinitis. Children with allergic rhinitis do not have fever, but often have allergic "shiners," nasal polyps, and pale edematous nasal mucosa.

31. Regarding URI's in children:

    1. The incidence is highest between the ages of 6 and 8 years.
    2. School-aged children normally experience 1–2 colds/year.
    3. Boys have more URIs than girls.
    4. Among children aged 1–4 years, those in day care have fewer URIs than those cared for only at home.

    A. 1, 2, 3
    B. 1, 3
    C. 2, 4
    D. 4 only
    E. All of the above

32. Which of the following causes pharyngitis most often?

    A. Mycoplasma Pneumoniae
    B. Rhinovirus
    C. Adenovirus
    D. Haemophilus Influenzae, untypeable
    E. Beta Hemolytic Strep

33. Which of the following are considered etiologic agents for the common cold in children?

    1. Parainfluenza viruses
    2. Group B beta hemolytic streptococci
    3. Respiratory syncytial virus
    4. Haemophilus Influenzae type B

    A. 1, 2, 3
    B. 1, 3
    C. 2, 4
    D. 4 only
    E. All of the above

34. Influenza viruses:

    1. Can cause primary pneumonia
    2. Cause epidemic respiratory infections
    3. Are spread from person to person via the respiratory route
    4. Confer lifelong immunity to all strains after one symptomatic infection

    A. 1, 2, 3
    B. 1, 3
    C. 2, 4
    D. 4 only
    E. All of the above

31. B. 1, 3

A viral URI typically lasts only 7 days with a minority lasting up to 2 weeks. As the URI resolves, the nasal secretions change from clear and thin to a thicker and yellow-green consistency.

32. C. Adenovirus

In children less than 2 years of age, the cause for pharyngitis is usually viral, whereas in children over 5 years of age Group A strep is the most common causative agent. Making the diagnosis of Strep phargyngitis is important because appropriate antibiotic treatment will prevent rheumatic fever as well as minimize the chance of local suppurative complications such as abscess formation. Diagnosis is with rapid antigen detection or throat culture. Antibiotic treatment does not, however, prevent the development of poststreptococcal glomerulonephritis.

33. B. 1, 3

The common cold in children is caused by a variety of viruses. It is not a bacterial infection and thus not treatable with antibiotics. Bacterial complications of viral URI's include sinusitis, otitis media, and pneumonia. There is not therapy for the common cold save symptomatic measures and most over the counter medications sold for URI treatment have not been shown to be effective in reducing the symptoms.

34. A. 1, 2, 3

Influenza A viruses are responsible for epidemics. These epidemics follow a shift in one of the major antigens, neuraminidase, or hemagglutinin. The clinical picture in young children is milder than that seen in adults. Young children may exhibit bronchitis, laryngotracheitis, and/or mild upper respiratory tract symptoms. Older children and adults have high fever of abrupt onset, myalgias, chills, and cough. The cough and congestion may last for 2 weeks.

Chapter 3
Surgery

R.S. Holzman et al., *Pediatric Anesthesiology Review: Clinical Cases for Self-Assessment*,
DOI 10.1007/978-1-4419-1617-4_3, © Springer Science+Business Media, LLC 2010

1. Which of the following organisms are associated with sepsis occurring after abdominal surgery?

   A. Haemophilus influenzae type B
   B. Neisseria gonorrhea
   C. Staphylocci
   D. Enteric gram negative rods

2. Gastroschisis differs from omphalocele in the following way(s):

   1. Gastroschisis is usually a 2–4 cm defect, often with a right paramedian location.
   2. In infants with gastroschisis, the bowel is not covered by membranes.
   3. Omphalocele is associated with a greater incidence of non-GI anomalies such as congenital heart disease, bladder extrophy, and/or cloaca.
   4. A silo is often used in closure of larger defects.

     A. 1, 2, 3
     B. 1, 3
     C. 2, 4
     D. 4 only
     E. All of the above

3. Which is the most common type of esophageal atresia?

   A. Esophageal atresia (EA) with a posterior tracheoesophageal fistula (TEF) near the carina
   B. "H"-type EA/TEF
   C. Esophageal connection to the trachea with a second, more distal TEF
   D. Esophageal connection to the trachea without a distal TEF

4. The VACTERL complex includes a tracheoesophageal anomaly and

   1. PDA, ASD, or VSD
   2. Renal defects
   3. Abnormalities of the bones of the forearm
   4. Spinal dysraphism

     A. 1, 2, 3
     B. 1, 3
     C. 2, 4
     D. 4 only
     E. All of the above

1. D. Enteric gram negative rods

The administration of prophylactic antibiotics in the OR and in the perioperative period is an important measure in reducing the incidence of infection. Overuse of antibiotics has been implicated as a cause for the development of *Clostridium difficile* toxin-associated diarrhea.

2. A. 1, 2, and 3

Omphalocele is a midline defect of variable size involving the omphalos (Greek: "navel"). Omphalocele is associated with chromosomal abnormalities, other GI defects (35%), cardiac defects (20%), and also cloacal extrophy. Only 10% of patients with omphalocele are born preterm. Omphalocele is part of the Beckwith–Wiedeman Syndrome (macroglossia, hyperinsulinism, hypoglycemia, and gigantism). Omphalocele results when the intestines fail to return into the abdomen from the umbilical coelom. With omphalocele, the bowel is covered with membranes, decreasing fluid loses. In gastroschisis, a part of the small intestine herniates through the abdominal wall. Sixty percent of patients with gastroschisis are born prematurely. A few affected patients have jejunal atresia but other anomalies are not seen with this condition. Repair of either defect may involve a "silo" if the extruded intestines do not fit into the smaller abdominal cavity.

3. A. Esophageal atresia (EA) with a posterior tracheoesophageal fistula (TEF) near the carina

TEF is the failure of the linear division of the trachea and esophagus during embryogenesis. The most common type (85–90%) is a proximal blind pouch with a distal TEF. All patients present with aspiration at birth with respiratory distress and inability to handle oral secretions. Mortality is approximately 3% in term infants but can be much higher in preterm newborns and in those with other congenital anomalies. Forty percent of infants born with TEF have associated anomalies, with cardiovascular anomalies being seen most often. TEF is also seen as part of the VATER (vertebral anomalies, anal atresia or arterial anomalies, TEF, renal anomalies) or VACTERL (vertebral anomalies, anal atresia or arterial anomalies, TEF renal anomalies, limb anomalies) associations.

4. E. All of the above

The VATER association includes vertebral anomalies, imperforate anus or arterial anomalies, TEF, and renal anomalies. A single umbilical artery is often seen. In VACTERL, the L stands for limb anomalies. An association does not have a single known etiology. The evaluation of an infant with TEF should include a search for the anomalies in the VACTERL association.

5. Regarding acute appendicitis in children:

    1. In well over 50% of children younger than 2 years of age the appendix is found perforated at operation.
    2. More males than females develop acute appendicitis.
    3. It is unusual for the child with acute appendicitis to have an appetite.
    4. Among school-aged children, the diagnosis is more often missed in girls than in boys.

       A. 1, 2, 3
       B. 1, 3
       C. 2, 4
       D. 4 only
       E. All of the above

6. Midgut volvulus:

    1. Occurs when the bowel twists upon itself
    2. Occurs when incomplete intestinal rotation leads to a shortened mesentery
    3. Leads to vascular compromise of the bowel
    4. Is seen in over 60% of neonates with malrotation

       A. 1, 2, 3
       B. 1, 3
       C. 2, 4
       D. 4 only
       E. All of the above

7. Duodenal atresia:

    1. Often presents with vomiting which may or may not be bilious
    2. Is often accompanied by other intestinal obstructions in both the small and large intestine
    3. Is associated with trisomy 21
    4. Generally does not present until 1–2 months of life

       A. 1, 2, 3
       B. 1, 3
       C. 2, 4
       D. 4 only
       E. All of the above

5. A. 1, 2, 3

The annual incidence of acute appendicitis is 4:1,000. In adolescent girls, the diagnosis is more difficult because other causes of abdominal pain such as ovarian cysts, ovulatory pain, menstrual pain, and pelvic inflammatory disease mimic appendicitis. Other diagnoses in the differential include: gastroenteritis, mesenteric adenitis, inflammatory bowel disease, RUL pneumonia, and urinary tract pathology.

6. E. All of the above

In 70% of patients with malrotation and volvulus, the presentation is within the neonatal period and in half of these the presentation is in the first 10 days of life. The balance of cases can present at any time, even into adulthood. Malrotation is twice as common in boys as girls. Presentation includes distention and bilious vomiting. X-ray studies (plain film or upper GI contrast study) confirm the diagnosis. In malrotation, the duodenum is seen in an abnormal position, with the duodenojejunal junction located to the right of the spine.

7. B. 1, 3

Duodenal atresia occurs in 1:20,000 live births. Common findings in affected infants include abdominal distention and jaundice. Maternal polyhydramnios is also often found. Associations in addition to trisomy 21 are congenital heart disease, TEF, and renal anomalies.

8. Intussusception:

1. Has a peak incidence in infants less than 1 year of age
2. Presents with colicky abdominal pain, bloody (currant jelly) stools and vomiting
3. May be reduced with a carefully performed enema
4. Is nearly always caused by a "lead point" such as a polyp or duplication

    A. 1, 2, 3
    B. 1, 3
    C. 2, 4
    D. 4 only
    E. All of the above

9. Hirschsprung's disease, the absence of normal enteric ganglionic neurons,

1. Has a much higher incidence in caucasians
2. Is limited to the rectum and sigmoid in over 50% of cases
3. Is initially managed with stool softeners since some cases spontaneously resolve
4. Rarely involves not only the rectum and sigmoid, but the entire colon

    A. 1, 2, 3
    B. 1, 3
    C. 2, 4
    D. 4 only
    E. All of the above

10. Hirschsprung's disease can be diagnosed by:

1. Rectal manometry
2. Surgical rectal biopsy
3. Suction biopsy
4. Barium enema

    A. 1, 2, 3
    B. 1, 3
    C. 2, 4
    D. 4 only
    E. All of the above

8. A. 1, 2, 3

Intussusception is seen in children from the age of 3 to 18 months. The incidence varies from 0.5 to 4/1,000 live births. In almost all children under 1 year of age, no clear cause is found. The nonspecific signs of vomiting and colicky pain are nearly always part of the presentation. Later in the course of the illness, fever and lethargy are seen and finally the child may pass a currant jelly stool. A carefully done barium enema is used as a diagnostic and therapeutic tool. Excessive pressure in the performance of the enema will perforate the bowel. Up to 50% of patients with intussusception are successfully treated with hydrostatic reduction.

9. C. 2, 4

Hirschprung's disease is a functional obstruction of the colon or rectum that results from failure of migration of ganglion cells in the developing colon. It is the cause for up to 25% of all cases of bowel obstruction in the newborn and is seen more often in males. The aganglionic segment does not permit normal colonic motility. More than 80% of cases involve only the rectum and a small part of the colon. Management is surgical since the aganglionic segment is permanently contracted. Generally, a colostomy is performed at the level of normal innervation (the so-called leveling colostomy) with a later colonic or ileal pull-through.

10. E. All of the above

The diagnosis should be suspected in any newborn who does not pass meconium within the first day of life. A frozen section can be done with the biopsy material which is stained for acetylcholine to identify abnormal nerve trunks. H&E stains confirm the absence of ganglion cells.

11. Other than organomegaly, which of the following may cause abdominal distention in the neonate?

    1. Pneumoperitoneum
    2. Intestinal obstruction
    3. Ascites
    4. Pyloric stenosis

       A. 1, 2, 3
       B. 1, 3
       C. 2, 4
       D. 4 only
       E. All of the above

12. Abdominal masses in the newborn:

    1. Are generally not malignant
    2. Are retroperitoneal in approximately 66% of cases
    3. If retroperitoneal, are most often renal in origin
    4. If due to a tumor, are most likely abdominal teratomas

       A. 1, 2, 3
       B. 1, 3
       C. 2, 4
       D. 4 only
       E. All of the above

13. Which of the following have been implicated as having a role in the development of necrotizing enterocolitis (NEC)?

    1. Intestinal ischemia
    2. Bacterial colonization of the bowel
    3. Feeding
    4. Multiple births

       A. 1, 2, 3
       B. 1, 3
       C. 2, 4
       D. 4 only
       E. All of the above

11. A. 1, 2, 3

Hepatomegaly or hepatosplenomegaly is a possible cause of abdominal distention in the newborn. Pneumoperitoneum is usually a result of GI tract perforation, often in preterm newborns. Among the causes of neonatal ascites, urinary ascites is the most common, followed by cardiac and idiopathic. Pyloric stenosis is an incomplete obstruction at the gastric outlet not associated with ascites.

12. E. All of the above

Approximately 10–15% of abdominal masses in the newborn are due to malignant tumors. Types of renal masses seen in newborns include hydronephrosis, polycystic disease, renal vein thrombosis, Wilms' tumor, and mesoblastic nephroma. Other retroperitoneal masses seen in this age group include neuroblastoma, ganglioneuroma, and sacrococcygeal teratoma.

13. A. 1, 2, 3

NEC is the most common gastrointestinal emergency in the infant. The incidence ranges from 1 to 4% of all NICU admissions, with a higher incidence in infants with birth weights <1,000 gm. The most commonly implicated etiologic factors are an ischemic insult to the gut, the presence of intraluminal bacteria or viruses and substrate (formula or milk). Approximately 93% of infants who develop NEC have been fed enterally. Because of the role of bacteria in NEC, antibiotics are often part of the therapy.

14. Which of the following are associated with intestinal ischemia?

    1. Polycythemia
    2. Umbilical vessel catheterization
    3. Congestive heart failure
    4. An open patent ductus arteriosus

       A. 1, 2, 3
       B. 1, 3
       C. 2, 4
       D. 4 only
       E. All of the above

15. Patients with extra hepatic biliary atresia (incidence = 1/8–10,000 live births):

    1. Will be cured for life if a Kasai operation is done within the first 3 weeks of life
    2. Are generally well initially and then develop jaundice at 3–6 weeks of age
    3. Should be started on phenobarbital to induce liver enzymes in the remaining normal liver
    4. Will likely die within the first year of life without surgical intervention

       A. 1, 2, 3
       B. 1, 3
       C. 2, 4
       D. 4 only
       E. All of the above

16. In pyloric stenosis:

    1. The child develops metabolic alkalosis due to continued vomiting of gastric contents.
    2. There is nonbilious vomiting which may contain "coffee grounds" material.
    3. The child may develop hypochloremia.
    4. The diagnosis is best made with a barium swallow.

       A. 1, 2, 3
       B. 1, 3
       C. 2, 4
       D. 4 only
       E. All of the above

14. E. All of the above

Mesenteric blood flow in the newborn is affected by a variety of factors in addition to those mentioned. During hypoxia, the so-called "diving reflex" shunts blood from the mesenteric, renal, and peripheral vascular systems to the brain and heart. Polycythemia and also exchange transfusions have been implicated in intestinal ischemia. Other possible etiologies for NEC are RDS, hypotension, hypothermia, and birth asphyxia. The presentation of NEC may include abdominal distention, vomiting and gastric residual, lethargy, hypotension, apnea, and temperature instability. Lab findings include pneumatosis intestinalis on X-ray, thrombocytopenia, blood and/or reducing substances in the stool, and metabolic acidosis.

15. C. 2, 4

This condition is defined as atresia or hypoplasia of any part of the extrahepatic biliary system. The most common form includes atresia up to the porta hepatis and even intrahepatic ducts. Approximately 15% of affected children have other defects. Clinical presentation includes jaundice in the second–third week of life, acholic stools, enlarged, hardened liver, and splenomegaly. Conjugated bilirubin is elevated along with alkaline phosphatase, gamma-glutamyl transferase, and transaminases.

16. A. 1, 2, 3

Pyloric stenosis is much more common in males. It is seen in 1:150 males and 1:750 females. The presentation includes progressive, relentless vomiting generally starting between the second and fourth week of life with a range of 2–12 weeks. Typical electrolyte abnormalities seen in infants with pylorioc stenosis include hypochloremia, hypokalemia, hyponatremia along with azotemia. The severity of the child's condition is graded by the degree of hypochloremia. An infant with more severe dehydration will have, in addition to the metabolic acidosis [alkalosis], a paradoxical aciduria. The kidney, in an effort to maintain intravascular volume, absorbs as much sodium as possible but the only anion available to absorb is bicarbonate. Thus, the urine is acidic despite the systemic alkalosis. Prior to surgical repair, the child should be adequately hydrated and the electrolyte abnormalities corrected. Given the nature of the pathology, gastric outlet obstruction leading to intractable vomiting, administration of contrast is a poor way to make the diagnosis. Ultrasound or air contrast plain X-rays are more current diagnostic tools.

Na⁺ is reabsorbed from kidney in an attempt to maintain the intravascular volume.

HCO₃⁻ is the only anion to match ∴ the urine becomes ACIDIC

17. Pyloric stenosis, the most frequently occurring cause of gastric obstruction in the newborn,

    1. Is seen in approximately 1/25,000 live births
    2. Is equally common in all races and ethnic groups
    3. Is seen with the same frequency in males and females
    4. Is seen in infants as young as 2 weeks and as old as 12 weeks

      A. 1, 2, 3
      B. 1, 3
      C. 2, 4
      D. 4 only
      E. All of the above

18. Regarding children in MVA's who have a history or physical exam indications of lap-belt injury:

    1. These injuries are most common in children under the age of 1 year.
    2. There may also be damage to the spinal cord in these children.
    3. Diagnostic peritoneal lavage is always indicated.
    4. Hollow viscus injury may not be apparent for 12–24 h.

      A. 1, 2, 3
      B. 1, 3
      C. 2, 4
      D. 4 only
      E. All of the above

19. In the evaluation of the child who has suffered blunt abdominal trauma, organ damage may be indicated by:

    1. Left shoulder pain
    2. Hematuria
    3. Flank ecchymoses
    4. Bilious emesis

      A. 1, 2, 3
      B. 1, 3
      C. 2, 4
      D. 4 only
      E. All of the above

17. D. 4

The incidence of pyloric stenosis is 1:2,500 live births. It is seen predominately in whites and is most common in firstborn males. The average age of onset is 3–4 weeks with a range of 2–12 weeks. Interestingly, this anomaly is not seen at birth and in cases where it is managed medically, the hypertrophic pyloris eventually (after 4–6 weeks) returns to normal and the child stops vomiting, all without surgical intervention. Pyloric stenosis is a common reason for surgery in the neonatal period.

18. C. 2, 4

Injuries to the pancreas can result from either lap-belt injury or bicycle handlebars. Injury to the pancreas is difficult to diagnose. Elevations in amylase and lipase may not be seen until 1–2 days after the injury. Rapid deceleration while in a lap belt may also damage the intestines with perforation or even transection possible. If there is intestinal damage, in addition to a bruise over the abdomen in the area of the lap belt, back pain may be a symptom.

19. E. All of the above

The spleen is the abdominal organ most often damaged following blunt abdominal trauma in children. Kehr's sign, left shoulder pain resulting from pressure on the left upper quadrant, is suggestive of splenic injury. The severity of splenic injury is graded by CT from 1 to 5. Grade 1 is a tear in the capsule while grade 5 indicates a completely ruptured spleen. Renal damage following blunt abdominal trauma is relatively common in children. Abdominal CT with renal contrast will make the diagnosis in most cases. Flank pain and bruising and urinalysis with blood and protein should raise the suspicion of renal damage.

20. Gastroesophageal reflux (GER) in infants and young children can present with:

    1. Recurrent pneumonia
    2. Irritability
    3. Wheezing, stridor, or hoarseness
    4. Apnea

       A. 1, 2, 3
       B. 1, 3
       C. 2, 4
       D. 4 only
       E. All of the above

21. Treatment for GER includes:

    1. Thickened, small, and frequent feeds
    2. Magnesium sulfate to increase gastric pH
    3. H-2 receptor blockade
    4. Avoidance of high carbohydrate meals

       A. 1, 2, 3
       B. 1, 3
       C. 2, 4
       D. 4 only
       E. All of the above

22. Esophageal foreign bodies in children:

    1. Are best diagnosed with a barium swallow
    2. Often lodge at or just below the cricopharyngeus muscle
    3. Always require removal if they pass into the stomach
    4. May cause stridor in infants

       A. 1, 2, 3
       B. 1, 3
       C. 2, 4
       D. 4 only
       E. All of the above

20. D. All of the above

GER must not be confused with other causes of regurgitation in the newborn/infant such as pyloric stenosis, duodenal stenosis, annular pancreas, malrotation, or any of a host of metabolic diseases. Contrast studies and/or 12–24 h pH probe studies may confirm the diagnosis. Pneumonia and/or wheezing develop with aspiration of refluxed gastric contents, irritability is due to the pain of reflux esophagitis and apnea is a possible reaction to the presence of aspirated gastric contents in the trachea or larynx.

21. B. 1, 3

Medical treatment of GER is directed to lowering the pH of the gastric contents and decreasing the amount of reflux. In the well, thriving child with a small amount of post feeding reflux, observation and reassurance are all that is needed. In more severe cases, placing the child at an angle (30 degrees head-up) after feeding may limit the reflux as will the institution of frequent small feedings instead of larger ones.

22. C. 2, 4

A barium study of the esophagus may be useful in the evaluation of upper airway obstruction, often demonstrating posterior esophageal compression from a vascular ring. The cricopharyngeus muscle, located high in the esophagus, often stops a swallowed esophageal foreign body from progressing further. A foreign body which passes into the stomach will likely be passed through the entire GI tract so retrieval is often not undertaken unless it is indicated by the specific nature of the foreign body (such as an open safety pin).

23. Extra intestinal manifestations of inflammatory bowel disease (IBD) include:

    1. Growth retardation
    2. Peripheral arthritis
    3. Anemia
    4. Reactive airways disease

       A. 1, 2, 3
       B. 1, 3
       C. 2, 4
       D. 4 only
       E. All of the above

24. Common findings in patients with IBD (ulcerative colitis or Crohn's disease) include:

    1. Iron deficiency anemia
    2. First degree heart block
    3. Hypoalbuminemia
    4. Stool cultures positive for various enteric pathogens

       A. 1, 2, 3
       B. 1, 3
       C. 2, 4
       D. 4 only
       E. All of the above

25. Cleft lip:

    1. May be unilateral or bilateral
    2. Occurs with and without cleft palate
    3. Occurs in 1:600–1,000 live births
    4. Varies from being a small notch in the vermilion border to a complete separation

       A. 1, 2, 3
       B. 1, 3
       C. 2, 4
       D. 4 only
       E. All of the above

23. A. 1, 2, 3

Inflammatory bowel disease (IBD) is a term given to both ulcerative colitis and Crohn's disease. Ulcerative colitis is a chronic inflammatory illness limited to the mucosa and submucosa of the colon and rectum. The risk for cancer is estimated to be 10–20% per decade after the first 10 years of disease. Crohn's disease is a transmural inflammation involving any and all portions of the GI tract. Management of IBD centers around nutritional support, immunosupression and surgery. Extraintestinal manifestations of these illness differ, but in either, growth retardation and anemia, due to poor nutrition and GI blood loss, are regularly seen. Arthritis, arthralgias and various skin manifestations, such as erythema nodosum, are also seen in both diseases

24. B. 1, 3

The hypochromic, microcytic anemia and hypoalbuminemia seen in IBD are due to both iron loss through subtle GI bleeding and to poor nutrition. Infection of the GI tract is generally not part of the problem in IBD. Except in cases of dehydration, electrolytes are generally within normal limits.

25. E. All of the above

Recurrence patterns of this problem do not suggest a simple pattern of inheritance. Isolated cleft palate appears to be a separate entity from cleft lip with or without cleft palate. Isolated cleft palate has an incidence of 1:2,500 live births. Cleft lip with cleft palate is more common than either seen in isolation. The frequency is higher than 1:1,000 in Native Americans, Japanese and Chinese people and lower in African Americans. Other anomalies are seen in up to 25% of all patients with cleft lip, palate or both and more often in children with bilateral cleft lip. The Robin malformation sequence includes cleft palate as well as micrognathia and glossoptosis. Up to 20% of patients with the Robin sequence have cardiac anomalies such as ASD, VSD, or PDA.

26. Problems seen in children with cleft palate ± cleft lip include:

    1. Otitis media
    2. Feeding difficulties
    3. Malpositioned teeth and dental decay
    4. Problems with phonation

       A. 1, 2, 3
       B. 1, 3
       C. 2, 4
       D. 4 only
       E. All of the above

27. Chiari type II malformations, also called Arnold–Chiari Malformations,

    1. Are seen in nearly all patients with meningomyelocele
    2. May be asymptomatic
    3. Can be a cause of headache, particularly with coughing or straining
    4. Can be associated with vocal cord paralysis

       A. 1, 2, 3
       B. 1, 3
       C. 2, 4
       D. 4 only
       E. All of the above

28. Tests used to confirm the diagnosis of Chiari II malformation include:

    1. Sleep studies
    2. PET scan
    3. EEG
    4. MRI

       A. 1, 2, 3
       B. 1, 3
       C. 2, 4
       D. 4 only
       E. All of the above

26. E. All of the above

Cleft lip and palate often occur as isolated anomalies. Various techniques and equipment are available for feeding these infants and no single solution is suitable for all. The management team for these infants should include a maxillofacial surgeon, audiologist, speech pathologist, otolaryngologist, pedodontist, and geneticist.

27. E. All of the above

A Chirai II malformation is a bony defect that includes caudal displacement of the cerebellar vermis, fourth ventricle, and lower brainstem below the plane of the foramen magnum. Chiari II malformations are often asymptomatic. Presentation is often a headache, in particular after cough or with flexion/extension of the neck, lower cranial nerve signs and if the Chiari malformation has led to development of a syrinx, long tract signs such as lower extremity weakness.

28. D. 4

Chiari malformations are graded by the distance the CNS structures (cerebellar tonsils) extend below the foramen magnum on MRI, i.e., >6 mm in children <10 years old and >5 mm in older children. In an MRI study of adults, the prevalence of Chiari II using these diagnostic criteria was 0.5–1.0% and >70% of these patients were asymptomatic. A syrinx was noted in 30% of these subjects.

Chapter 4
Hematology/Oncology

R.S. Holzman et al., *Pediatric Anesthesiology Review: Clinical Cases for Self-Assessment,*
DOI 10.1007/978-1-4419-1617-4_4, © Springer Science+Business Media, LLC 2010

1. Clinical manifestations of sickle cell anemia include:

   1. Hand-foot syndrome, painful often symmetrical swelling of the hands and feet
   2. Painful, vaso-occlusive crises
   3. Acute chest syndrome
   4. More frequent bacterial infections

     A. 1, 2, 3
     B. 1, 3
     C. 2, 4
     D. 4 only
     E. All of the above

2. Sickle trait:

   1. Is found in approximately 8% of the African-American population in America
   2. Is found in approximately 3% of the Hispanic population in America
   3. Is found in <1% of racial groups in America other than Hispanic and African-American
   4. Is not associated with hemolytic anemia

     A. 1, 2, 3
     B. 1, 3
     C. 2, 4
     D. 4 only
     E. All of the above

3. The acute chest syndrome:

   1. Is the leading cause of death in sickle cell patients after the age of 10 years
   2. Is only seen in infants with SS disease
   3. Is a syndrome of hypoxemia, CXR infiltrates, and pulmonary infection/infarction
   4. Is best treated with nebulized bronchodilators and vigorous hydration

     A. 1, 2, 3
     B. 1, 3
     C. 2, 4
     D. 4 only
     E. All of the above

1. All of the above

Sickle hemoglobin differs from normal adult hemoglobin by one amino acid substitution, glutamic acid for valine, at position 6 on the beta chain. Individuals heterozygous for Hb S are resistant to falciparum malaria. Affected homozygous SS individuals have severe hemolytic anemia since the sickled cells are poorly deformable and brittle. Clinical manifestations are rarely seen before 6 months of age with the hand-foot syndrome often seen in 1–2-year-old children.

SS disease is a chronic hemolytic anemia with associated crises such as splenic sequestration crises, aplastic crises, and vaso-occlusive crises. Pain crises are the most common type of vaso-occlusive crisis. Below is a list of common clinical manifestations seen in SS disease:

- Cerebrovascular accidents
- Acute chest syndrome
- Priapism
- Gallbladder disease
- Hematuria
- Renal concentrating defect
- Cardiomyopathy
- Infections
- A variety of psychological problems including school failure and depression

2. E. All of the above

Individuals heterozygous for HbS typically have no signs or symptoms of sickle cell disease. Rarely, these individuals have painless hematuria. The diagnosis of sickle trait is made with hemoglobin electrophoresis. The RBCs in people with sickle cell trait contain 30–40% HbS, thus sickling does not occur under normal circumstances. In unusual conditions such as shock, very high altitude or extremely demanding exercise, a vaso-occlusive crisis may occur.

3. B. 1, 3

This clinical syndrome may occur as a complication of postoperative atelectaisis. Initially, the child may not appear severely ill, but the condition can progress rapidly. Early detection of any pulmonary compromise in a child with sickle cell disease, followed by vigorous treatment (CPT, incentive spirometry, etc.), is essential given the high mortality of children who develop the syndrome.

4. Regarding infection in children with sickle cell disease:

   1. Osteomyelitis is relatively common, particularly with Salmonella.
   2. Encapsulated organisms such as Pneumococcus and Haemophilus influenzae type b are common etiologic agents.
   3. Serious infections are particularly common in the first 5–6 years of life.
   4. With the newer vaccines, infections are no longer a problem for these children.

      A. 1, 2, 3
      B. 1, 3
      C. 2, 4
      D. 4 only
      E. All of the above

5. Therapy for vaso-occlusive crises includes:

   1. Adequate analgesia
   2. Antibiotics
   3. Adequate hydration
   4. Immobility
      A. 1, 2, 3
      B. 1, 3
      C. 2, 4
      D. 4 only
      E. All of the above

6. Acute lymphoblastic leukemia (ALL):

   1. Is the most common leukemia in childhood
   2. Has its peak incidence in children at 10 years of age
   3. May relapse in the bone marrow or CNS
   4. Is treated with total body irradiation

      A. 1, 2, 3
      B. 1, 3
      C. 2, 4
      D. 4 only
      E. All of the above

4. A. 1, 2, 3

The polyvalent pneumococcal vaccines currently available are poorly immunogenic in children under the age of 5 years. Prophylactic penicillin is effective in preventing serious pneumococcal infections in these younger children. Full immunization status is especially important in children with sickle cell disease.

5. B. 1, 3

Children with frequent painful pain crises are difficult to assess. Children afflicted with this chronic painful condition often have a flat affect making observer assessment of their degree of discomfort unreliable. Analgesics should not be withheld if the child reports pain, however. Treatment is directed toward preventing complications such as the acute chest syndrome, uncovering etiologies such as infections (osteomyelitis, pneumonia) and providing adequate hydration, nutrition, and comfort.

6. B. 1, 3

ALL occurs with slightly greater frequency in boys than girls. It is subclassified on the basis of immunologic, cytogenetic, and molecular genetic markers. The median ages for the various types of ALL range from <1 year to 7 years. Presenting signs and symptoms are usually nonspecific and include anorexia, lethargy, and irritability. Pallor, bleeding and fever, signs of bone marrow failure prompt medical attention. There are approximately 200 new cases of ALL/year. Based on survival, ALL is characterized into standard and high risk. Standard risk characteristics in addition to cytogenetic and immunologic factors include age 2–9, female gender, white race, absence of adenopathy, WBC count $<10 \times 10^9$, and absence of CNS disease.

7. Chemotherapeutic agents used in the treatment of standard risk ALL include:

1. Prednisone
2. Vincristine
3. Intrathecal methotrexate (MTX)
4. Bleomycin

   A. 1, 2, 3
   B. 1, 3
   C. 2, 4
   D. 4 only
   E. All of the above

8. Hodgkin's disease:

1. Has a bimodal age distribution with peak incidences in the second and fifth decades of life
2. Commonly presents with painless enlarged cervical lymph nodes
3. Often causes enlarged mediastinal lymph nodes, which may cause cough or other respiratory symptoms
4. Is sensitive to both chemotherapy and radiation

   A. 1, 2, 3
   B. 1, 3
   C. 2, 4
   D. 4 only
   E. All of the above

9. Acute cervical adenitis, inflammation of one or more lymph nodes in the neck, is caused by:

1. Staph Aureus
2. Atypical Mycobacteria
3. Group A Streptococcus
4. Adenoviruses

   A. 1, 2, 3
   B. 1, 3
   C. 2, 4
   D. 4 only
   E. All of the above

7. A. 1, 2, 3

Without treatment of sanctuaries, relapses in the CNS and testicles were common. Induction generally consists of vincristine, prednisone, and asparaginase, accompanied by intrathecal methotrexate, hydrocortisone, and Ara-C. CNS irradiation is effective in minimizing CNS disease but it also produces late neuro-psychiatric effects.

8. E. All of the above

The lymphadenopathy seen is usually in the cervical area but axillary and inguinal nodes are sometimes part of the presentation. Hepatosplenomagaly is rare. Fever, weight loss, and night sweats are seen. Staging is important in prognosis and in determining treatment. Disease-free survival rates from 60 to 90% are achieved, based on the staging at diagnosis.

9. A. 1, 2, 3

With chronic infection, signs such as erythema, warmth, and fluctuance are absent. Nodes associated with malignancy are firm and may be fixed to underlying structures or overlying skin. Another infectious cause of cervical adenitis is Kawasaki's Disease.

10. Relatively common noninfectious causes of cervical adenitis include:

   1. Hodgkins disease
   2. Non-Hodgkin's lymphoma
   3. Neuroblastoma
   4. Hemangiomas

     A. 1, 2, 3
     B. 1, 3
     C. 2, 4
     D. 4 only
     E. All of the above

11. Neuroblastoma, the most common extra cranial tumor of childhood and the most frequently diagnosed cancer in infants, presents in a variety of ways including:

   1. With a hard painless mass in the neck
   2. As an abdominal or thoracic mass
   3. With bone pain from skeletal and bone marrow metastases
   4. With seizures from CNS metastases

     A. 1, 2, 3
     B. 1, 3
     C. 2, 4
     D. 4 only
     E. All of the above

12. Wilms tumor of the kidney:

   1. Commonly presents with an asymptomatic flank mass
   2. Is often diagnosed in children at 2–4 years of age
   3. Is associated with hypertension in up to 60% of cases
   4. Often metastasizes to the lungs

     A. 1, 2, 3
     B. 1, 3
     C. 2, 4
     D. 4 only
     E. All of the above

10. B. 1, 3

The most common presentation of Hodgkin's Disease is painless, firm adenopathy. Cervical or supraclavicular nodes are commonly involved. Significant enlargement of the nodes in the anterior mediastinum leads to cough, respiratory distress, and cardiovascular embarrassment. This mediastinal involvement is seen the most in older children with Hodgkin's Disease. Hodgkin's Disease is staged using the Ann Arbor system:

Stage I	disease involves a single LN area or a single extralymphatic site.
Stage II	is more extensive but on one side of the diaphragm.
Stage III	disease is seen on both sides of the diaphragm.
Stage IV	the malignancy is disseminated, involving greater than one extralymphatic site.

Neuroblastoma has a very varied presentation. Abdominal pain and mass is a common presentation, but in children with localized disease, adenopathy is also seen.

11. A. 1, 2, 3

This tumor has a variable presentation since it may develop at any site of the sympathetic nervous system. It is generally discovered as a mass or masses on exam or on a radiologic scan. Treatment varies depending on the stage at diagnosis, as does the chance for survival. Overall cure rate, with all stages included, is approximately 50%.

12. E. All of the above   *(! American book)*

This tumor accounts for most renal cancer in children. The asymptomatic mass is often discovered by a parent. Surgical removal is indicated even in cases where pulmonary metastases have occurred. With chemotherapy following surgery, survival ranges from 50 to <90% depending on histology and stage.

13. Manifestations of graft versus host disease (GVHD) in children include:

    1. Maculopapular rash
    2. Generalized erythroderma with bullae and desquamation
    3. Liver dysfunction manifested by elevated bilirubin
    4. GI disturbances manifested primarily by diarrhea

    A. 1, 2, 3
    B. 1, 3
    C. 2, 4
    D. 4 only
    E. All of the above

14. Brain tumors:

    1. Are the most common solid tumor in children
    2. In children between the ages of 2 and 12 years are most often located in the posterior fossa
    3. May present with signs of increased intracranial pressure
    4. May present with focal neurological signs

    A. 1, 2, 3
    B. 1, 3
    C. 2, 4
    D. 4 only
    E. All of the above

15. Regarding posterior fossa tumors:

    1. They tend to present with symptoms of raised intracranial pressure.
    2. The most common histology, cerebellar astrocytoma, also has the best prognosis.
    3. Morning headache with associated vomiting may be part of the presentation.
    4. Medulloblastoma is the second most common posterior fossa tumor.

    A. 1, 2, 3
    B. 1, 3
    C. 2, 4
    D. 4 only
    E. All of the above

13. E. All of the above

GVHD occurs when there is a disparity of histocompatability antigens between the recipient of a bone marrow transplant and the donor marrow. Donor T lymphocytes damage various tissues in the host especially the skin, GI tract (mucositis), and liver. There are acute and chronic forms of the disease with chronic having a worse prognosis.

14. E. All of the above

Brain tumors are the second most common reported malignancy in children and adolescents. Surgery and radiation are the mainstays of treatment. CNS tumors may present with headache, worse in the morning. These tumors are classified by location (infratentorial, supratentorial) and histology.

15. E. All of the above

Infratentorial (posterior fossa) tumors predominate in children 4–14 years of age. Nearly one-half of pediatric brain tumors arise in the cerebellum, frequently astrocytomas and medulloblastomas. In another classification system medulloblastomas, which are poorly differentiated, very malignant tumors, are termed primitive neuroectodermal tumors (PNET).

Chapter 5
Cardiology

R.S. Holzman et al., *Pediatric Anesthesiology Review: Clinical Cases for Self-Assessment,*
DOI 10.1007/978-1-4419-1617-4_5, © Springer Science+Business Media, LLC 2010

1. Paroxysmal supraventricular tachycardia:

    1. Can cause low output congestive heart failure
    2. Can be treated with IV adenosine
    3. Can be prevented with PO digoxin
    4. Should be initially treated with verapamil

        A. 1, 2, 3
        B. 1, 3
        C. 2, 4
        D. 4 only
        E. All of the above

2. The ECG of a newborn or infant:

    1. Will show increased right ventricular forces
    2. Will show prominence R wave in V1
    3. Will show inverted T waves in lead V1
    4. Will show right bundle branch block pattern until 5 years of age

        A. 1, 2, 3
        B. 1, 3
        C. 2, 4
        D. 4 only
        E. All of the above

3. The most common cardiac lesions, exclusive of PDAs in premies, are (choose 2):

    A. ASD
    B. Tetralogy of Fallot (TOF)
    C. Hypoplastic left heart syndrome
    D. VSD
    E. Coarctation of the aorta (CoA)

4. A relatively large VSD:

    1. Will often present with dyspnea, feeding difficulty, and poor growth
    2. Presents at 1–3 months of age as pulmonary vascular resistance (PVR) decreases
    3. Will cause a Qp:Qs > 2:1
    4. Will present with a harsh holosystolic murmur and a loud P2

        A. 1, 2, 3
        B. 1, 3
        C. 2, 4
        D. 4 only
        E. All of the above

1. A. 1, 2, 3

SVT is a tachydysrhythmia which originates from above the bifurcation of the bundle of His. Onset is usually paroxysmal. In children, the rate is generally >230 beats/min and in infants the rate can exceed 300 beats/min. The QRS is narrow, often little different from the QRS seen during normal sinus rhythm. Predisposing factors for the development of PSVT are the preexcitation syndromes such as Wolf–Parkinson–White, congenital heart disease, and sympathomimetic medications such as atropine or glycopyrrolate.

2. A. 1, 2, 3

At birth, the RV and LV walls are of approximately equal thickness, thus the infant has relative RV hypertrophy with prominence of right and anterior forces.

3. A. ASD and D. VSD

Atrial septal defects (ASDs) come in four varieties: patent foramen ovale (PFO), secundum (at the fossa ovalis) ASDs, coronary sinus defects (absence of wall separating the coronary sinus and LA), and sinus venosus defects (immediately below the SVC opening). Sinus venosus defects are associated with partial anomalous pulmonary venous return.

4. E. All of the above

VSD is the most common congenital cardiac malformation in children with an incidence of approximately 2–3:1,000 live births. VSDs are often not apparent in the newborn because the relatively high pulmonary vascular resistance limits the right to left flow through the defect. Congestive heart failure (CHF) becomes clinically apparent as the infant grows and PVR decreases. The severity of the shunt is characterized by the Qp:Qs ratio. With a Qp:Qs>2, signs and symptoms of CHF are seen. CHF in infants and newborns presents with poor feeding, diaphoresis with feeding, effortless tachypnea, lethargy, and FTT. The typical murmur of a VSD is holosystolic, harsh, and best heard along the left sternal border.

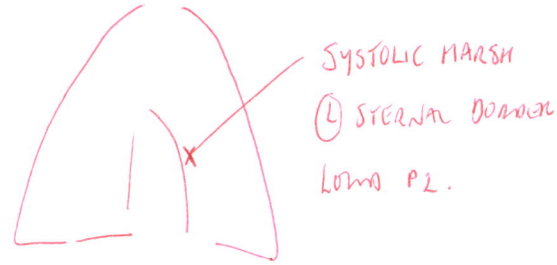

SYSTOLIC HARSH
(L) STERNAL BORDER
LONG P2.

5. Regarding ventricular septal defects (VSDs):

1. They occur with an overall incidence of 3–4/1,000 live births.
2. They undergo spontaneous closure in approximately 25% of cases.
3. Complications of repair are rare and include acquired complete heart block.
4. Most VSDs occur in association with other congenital anomalies.

    A. 1, 2, 3
    B. 1, 3
    C. 2, 4
    D. 4 only
    E. All of the above

6. Regarding ASDs:

1. They can be divided into primum, secundum, and sinus venosus based on location and etiology.
2. Secundum ASDs are the most common type.
3. Secundum ASDs often are asymptomatic in childhood.
4. There may be associated partial anomalous venous return with an ASD.

    A. 1, 2, 3
    B. 1, 3
    C. 2, 4
    D. 4 only
    E. All of the above

7. Which of the following organisms are associated with sepsis occurring after cardiac surgery?

    A. Haemophilus influenzae type b
    B. *Neisseria gonorrhoeae*
    C. *Staphylococci*
    D. Enteric gram negative rods

8. The so-called innocent murmur of childhood:

1. May be heard in up to 30% of children at some point in their lives
2. Is best heard in a localized area along the left lower sternal border
3. Is short, vibratory ejection-type murmur
4. Is generally heard in children between the ages of 3 and 7 years

    A. 1, 2, 3
    B. 1, 3
    C. 2, 4
    D. 4 only
    E. All of the above

5. A. 1, 2, 3

VSDs are classified by location in the septum. Membranous or perimembranous defects are the most common. These are located below the aortic valve and adjacent to the tricuspid valve. Other types of VSD include: AV canal type, subpulmonary, conoventricular, and muscular VSDs. Many VSDs undergo spontaneous closure with larger defects less likely to do so. Currently, repair is undertaken in infancy. The risk of heart block in the postoperative period is related to the size and location of the patch used to repair the defect.

6. E. All of the above

Isolated secundum ASDs, which represent 80% of all ASDs, generally do not present in infancy. Children with this defect generally are in sinus rhythm. Primum ASDs are often associated with a cleft mitral valve. Sinus venosus and coronary sinus ASDs are actually defects in the embryologic sinus venosus. The murmur noted in children with relatively large ASDs is a pulmonary flow murmur with associated fixed splitting of S2. Patients with unrepaired ASDs often do relatively well into their 20s when progressive cyanosis and dyspnea develop.

7. C. *Staphylococci*

8. E. All of the above

The history is unremarkable in these children since they have no cardiac disease. Murmurs are more frequently heard in children during febrile episodes. The cause of the murmur is unknown. Some speculate that it is heard only in childhood because the relatively thin chest wall of young children transmits extra cardiac sounds more easily.

9. Congestive heart failure in childhood may present:

1. Chronic cough
2. As failure to thrive
3. With respiratory distress during feedings
4. With the child's complaint that it is difficult to keep up with peers during play

   A. 1, 2, 3
   B. 1, 3
   C. 2, 4
   D. 4 only
   E. All of the above

10. Tetralogy of Fallot:

1. Is the most common cyanotic congenital cardiac lesion presenting after 2 weeks of age
2. Includes pulmonary stenosis, VSD, overriding aorta, and RVH
3. May have infundibular and valvar pulmonary stenosis
4. Is inherited as an autosomal dominant

    A. 1, 2, 3
    B. 1, 3
    C. 2, 4
    D. 4 only
    E. All of the above

11. So-called Tet spells:

1. Occur in infants with unrepaired Tetralogy of Fallot
2. Are the result of increased tone in the infundibulum of the RV outflow tract
3. Result in intense cyanosis and diminution of the systolic ejection murmur as pulmonary blood flow dramatically decreases
4. Can be treated with IV fluid administration and/or increasing SVR

   A. 1, 2, 3
   B. 1, 3
   C. 2, 4
   D. 4 only
   E. All of the above

12. The most common congenital cardiac defect presenting with cyanosis in the newborn is:

   A. Transposition of the great arteries (TGA)
   B. Patent ductus arteriosus (PDA)
   C. Hypoplastic left heart syndrome (HLHS)
   D. Tetralogy of Fallot (TOF)
   E. Truncus arteriosus

9. E. All of the above

CHF presents in infancy with tachycardia, tachypnea, poor feeding, and failure to thrive. In older children, decreased exercise tolerance is noted, as in adults. Recurrent respiratory infections are common, although rales are not heard until later in the course of CHF.

10. A. 1, 2, 3

TOF is found in approximately 6–10% of infants with cyanotic congenital heart disease. TOF has no known inheritance pattern but it is found in association with a number of syndromes such as Goldenhar (oculoauriculovertebral hypoplasia), VACTERL (vertebral anomalies, esophageal atresia with tracheoesophageal fistula, radial dysplasia, renal anomalies, imperforate anus, cardiac defects), CHARGE (choanal atresia, heart defects, deafness, genital hypoplasia in males, coloboma), and Klippel-Feil (short neck, limited neck motion, low occipital hairline).

11. E. All of the above

With repair of TOF now routinely performed in the neonate and infant, "tet spells" are rare.

12. A. Transposition of the great arteries (TGA)

Without mixing of the two parallel circulations, the newborn with TGA cannot survive. The presentation of TGA is affected by the presence of other anomalies such as a VSD, left ventricular outflow tract obstruction (LVOTO), or subpulmonic stenosis. Newborns with intact ventricular septa rely on the presence of a PFO or PDA to mix oxygenated and deoxygenated blood.

13. A newborn with isolated TGA may present with:

    1. Cyanosis
    2. Tachypnea without dyspnea or respiratory distress
    3. Normal peripheral pulses
    4. An ECG showing right ventricular hypertrophy, indistinguishable from that a newborn with a normal heart

    A. 1, 2, 3
    B. 1, 3
    C. 2, 4
    D. 4 only
    E. All of the above

14. Which of the following may be done to newborns with TGA to improve arterial SpO_2?

    1. A Rashkind–Miller procedure
    2. Administration of milrinone
    3. Prostaglandin E1 administration
    4. Dilation of the ductus arteriosus in the cath lab

    A. 1, 2, 3
    B. 1, 3
    C. 2, 4
    D. 4 only
    E. All of the above

15. Regarding the ductus arteriosus:

    1. More than 90% of fetal RV output passes through the ductus.
    2. If it remains open postnatally, it has flow through it both during systole and diastole.
    3. It closes functionally during the first day of life in most term infants.
    4. Spontaneous closure of a persistently open PDA is unlikely after the age of 6 months.

    A. 1, 2, 3
    B. 1, 3
    C. 2, 4
    D. 4 only
    E. All of the above

13. E. All of the above

In newborns with TGA and IVS (intact ventricular septum), there often is no murmur present. A CXR may be normal but approximately 30% show an "egg on a string" pattern of the cardiothymic shadow.

14. B. 1, 3

Maneuvers which enhance mixing of the parallel circulations improve the situation in newborns with TGA. Prostaglandins keep the PDA open and the Rashkind procedure involves creation of an atrial septostomy using a specially designed catheter.

15. E. All of the above

In full-term infants, persistent patent ductus arteriosus accounts for approximately 10% of congenital heart disease. PDAs are much more common in the premature newborn. (see question/answer 18, 19 in newborn medicine). Commonly, the PDA is picked up when a murmur is heard in an asymptomatic child who is being examined for another reason. The typical murmur is continuous (machine-like) and heard best in the midclavicular line between the first and second interspace.

16. Endocardial cushions contribute to which of the following cardiac structures?

    1. The lower part of the atrial septum
    2. The part of the ventricular septum where the AV valves insert
    3. Tissue that forms part of the mitral and tricuspid valves
    4. Part of the intraventricular conduction system

       A. 1, 2, 3
       B. 1, 3
       C. 2, 4
       D. 4 only
       E. All of the above

17. Common atrioventricular canal defects (CAVC):

    1. Result in communication between all four cardiac chambers
    2. Have abnormal mitral and/or tricuspid valves
    3. Often present in a manner similar to large VSDs
    4. Predispose the child to the early development of pulmonary vascular obstructive disease (PVOD)

       A. 1, 2, 3
       B. 1, 3
       C. 2, 4
       D. 4 only
       E. All of the above

18. In Total Anomalous Pulmonary Venous Return (TAPVR):

    1. These are often divided into several types based upon the site of pulmonary venous drainage.
    2. All the pulmonary veins drain into the systemic venous system, not the left atrium.
    3. There often is pulmonary venous obstruction.
    4. There is an ASD or PFO allowing a right to left shunt to compensate for the left to right shunt resulting from the TAPVR.

       A. 1, 2, 3
       B. 1, 3
       C. 2, 4
       D. 4 only
       E. All of the above

16. A. 1, 2, 3

AV canal defects, also called endocardial cushion defects, involve a primum ASD, defects in one or more of the AV valves, and also a defect in the ventricular septum.

17. E. All of the above

AV canal defects have variable anatomy. The atrial and ventricular septa and AV valves are affected in many different ways. Down syndrome is frequently associated with CAVC defects. Two dimensional ECHO demonstrates absence of the atrial septum while pulsed doppler ECHO demonstrates the presence of AV valve regurgitation.

18. E. All of the above

TAPVR is classified into four types. In decreasing order of frequency they are supracardiac, cardiac, infracardiac, and mixed. Obstruction of the anomalous venous drainage leading to pulmonary congestion may occur at any point along the anomalous venous pathway. Obstruction almost always occurs in the infracardiac type.

19. Regarding the locations of the pulmonary venous drainage in TAPVR:

   1. Supracardiac, the most common, involves drainage into an anomalous vein which eventually empties into the SVC.
   2. With intracardiac TAPVR, venous drainage is directly into the RA or coronary sinus.
   3. With infracardiac TAPVR, a vein passes through the diaphragm.
   4. Mixed TAPVR, a combination of the other types, is the least common.

      A. 1, 2, 3
      B. 1, 3
      C. 2, 4
      D. 4 only
      E. All of the above

20. Coarctation of the aorta (CoA):

   1. Is a congenital narrowing of the aorta near the insertion of the ductus arteriosus
   2. Is commonly associated with VSD or hypoplastic left heart syndrome (HLHS)
   3. May cause reduced lower body perfusion
   4. Produces aortic insufficiency

      A. 1, 2, 3
      B. 1, 3
      C. 2, 4
      D. 4 only
      E. All of the above

21. Newborns and infants presenting with coarctation of the aorta:

   1. Generally have more severe coarctation
   2. May have metabolic acidosis as a result of poor lower body perfusion
   3. May present with signs of LV failure
   4. Have an extensive network of collaterals

      A. 1, 2, 3
      B. 1, 3
      C. 2, 4
      D. 4 only
      E. All of the above

19. E. All of the above

The presence and degree of venous obstruction and the degree of intra atrial mixing determine the severity of clinical symptoms. Infants with obstruction in the anomalous venous connections develop cyanosis and respiratory distress early in life. Infants without obstruction and a nonrestrictive inter atrial communication may have only minimal symptoms during the first year of life.

20. A. 1, 2, 3

The aortic narrowing seen in CoA is located in the descending thoracic aorta just across from the insertion of the ductus arteriosus. This anomaly has a 2:1 male predominance. The major problem associated with CoA is increased LV afterload. For CoA to become clinically significant, the aortic diameter must be decreased by at least 50%. Pulses and measured blood pressure in the lower extremities are diminished compared with the upper extremities.

21. E. All of the above

Newborns with CoA may appear well initially, but cardiac failure and respiratory distress quickly develop as the ductus closes. Prostaglandin administration may improve the situation as the dilated ductus allows improved lower extremity and renal perfusion.

22. Children with coarctation of the aorta:

   1. Have had time to develop collateral flow through intercostal and other arteries
   2. Usually require cardiopulmonary bypass for surgical repair
   3. May have systemic hypertension
   4. Are often managed medically until adulthood

     A. 1, 2, 3
     B. 1, 3
     C. 2, 4
     D. 4 only
     E. All of the above

23. The hypoplastic left heart syndrome can include:

   1. Hypoplasia of the LV and RA
   2. Mitral atresia
   3. Coronary, carotid, and subclavian flow via retrograde filling of a small ascending aorta from the ductus
   4. RV hypertrophy

     A. 1, 2, 3
     B. 1, 3
     C. 2, 4
     D. 4 only
     E. All of the above

24. What happens to newborns with HLHS when the PDA closes?

   1. There is improved systemic blood pressure.
   2. There is reduced coronary flow.
   3. There is increased systemic flow.
   4. There is decreased systemic flow.

     A. 1, 2, 3
     B. 1, 3
     C. 2, 4
     D. 4 only
     E. All of the above

22. B. 1, 3

Children with isolated CoA often have no specific complaints. With a careful history, the child may report leg cramps. The coarctation may be discovered during an evaluation of systemic hypertension. The ECG may show no changes or LVH by voltage criteria may be seen. The pathognomonic CXR finding of rib notching, due to rib erosion by the enlarged collateral vessels, is rarely seen in children younger than 5–6 years of age.

23. A. 1, 2, 3

HLHS is seen in 3–4:10,000 live births. There is a spectrum of anomalies in this left-sided obstructive lesion. The LV and ascending aorta are underdeveloped. The mitral valve is often involved, exhibiting stenosis, hypoplasia, or atresia. The RV provides both pulmonary and systemic flow in HLHS. There is a L to R shunting of pulmonary venous return at the atrial level and a R to L shunting of RV output at the PDA, with the ascending aorta and its vessels (carotids, subclavian, and coronaries) perfused retrograde via flow from the PDA.

24. C. 2, 4

The PDA allows the RV output to flow to the pulmonary circuit, the systemic circuit and retrograde into the ascending aorta. Once the diagnosis of HLHS is made, prostaglandin should be infused to keep the PDA open and the newborn monitored for the development of metabolic acidosis.

25. In HLHS, systemic flow is affected by:

    1. SVR
    2. PaO_2
    3. PVR
    4. pH

        A. 1, 2, 3
        B. 1, 3
        C. 2, 4
        D. 4 only
        E. All of the above

26. Which of the following CHD diagnoses is matched with the past or present appropriate surgical procedure?

    1. TOF-BT shunt
    2. TGA Switch
    3. HLHS – Stage I – Glenn–Fontan
    4. VSD-PA band

        A. 1, 2, 3
        B. 1, 3
        C. 2, 4
        D. 4 only
        E. All of the above

27. The Fotan operation, also called total cavopulmonary connection,

    1. Directs systemic venous return to the PA
    2. Is the surgical procedure for many patients with single ventricle physiology
    3. Is generally performed at 1–2 years of age
    4. Is generally preceded by a bidirectional Glenn procedure

        A. 1, 2, 3
        B. 1, 3
        C. 2, 4
        D. 4 only
        E. All of the above

25. E. All of the above

The ratio of systemic to pulmonary vascular resistances is crucial in determining flows into these vascular beds. Excessive pulmonary flow will lead to underperfusion of the body. Hyperventilation and oxygen administration may increase SpO_2 but lead to systemic hypoperfusion and the development of metabolic acidosis. Chromosomal abnormalities have been reported in 11% of infants with HLHS and autopsies have revealed neurologic abnormalities in 29% of these patients.

26. E. All of the above

Palliation of TOF is no longer done as a routine, but if done, the goal is to achieve an increase in pulmonary blood flow. A Blalock–Taussig shunt (B–T shunt) diverts subclavian artery flow to the pulmonary circulation, either using a gortex graft or by an end-to-side anastamosis of the subclavian artery to the PA.

Transposition of the great arteries (TGA) is treated surgically with a so-called "switch operation" in which the PA and Aorta are moved to the appropriate ventricular outflow tract. It is very important to know the coronary arterial anatomy beforehand. The coronaries are removed from the aortic root along with a small area of surrounding tissue and moved to the newly "switched" aorta.

Hypoplastic left heart syndrome accounts for 1% of all CHD. There is a small LV, mitral valve, aortic valve, and aortic arch. A stage I procedure is done in the newborn period. Systemic flow is carried by the PDA and coronary flow is retrograde in the small aortic arch. The Stage I procedure involves creation of a neoaorta from the hypoplastic aortic arch, main PA, and homograft. A large ASD is created and pulmonary blood flow is via a modified (graft material) B–T shunt.

Ventricular septal defects often become clinically apparent in the third month of life, when PVR decreases substantially and the higher left ventricular pressures divert more and more blood to the lower pressure right ventricle, leading to CHF. The degree of shunt is characterized by the ratio of systemic to pulmonary flow (Qp:Qs). A 2:1 shunt or greater is associated with CHF. Currently, most VSDs are repaired primarily in the OR or with a device in the cardiac catheterization lab. A PA band was used previously as a temporary means to increase resistance to pulmonary flow, thus decreasing the shunt.

27. E. All of the above

The Fontan procedure involves so-called passive flow of systemic venous return into the pulmonary circuit. This requires a transpulmonary gradient of 3–8 mmHg. This can be achieved if the CVP (PA) pressure is kept at 12–15 mmHg with an LVEDP of 5–10 mmHg. In addition, the cardiac rhythm must be kept in sinus, and ventricular performance must often be supported pharmacologically.

Chapter 6
The Musculoskeletal System

R.S. Holzman et al., *Pediatric Anesthesiology Review: Clinical Cases for Self-Assessment,*
DOI 10.1007/978-1-4419-1617-4_6, © Springer Science+Business Media, LLC 2010

1. Cerebral palsy, a movement and posture disorder,

   1. Is seen in 1–2/1,000 children, making it the most common childhood movement disorder
   2. Is initially diagnosed when the child exhibits delayed motor development
   3. Does not have an identifiable risk factors in most cases
   4. Has a changing clinical picture despite the static nature of the neurologic damage

      A. 1, 2, 3
      B. 1, 3
      C. 2, 4
      D. 4 only
      E. All of the above

2. Even though many cases of cerebral palsy (CP) do not have an identified etiology, there are known associations such as:

   1. Birth asphyxia
   2. Prematurity
   3. IUGR (intrauterine growth restriction)
   4. Family history

      A. 1, 2, 3
      B. 1, 3
      C. 2, 4
      D. 4 only
      E. All of the above

3. Children with CP may also have which of the following:

   1. Seizures
   2. Normal intellect
   3. Mental retardation
   4. Communication disorders, hearing, and visual dysfunction

      A. 1, 2, 3
      B. 1, 3
      C. 2, 4
      D. 4 only
      E. All of the above

1. E. All of the above

This condition is the result of an anomaly or insult to the immature CNS, but in many, if not most cases, a specific antecedent event or cause cannot be identified. The term static encephalopathy is often used synonymously with cerebral palsy. The incidence of CP is 7:1,000 live births and prevalence is 5:1,000 of the population. Cognitive impairment is not a consistent feature of CP, although many affected children do have a lower than normal IQ. Between 30 and 70% of children with CP do have impaired intellect. Many children with CP also have seizures. CP is described by the clinical appearance:

- Spastic diplegia
- Spastic quadriplegia
- Spastic hemiplegia
- Extrapyramidal
- Atonic
- Mixed

2. A. 1, 2, 3

The association of CP with prematurity is changing as neonatal care improves. The incidence is decreasing in heavier preterm newborns but VLBW (very low birth weight) infants have a higher incidence.

Clinical types of CP:

Spastic diplegia. Lower extremity involvement, seen in low birth weight infants, after intraventricular hemorrhage. Severe mental deficits less common than in other types.

Spastic quadraplegia. All four extremities involved. More severe mental deficiencies, seizures likely. Scoliosis, feeding problems more common.

Extrapyramidal. Decreased tone, choreoathetosis seen. Fewer seizures and more normal development seen in these patients.

Atonic. Hypotonia, brisk reflexes seen only in this type, severe cognitive delays.

3. E. All of the above

Overall, approximately 60% of CP patients have mental retardation (MR). Children with spastic forms have a higher incidence of MR which increases with the number of limbs involved. Learning disorders, deafness, and sensory impairment are also seen in these children. Impaired oromotor function may lead to difficulties with speech or aspiration pneumonia. One-third of children with CP have seizures.

4. Treatments for CP include:

1. Braces and/or splints
2. Intramuscular injections of Botulinum toxin and/or phenol
3. Surgery
4. Neuraxial administration of baclofen to decrease spasticity

   A. 1, 2, 3
   B. 1, 3
   C. 2, 4
   D. 4 only
   E. All of the above

5. Septic arthritis:

1. Is slightly more common than hematogenous osteomyelitis in children
2. Occurs more often in infants and young children
3. May present in infancy with fever, poor feeding, and subtle asymmetry of soft tissue folds
4. In infants most often involves the hip

   A. 1, 2, 3
   B. 1, 3
   C. 2, 4
   D. 4 only
   E. All of the above

6. Talipes equinovarus congenita (clubfoot):

1. Has an incidence of 1:1,000
2. May be bilateral or unilateral
3. May be treated conservatively until the second birthday
4. May be effectively treated with casting in up to 70% of cases

   A. 1, 2, 3
   B. 1, 3
   C. 2, 4
   D. 4 only
   E. All of the above

4. E. All of the above

Treatments are directed toward maximizing motor function. Physical therapy and positioning techniques may delay the development of contractures. bracing is most often used for foot and ankle problems. Botulinum toxin or phenol injection may temporarily decrease spasticity.

5. E. All of the above

The role of arthrotomy vs. needle aspiration in the treatment of septic arthritis is controversial although many would opt for arthrotomy in cases involving the hip joint. IV antibiotics should be given for 4–6 weeks. The differential diagnosis of an infant with fever, joint pain, and elevated WBC count includes juvenile rheumatoid arthritis, cellulitis, and toxic synovitis.

6. A. 1, 2, 3

Clubfoot is more common in males. Casting, if done early (in the neonatal period), with the casts being changed every few days, may successfully treat mild forms of talipes equinovarus (from the Latin talus [ankle] + pes [foot]; equino indicates the heel is elevated like a horse's and varus indicates it is turned inward) in about one-third of cases.

7. Which of the following are associated with or characteristic of Osteogenesis Imperfecta?

   1. Defects in collagen formation
   2. Bones with thin cortices
   3. Deafness
   4. B-cell immunodeficiencies

      A. 1, 2, 3
      B. 1, 3
      C. 2, 4
      D. 4 only
      E. All of the above

8. Regarding developmental dysplasia of the hip (DDH) formerly called congenital dislocated hips (CDH):

   1. It can be diagnosed in the newborn with the Barlow and Ortolani tests.
   2. In the newborn is diagnosed with plain X-rays of the hips.
   3. It is more common in girls and newborns who were born with breech presentations.
   4. It is treated with surgery followed by bracing for 6 months.

      A. 1, 2, 3
      B. 1, 3
      C. 2, 4
      D. 4 only
      E. All of the above

9. Slipped capital femoral epiphysis (SCFE):

   1. Is more common in males
   2. Often presents with limp
   3. Is often accompanied by obesity
   4. Is commonly bilateral

      A. 1, 2, 3
      B. 1, 3
      C. 2, 4
      D. 4 only
      E. All of the above

7. A. 1, 2, 3

OI is a group of disorders characterized by brittle bones. Stills classification system has six types, with varying degrees of bone fragility, different associated findings and inheritance patterns. Associated findings in these patients include middle-ear deafness, blue sclerae, short stature, and thin skin.

8. B. 1, 3

DDH occurs more frequently in firstborns. More than 20% of children with DDH have a positive family history and it occurs six times more frequently in girls than in boys. The degrees of hip dysplasia (in order of increasing severity) are dislocatable, subluxable, and dislocated hips. X-rays are of little value as a diagnostic aid before 6 months of age since bony changes are not apparent. Ultrasonography is used in some centers and in Europe but interpretation is difficult.

9. A. 1, 2, 3

In SCFE, the femur is rotated externally from under the epiphysis. About one fourth of children have bilateral involvement, but not simultaneously. Obesity is commonly seen in affected children. In Legg–Calve–Perthe's disease (LCP), which is seen in younger (4–8 years) children than SCFE, there is ischemic necrosis of the proximal femoral epiphysis and later resorption. With subsequent reossification, there may be collapse of the femoral head. As a group, affected children have shorter stature and delayed bone age compared with their peers.

10. Scoliosis:

    1. Is defined as a lateral curvature of the spine
    2. May compromise pulmonary function
    3. Has both congenital and acquired etiologies
    4. Involves rounding of the back in the thoracolumbar area of the spine

       A. 1, 2, 3
       B. 1, 3
       C. 2, 4
       D. 4 only
       E. All of the above

11. Which of the following organisms are associated with sepsis occurring after orthopedic surgery?

    A. Haemophilus influenzae type b
    B. *Neisseria gonorrhoeae*
    C. *Staphylococci*
    D. Enteric gram negative rods

12. Juvenile rheumatoid arthritis:

    1. Has a prevalence of 60–100/1,000,000
    2. Is much more common in females
    3. Is divided into three subtypes: systemic onset, polyarticular, and pauciarticular
    4. Generally first presents in young children, before the age of 6–7 years

       A. 1, 2, 3
       B. 1, 3
       C. 2, 4
       D. 4 only
       E. All of the above

10. A. 1, 2, 3

Types of scoliosis include idiopathic (80%), congenital (5%), neuromuscular (10%), and miscellaneous (5%). Miscellaneous causes include genetic disorders and connective tissue diseases. Although idiopathic scoliosis requiring correction is much more common in girls than boys, mild curves are found equally in both genders. Scoliosis curves >25° are likely to increase if the child is still growing. Curves of 40–50° will increase even if growth is complete and curves >75° will affect pulmonary function.

Congenital scoliosis can be complete or partial and is often associated with other congenital anomalies. Associated anomalies include renal agenesis or obstructive uropathy, congenital heart disease, or spinal dysraphism. Congenital scoliosis is seen in children with VATER or Klippel–Feil Syndrome and meningomyelocele.

11. C. *Staphylococci*

While perioperative antibiotics are important in the prevention of postoperative sepsis, overuse or extended administration of antibiotics has been implicated in the increased incidence of *Clostridium difficile* toxin-related diarrhea.

12. E. All of the above

JRA is one of the more common chronic illnesses of children. This disease affects approximately 200,000 children in the USA. It commonly presents at either 1–3 years of age or in adolescence. Girls are affected twice as frequently as boys with both polyarticular and pauciarticular forms, while the sex incidence is equal in systemic-onset disease. Affected children often have growth retardation, anemia, and chronic uveitis. Severity is based on the degree of impairment in tasks of life. Treatment includes NSAIDs, steroids, gold to decrease inflammation, physical therapy, occupational therapy and surgery to preserve function, and counseling and nutritional support. Differential diagnosis includes systemic lupus erythematosus, Lyme disease, or Kawasaki disease.

Clinical types:

Systemic. Ill appearance associated with high fevers, irritability, rash, splenomegaly.

Polyarticular. Involvement of >5 joints for 6 months or more. Subdivided into seronegative or seropositive. More common in girls.

Pauciarticular. Peak age at 2 years; large joints are generally involved.

Chapter 7
General Pediatrics

R.S. Holzman et al., *Pediatric Anesthesiology Review: Clinical Cases for Self-Assessment,*
DOI 10.1007/978-1-4419-1617-4_7, © Springer Science+Business Media, LLC 2010

1. Which of the following are considered risk factors for the development of tuberculosis in children?

   1. HIV infection
   2. Exposure to an infectious adult
   3. Malnutrition
   4. Passive exposure to cigarette smoke

      A. 1, 2, 3
      B. 1, 3
      C. 2, 4
      D. 4 only
      E. All of the above

2. Tuberculosis infection may involve which of the following organs/systems?

   1. The lungs
   2. The bones
   3. The CNS
   4. The kidneys

      A. 1, 2, 3
      B. 1, 3
      C. 2, 4
      D. 4 only
      E. All of the above

3. What percentage of immunocompetent adults infected with tuberculosis will develop active disease during their lives?

   A. 100%
   B. 50%
   C. 25%
   D. 5%
   E. 2%

4. Which of the following factors may affect the accuracy of the Mantoux test (the intradermal injection of 5 TU of PPD in 0.1 mL diluent):

   1. Concurrent penicillin treatment
   2. The presence of other infections
   3. Presence of fever >38°C
   4. Prior BCG vaccination

      A. 1, 2, 3
      B. 1, 3
      C. 2, 4
      D. 4 only
      E. All of the above

1. A. 1, 2, 3

TB in the USA is unfortunately becoming more common in adults as well as in children. It is an important cause of mortality worldwide. In the USA, infection of children often results from exposure to an untreated individual with active disease. Reservoirs of TB include people with HIV/AIDS, the homeless, patients living in overcrowded conditions, and new immigrants.

2. E. All of the above

TB infection can involve most organ systems. It most commonly affects the lungs. Superficial lymph node infection is a common manifestation of TB infection. The major cause of death in children from TB is meningitis. Cerebrospinal fluid findings in TB meningitis include a predominance of lymphocytes in low numbers (50–500 cells/μL), low glucose, and elevated protein. The TB organism is seen in less than 50% of cases and CSF cultures become positive only after several weeks. Miliary tuberculosis, so called because the small lesions found throughout the body resemble millet seeds, is due to blood-borne spread of the organism.

3. D. 5%

Predisposing factors for the development of serious disease in patients infected with TB include young age, pregnancy, and decreased vigor of immune response (HIV/AIDS, poor nutrition, steroid treatment).

4. E. All of the above

Patients previously immunized by Bacille Calmette-Guerin (BCG) will show a positive PPD. The BCG vaccine, derived from a mycobacterium related to TB, activates cell-mediated immunity. Since the many vaccines derived from strains of the bacterium differ from one another in antigenicity, the immune response to the vaccines is quite variable.

5. Group A beta Hemolytic Streptococci cause:

1. Scarlet fever
2. Tonsillitis
3. Impetigo
4. Erysipelas

    A. 1, 2, 3
    B. 1, 3
    C. 2, 4
    D. 4 only
    E. All of the above

6. Which one of the following is true regarding the nonsupportive complications of group A beta hemolytic infections?

    A. Rheumatic fever may develop after tonsillitis.
    B. Neither nephritis nor rheumatic fever develops after impetigo.
    C. Rheumatic fever is caused by the same strains of the organism as nephritis.
    D. Nephritis develops only after scarlet fever rashes.

7. *Helicobacter pylori* (*H. pylori*):

1. Has been cultured from children with hypertrophic pyloric stenosis
2. Has been implicated as a cause of chronic abdominal pain in children
3. Generally causes watery, but not bloody diarrhea
4. Is considered a contributing factor in the pathogenesis of peptic ulcer

    A. 1, 2, 3
    B. 1, 3
    C. 2, 4
    D. 4 only
    E. All of the above

8. Colitis due to infection with toxigenic *Clostridium difficile*:

1. Is due to overgrowth of the organism after antibiotic therapy
2. Is characterized by watery, often bloody diarrhea
3. Is due to the toxins produced by *C. difficile*
4. Can also be caused by ingestion of preformed toxin found in poorly refrigerated food

    A. 1, 2, 3
    B. 1, 3
    C. 2, 4
    D. 4 only
    E. All of the above

5. E. All of the above

This gram-positive organism, also called Strep pyogenes, can be divided into over 60 subtypes based on surface protein, such as the M proteins. Impetigo is most common in younger children, tonsillitis/pharyngitis in school-aged children.

6. A. Rheumatic fever may develop after tonsillitis

Many serologic types of group A Strep infecting the throat can be associated with rheumatic fever. Nephritis, in contrast, is related to a limited number of types and may occur following skin infections while rheumatic fever only follows pharyngitis.

7. C. 2, 4

Infection with this bacterium is associated with ulcer disease, acute gastritis, and chronic abdominal pain. *H. pylori* is responsible for at least 50% of duodenal and gastric ulcers in adults but it is the cause of a lower percentage of ulcers in children. In some patients with chronic abdominal pain, eradication of *H. pylori* has been associated with diminution of the pain.

8. A. 1, 2, 3

Antibiotic-associated diarrhea is due to toxins produced by *C. difficile*. Overgrowth of the bacteria occurs when antibiotic treatment suppresses normal flora in the GI tract. Symptoms continue for 7–10 days after stopping the antibiotic therapy. In more severe cases, IV and/or enteral vancomycin therapy may be needed. Food poisoning is caused by ingestion of *C. perfringens* capable of forming spores. Botulism is a form of food poisoning caused by ingestion of the neurotoxin made by *C. botulinum*.

9. Regarding the clinical manifestations of bacterial meningitis beyond the neonatal period:

   1. Focal neurologic signs are seen in 10–15% of cases.
   2. If seizures occur, it is very likely that the child will be left with a permanent seizure disorder.
   3. Fever need not be present.
   4. Photophobia, due to inflammation of the optic nerve, may lead to permanently impaired vision.

   A. 1, 2, 3
   B. 1, 3
   C. 2, 4
   D. 4 only
   E. All of the above

10. Regarding the prognosis of bacterial meningitis beyond the neonatal period:

    1. Some degree of hearing loss is seen in approximately 10% of survivors.
    2. Neurologic abnormalities seen shortly after the onset of meningitis may resolve over time.
    3. The mortality rate is 1–5%.
    4. Brain abscesses are commonly seen during the course of antibiotic therapy.

    A. 1, 2, 3
    B. 1, 3
    C. 2, 4
    D. 4 only
    E. All of the above

11. The Hemolytic–Uremic syndrome:

    1. Typically has a prodrome of 3–5 days of diarrhea
    2. May include neurologic dysfunction such as seizures or coma in its presentation
    3. May include hypertension as part of its presentation
    4. Generally is treated with supportive care (careful fluid and electrolyte management, dialysis, and transfusion as needed)

    A. 1, 2, 3
    B. 1, 3
    C. 2, 4
    D. 4 only
    E. All of the above

9. B. 1, 3

Fever is often part of the presentation of bacterial meningitis in children. Lethargy, vomiting, and decreased level of consciousness may also be part of the presentation.

10. A. 1, 2, 3

The worst prognosis is seen in younger children with higher bacterial counts in the CSF. Cerebral or spinal cord infarction, another unusual complication seen in children with bacterial meningitis, can be diagnosed by CT.

11. E. All of the above

HUS is primarily a disease of young children. HUS is characterized by hemolytic anemia, thrombocytopenia, and renal dysfunction. Prognosis for survival is very good and long-term morbidity such as hypertension and mild azotemia is seen in <10% of cases. Many causes and associations have been noted. The syndrome can be seen as a result of a toxin-producing *E. coli*, following a prodrome of diarrhea. Treatment is mainly supportive, with careful fluid and electrolyte management.

12. Children with the hemolytic uremic syndrome (HUS):

   1. May have had infection with *E. Coli*, *Shigella*, or *Salmonella*
   2. Have anemia, thrombocytopenia, and low WBC counts due to bone marrow failure
   3. Are generally younger than 5 years of age
   4. Are best treated with IV immunoglobulin

      A. 1, 2, 3
      B. 1, 3
      C. 2, 4
      D. 4 only
      E. All of the above

13. In children with a temperature greater than 39°C without a source for the fever:

   1. Bacteremia will likely occur in 1–5% of cases.
   2. Bacteremia, if it occurs, will most often be due to *Streptococcus* Pneumonia.
   3. The risk for occult bacteremia is greatest among those younger than 24 months.
   4. Almost all of the children who have bacteremia will develop purulent complications.

      A. 1, 2, 3
      B. 1, 3
      C. 2, 4
      D. 4 only
      E. All of the above

14. Which of the following are seen relatively often in children with immunodeficiencies?

   1. Growth failure
   2. Chronic diarrhea
   3. Skin rashes
   4. Recurrent or chronic infections

      A. 1, 2, 3
      B. 1, 3
      C. 2, 4
      D. 4 only
      E. All of the above

12. B. 1, 3

Treatment of children with HUS is supportive. The low red cell and platelet counts are due to hemolysis and increased destruction, respectively. The hemoglobin at presentation may be as low as 2 gm/dL and platelet count <100,000/mm^3.

13. A. 1, 2, 3

Children who present with fever without a source often have viral illnesses, but in children <36 months of age, a WBC count with differential count may help identify those with a much greater likelihood of bacteremia.

14. E. All of the above

Immunodeficiencies can be primary or secondary. Primary immunodeficiencies can involve defects in B cells, complement, T cells, or neutrophils. Secondary immunodeficiencies can result from malnutrition, viral infections, metabolic disorders (diabetes mellitus, sickle cell disease, uremia) or malignancies, and cancer chemotherapy.

15. Scabies:

    1. Is characterized by beefy red skin with satellite lesions
    2. Has 1–2 mm red papules which may be excoriated or crusted
    3. Is caused by contact with an allergen
    4. Is a pruritic rash, particularly at night

      A. 1, 2, 3
      B. 1, 3
      C. 2, 4
      D. 4 only
      E. All of the above

16. Urticaria (hives) in children may be associated with:

    1. Airway edema
    2. Contact with a food or chemical
    3. Exposure to cold
    4. Exercise

      A. 1, 2, 3
      B. 1, 3
      C. 2, 4
      D. 4 only
      E. All of the above

17. Urticaria:

    1. Is an evanescent rash consisting of red-pink wheals
    2. May be treated with PO diphenhydramine
    3. Is commonly associated with beta Streptococcal infections
    4. Is especially common in children with abnormalities in T-cell function

      A. 1, 2, 3
      B. 1, 3
      C. 2, 4
      D. 4 only
      E. All of the above

18. The first teeth to erupt, the lower central incisors, do so at the age of:

    A. 4 months
    B. 7 months
    C. 12 months
    D. 15 months

15. C. 2, 4

Scabies is an intensely pruritic rash and its preferred sites are interdigital spaces, wrists, elbows, and ankles. Other common rashes seen in infants and children include Candida albicans which commonly complicates diaper dermatitis (which does not have the same beefy red appearance and satellite lesions) and Tinea corporis, which is well described by its common name, ringworm.

16. E. All of the above

Urticaria is characterized by a localized or generalized erythematous, raised rash with lesions of various sizes.

17. A. 1, 2, 3

Up to 20% of the general population experience urticaria at some point in their lives. Angioedema is a different lesion involving deeper skin layers or submucosa which involves the periorbital and perioral areas, lips, tongue, respiratory tract, hands, feet, and GI tract.

Hereditary angioedema (HAE) is a different condition, transmitted as an autosomal dominant trait. HAE results from partial deficiency of C1 esterase, an enzyme that inhibits the first part of the complement system. This deficiency allows activation of the complement system with resultant symptoms such as angioedema. This edema, without urticaria, can involve the airway.

18. B. 7 months

Deciduous teeth erupt as follows:

6–7 months.	Upper (first) and lower incisors
7–9 months.	Upper and lower (first) lateral incisors
16–18 months.	Bicuspids
12–14 months.	First molars
20–24 months.	Second molars

Permanent teeth begin erupting at 67 years of age with incisors first, then molars, followed by bicuspids.

19. Which of the following is the most common form of child maltreatment?

    A. Physical abuse
    B. Neglect
    C. Sexual abuse
    D. Emotional abuse

20. Sudden infant death syndrome (SIDS) has been associated with:

    1. Inadequate nutrition
    2. Recent immunization
    3. Maternal smoking
    4. Concurrent upper respiratory infection

        A. 1, 2, 3
        B. 1, 3
        C. 2, 4
        D. 4 only
        E. All of the above

21. SIDS:

    1. Is the most common cause of death in the first 2 weeks of life
    2. Accounts for 35% of postperinatal deaths/year in the USA
    3. Occurs with the same frequency in all ethnic groups
    4. Has no pathongomonic markers at autopsy

        A. 1, 2, 3
        B. 1, 3
        C. 2, 4
        D. 4 only
        E. All of the above

22. An apparent life-threatening event (ALTE):

    1. Would have previously been called a near-miss SIDS event
    2. Is more likely to occur following immunizations
    3. May present with pallor, cyanosis, limpness and apnea
    4. Would be much more likely to occur in first-born children

        A. 1, 2, 3
        B. 1, 3
        C. 2, 4
        D. 4 only
        E. All of the above

19. B. Neglect

Each year in the USA, there are approximately 1 million confirmed cases of abuse or neglect of children. The true incidence of abuse and neglects is almost certainly much greater than the 1 million confirmed reports, however. Physicians are required by law in all states to report all cases of suspected child abuse. Cultural and geographic norms vary greatly but a working definition of abuse is parental (or guardian) behavior that damages the normal physical and psychological development of a child.

20. B. 1, 3

SIDS occurs almost exclusively in the second through fifth months of life with the peak in the mid-point of that time period. The incidence does not differ much in various seasons or in different climates.

21. E. All of the above

The diagnosis is often one of exclusion. The incidence appears to be stable. In some cases of SIDS, there may have been suffocation by an adult, but this is difficult to prove.

22. B. 1, 3

Although infants who suffer an ALTE requiring intervention may seem to have a slightly higher chance of dying from SIDS, most infants who do succumb to SIDS have not had a prior ALTE.

23. Which of the following conditions are often associated with ALTEs?

    1. Gastroesophageal reflux (GER)
    2. Acute upper respiratory infections (URI)
    3. Seizures
    4. Failure to thrive (FTT)

       A. 1, 2, 3
       B. 1, 3
       C. 2, 4
       D. 4 only
       E. All of the above

24. In children with obstructive sleep apnea syndrome (OSAS), also called sleep disordered breathing:

    1. The physical exam during wakefulness may be entirely normal.
    2. There is anatomical narrowing of the upper airway.
    3. There is abnormal neuromuscular control of upper airway patency.
    4. The complications which may develop include FTT, hyperactivity, and poor school performance.

       A. 1, 2, 3
       B. 1, 3
       C. 2, 4
       D. 4 only
       E. All of the above

25. Myelomeningocele:

    1. Is the most common severe form of neural tube defect
    2. Occurs less often in children of mothers who took supplemental folate in the periconceptional time period
    3. May be located anywhere along the neuaxis
    4. Is associated with a Chiari type II defect in 80% of cases

       A. 1, 2, 3
       B. 1, 3
       C. 2, 4
       D. 4 only
       E. All of the above

23. A. 1, 2, 3

While these conditions are seen with higher frequency in infants who have suffered an ALTE, they are not seen more often in infants who have succumbed to SIDS. The pathologic hallmark of SIDS is that there is no pathognomic finding for SIDS.

24. E. All of the above

In addition to the problems mentioned, nighttime hypoxemia with resultant pulmonary hypertension and cor pulmonale can develop in children with sleep disordered breathing. Sleep studies are used to confirm the diagnosis. A history of nighttime snoring is not sufficient to diagnose sleep disordered breathing.

25. E. All of the above

The caudal neuropore closes by the 4th–5th week of gestation. Failure of this closure to occur leads to the development of a variety of congenital anomalies including spina bifida occulta, spina bifida cystica, meningocele, and myelomeningocele. Spina bifida occulta is seen in 10% of the population and generally causes no symptoms. Spina bifida cystica, a sac-like lesion associated with unfused vertebrae, is seen in 0.1% of people. Myelomeningocele is seen in approximately 0.1% of live births. The location within the cord determines the clinical picture of this condition. Affected children undergo repair within 1–2 days of life, and commonly ventriculoperitoneal shunt placement shortly thereafter. The problems (orthopedic, urological, gastrointestinal) persist throughout life. Most children with myelomeningocele have normal intellect.

26. Tetanus immunization is usually done in combination with other immunizing agents (DTP, Td, DT). Active immunization with tetanus toxoid:

    1. Provides 10 years of immunity
    2. Is given with pertussus in children only until 7 years of age
    3. Is unnecessary in persons with superficial clean wounds who have received their last tetanus toxoid within the past 10 years
    4. Should be given to persons with more serious and dirty/animal wounds if their most recent tetanus toxoid dose was given more than 5 years ago

       A. 1, 2, 3
       B. 1, 3
       C. 2, 4
       D. 4 only
       E. All of the above

27. Which of the following statements are true regarding current vaccines given to children?

    1. Paralytic polio is very rarely (1 in 2.6 million) caused by oral polio vaccine (OPV) in either vaccine recipients or contacts.
    2. Although measles vaccine may cause fever in 15% of recipients, more serious side effects are exceedingly rare.
    3. Mumps vaccine may rarely cause orchitis.
    4. Local reactions may occur in up to 25% of recipients of Haemophilus influenzae type b vaccine.

       A. 1, 2, 3
       B. 1, 3
       C. 2, 4
       D. 4 only
       E. All of the above

28. Therapy for suspected tetanus infection includes:

    1. Penicillin G to kill the C. tetani
    2. Tetanus immune globulin to neutralize circulating toxin before it binds to neuronal membranes
    3. Active immunization with tetanus toxoid
    4. Dialysis to remove toxin if the patient deteriorates, developing more and more severe muscle spasms

       A. 1, 2, 3
       B. 1, 3
       C. 2, 4
       D. 4 only
       E. All of the above

26. E. All of the above

Tetanus is fortunately very rare in the USA. The bacterium Clostridium tetanii produces two toxins but only one, tetanospasmin, produces disease. It is a very potent neurotoxin. Generalized tetanus, the most common presentation, involves trismus, nuchal rigidity, difficulty swallowing as well as headache. Subsequently, affected individuals develop generalized, uncoordinated muscle spasms. These muscle spasms can lead to fractures, dysphagia, and even respiratory failure.

27. E. All of the above

Treatment involves inactivation of the circulating toxin, treatment of the infection to stop toxin production, and supportive care as needed. If there is significant tissue necrosis, IV antibiotics will not reach therapeutic levels and these wounds must be debrided. In very severe cases, amputation should be considered.

28. A. 1, 2, 3

Tetanus is caused by an exotoxin produced by C. tetani. TIG has no effect on toxin which has already bound to neural tissue and does not cross the blood brain barrier.

29. Regarding pertussis infection in the USA:

    1. Mortality is highest among infants.
    2. The attack rate of approximately 1 per 1,000,000 is due to high vaccinate rate.
    3. Approximately 50% of reported cases are in children <1 year of age.
    4. It is extremely contagious among nonimmunized children.

       A. 1, 2, 3
       B. 1, 3
       C. 2, 4
       D. 4 only
       E. All of the above

30. The clinical manifestations of pertussis include:

    1. Severe paroxysms of coughing, particularly at night
    2. A characteristic inspiratory sound (whoop) between coughing spells
    3. A calm appearance between coughing spells
    4. Normal temperature throughout the illness.

       A. 1, 2, 3
       B. 1, 3
       C. 2, 4
       D. 4 only
       E. All of the above

31. Complications of pertussus infection include:

    1. Bronchopleural fistula
    2. Seizures and mild, transient encephalitis
    3. Coagulopathy
    4. Pneumonia

       A. 1, 2, 3
       B. 1, 3
       C. 2, 4
       D. 4 only
       E. All of the above

29. E. All of the above

Herd immunity ("community immunity" – when the vaccination of a portion of the population (or herd) provides protection to unvaccinated individuals) keeps the incidence of the illness low, protecting those infants who are not fully immunized.

30. A. 1, 2, 3

Morbidity and mortality of infants is due to the severe paroxysms of coughing. The infant with these severe coughing spells cannot feed and may aspirate during attempted feeds. Temperature elevations to 40°C are part of the illness. WBC counts in pertussis may be so high that the diagnosis of Acute Lymphoblastic Leukemia (ALL) may be considered.

31. C. 2, 4

Pneumonia is often due to bacterial superinfection, not the *B. pertussis* organism itself. Treatment is generally empiric since the infectious organism may not be recovered from the child.

32. Regarding reactions to pertussus immunization:

    1. Temperature elevations >38°C are seen in approximately 50% of vaccine recipients.
    2. Seizures occur in approximately 1 of 2,000 vaccine recipients.
    3. Reactions seem more common and perhaps more severe in children who are older than 7 years when vaccinated.
    4. Evidence for pertussis vaccine encephalopathy or SIDs following the vaccine has not been found.

       A. 1, 2, 3
       B. 1, 3
       C. 2, 4
       D. 4 only
       E. All of the above

33. Regarding vaccination against polio:

    1. The IPV is contraindicated in immunocompromised children.
    2. Lifelong, but type-specific immunity is conferred by both recognized infection and vaccination.
    3. Paralytic polio has never been seen in a contact of a recipient of OPV.
    4. OPV and BP are trivalent and provide immunity to three virus types.

       A. 1, 2, 3
       B. 1, 3
       C. 2, 4
       D. 4 only
       E. All of the above

34. Influenza vaccine is recommended for:

    1. Children with diabetes
    2. Children with asthma
    3. Children with seizures
    4. All children below the age of 3 years

       A. 1, 2, 3
       B. 1, 3
       C. 2, 4
       D. 4 only
       E. All of the above

32. E. All of the above

The vaccine has been suspected as an etiologic agent in various forms of encephalopathy or developmental delay, but a causative link has never been proved despite numerous reviews of databases both in the USA and the UK.

33. C. 2, 4

Inactivated polio vaccine is one of several inactivated virus vaccines. The others given in childhood are hepatitis A (HAV) and influenza. Other types of vaccines in use are made up of immunogenic components of the organism such as pertussis, *Haemophilus influenzae* type b (HIB), and *Strep pneumoniae*. Attenuated live virus vaccines in use include measles, mumps, rubella, and varicella.

34. A. 1, 2, 3

The vaccine is recommended for children with medical conditions that may lead them to suffer a more severe form of influenza should they contract the illness. Influenza is passed from person to person via the respiratory route. Infection with influenza is associated with considerable morbidity and mortality. After infection, there is a 2–3-day incubation period prior to the onset of symptoms. Generally in adults and older children the onset is sudden, with high fevers, headache, myalgias, and chills. This lasts for several days followed by a 2–4-week period of more prominent respiratory symptoms including a prominent dry cough. In young children, influenza infection presents in a manner similar to other viral respiratory illnesses, with fever, cough, coryza, and fussiness. Serious morbidity in otherwise well individuals is due to bacterial respiratory superinfections.

35. In which of the following groups are accidents NOT the leading cause of death?

    A. 10–14-year-old males
    B. 10–14-year-old females
    C. 14–19-year-old males
    D. 14–19-year-old females
    E. None of the above
    F. All of the above

36. Which of the following milestones are appropriate for a 6-month-old with normal development?

    1. Able to feed her/himself
    2. Able to sit unsupported
    3. Speaks single syllables or imitates speech sounds
    4. Beginning walking

       A. 1, 2, 3
       B. 1, 3
       C. 2, 4
       D. 4 only
       E. All of the above

37. Which of the following milestones are appropriate for a 12-month-old with normal development?

    1. Beginning walking
    2. Wave bye-bye
    3. Have a 1–3 word vacabulary
    4. Play ball with parent

       A. 1, 2, 3
       B. 1, 3
       C. 2, 4
       D. 4 only
       E. All of the above

35. E. None of the above

The cause for mortality in children varies by age. The four most common causes are:

Birth to 1 year of age	
Perinatal factors	50%
Congenital anomalies	20%
Infections	4%
Cardiac disease	3%
1–4 years of age	
Injuries	40%
Congenital anomalies	13%
Infections	8%
Cancer	8%
5–14 years of age	
Injuries	55%
Cancer	15%
Cardiac disease	4%
Congenital anomalies	4%
15–25 years of age	
Injuries	75%
Cancer	6%
Cardiac disease	4%
Infections	2%

36. A. 1, 2, 3

Another important developmental milestone for anesthesiologists and other medical professionals to note is the beginning of stranger anxiety. Most 6–8-month-old infants will easily go to a smiling stranger but at around 8–9 months, most will be quite fearful of people with whom they are not very familiar.

37. E. All of the above

At this age, most language will be intelligible only to the parents or close family members. Phrases and sentences that strangers will understand will not be articulated until 2–4 years of age. A solid understanding of growth and development is a crucial part of caring for children and an invaluable aid in establishing rapport with these young people.

Part II
Consultations in Pediatric Anesthesia

Chapter 1
Prematurity/Extreme Prematurity

A 2-week-old male, 900 g, born at 27 weeks gestational age is scheduled emergently for exploratory laparotomy for free air in the abdomen. Vital signs are BP = 50/30 mmHg, P = 185 bpm, T = 36.2°C. His hemoglobin is 13.0 g/dL. He is intubated with a 2.5 mm oral endotracheal tube. Ventilator settings are FiO_2 = 0.5, RR = 30/min, PEEP = 3 cm H_2O, PIP = 28 cm H_2O.

R.S. Holzman et al., *Pediatric Anesthesiology Review: Clinical Cases for Self-Assessment,* DOI 10.1007/978-1-4419-1617-4_1, © Springer Science+Business Media, LLC 2010

Preoperative Evaluation

1. Is this patient premature? Why? What organ systems are you concerned about in caring for the preterm newborn in the operating room?

2. Does this patient have surfactant in his lungs? If not, when will it develop? Would the administration of artificial surfactant influence your anesthetic plan?

3. How can you evaluate the status of the central nervous system (CNS)? What signs and symptoms would you look for with regard to intraventricular hemorrhage? What factors contribute to the onset of intraventricular hemorrhage? How will it affect your anesthetic management?

Preoperative Evaluation

1. Infants born before the 37th week of gestation are considered premature [1]. The third trimester is the time when most organ systems mature. Of particular importance is the immaturity of the pulmonary, central nervous, renal, and hepatic systems. Gas exchange and management of mechanical ventilation require exquisite attention to detail in these tiny patients. CNS immaturity and the possible deleterious effects not only of hypoxia and metabolic derangements but also of the anesthetic, hypnotic, and analgesic agents themselves is an evolving issue. Preterm infants do not maintain fluid and electrolyte balance well, requiring care in the administration of IV fluids and electrolytes. Liver immaturity, both in synthetic and metabolic capacities, can result in much longer duration of action of IV agents.

2. An infant born at 27 weeks will almost certainly be deficient in pulmonary surfactant and develop respiratory distress syndrome (RDS) [2]. Surfactant is produced by type II pneumocytes. The amount and composition of the surfactant changes throughout gestation. Lamellar bodies are first seen in type II pneumocytes at 20–24 weeks gestation. There is progressive accumulation of saturated phosphatidylcholine in the lung tissue until term. The surfactant present in the lungs of term newborns is composed as follows: 50% saturated phosphatidylcholine, 20% unsaturated phosphatidylcholine, 14% other lipids, 8% phosphatidylglycerol, and 8% surfactant proteins (SP-A through SP-D). The immature lung has decreased surfactant function, much less phosphatidylglycerol and more phosphatidylinisitol. Administration of artificial surfactant following delivery is very beneficial, decreasing surface tension in the alveoli as natural surfactant does in the term newborn. If surfactant were administered, it should be expected that the compliance of the lungs would increase to closer to that seen in term newborns. When ventilating for a newborn treated with surfactant it is important to consider this improved compliance.

3. Periventricular–intraventricular hemorrhage (IVH) is a common occurrence in the preterm newborn and the most serious CNS lesion encountered in the newborn period [3]. It is a major cause of death in preterms. In at least 90% of cases, the hemorrhage occurs in the first week of life. The incidence and severity if periventricular–intraventricular hemorrhage occurs varies inversely with gestational age. IVH is graded I–IV based upon the radiographic appearance of the extent of the hemorrhage, from an isolated germinal matrix hemorrhage to intraventricular and parenchymal hemorrhage.

Grade I: Subependymal and/or germinal matrix hemorrhage
Grade II: Subependymal hemorrhage also into lateral ventricles
Grade III: Grade II plus ventricular enlargement
Grade IV: Intraparenchymal hemorrhage

4. How can you diagnose persistent patency of the ductus arteriosus? Is this significant for anesthetic management? Why/why not?

5. Does this patient need a work-up for D.I.C.? Why? Will an assessment of fibrin split products help? Why/why not?

Clinically, the occurrence of an IVH may be suggested by sudden cardiovascular instability or, if the IVH itself goes unnoticed, hydrocephalus may occur later. Numerous causes for IVH have been proposed, but it is often difficult to establish a definite cause and effect relationship. Loss of autoregulation of cerebral blood flow in these patients and rapid changes in cerebral blood flow and pressure are likely involved. Possible specific causes include neonatal asphyxia with low blood pressure, rapid volume expansion, changes in serum osmolarity, abnormal coagulation, hypoxemia, hypercarbia, and large swings in systemic BP with excessive agitation in resisting mechanical ventilation.

4. PDA is nearly a normal finding in the preterm [4]. In the fetus, the ductus arteriosus is essential for adequate circulation and oxygen delivery. In postnatal life, a PDA may lead to inadequate forward systemic flow and CHF from excessive pulmonary blood flow. Clinically, bounding pulses, tachypnea, cardiomegaly, and signs of pulmonary overcirculation are seen when the ductus is opened. A functionally closed ductus in a patient such as the one in this case can be reopened by excessive fluid administration. This makes fluid administration in these critically ill infants challenging. Excessive fluid administration can lead to significantly worsened gas exchange and also decreased systemic flow whereas inadequate preload will also lead to decreased LV output.

5. NEC is often associated with a coagulopathy. Thrombocytopenia is commonly seen as NEC worsens. In patients suspected of having NEC, serial platelet counts are followed as a measure of disease severity. The laboratory diagnosis of DIC can be difficult since, in the newborn, several tests of coagulation may be outside of the reference range [5, 6]. For example, D-dimers are often found in preterm newborns without DIC. In the clinical setting of NEC, thrombocytopenia, microangiopathic hemolytic anemia, and prolonged PT are indicative of DIC. Treatment of this infant's coagulopathy will involve transfusion of PRBCs, platelets and also coagulation factors either in the form of FFP or cryoprecipitate. In the NICU, exchange transfusion may also be undertaken.

Intraoperative Course

1. Does this patient need an arterial line? Why/why not? A central line? Why? What site will you use to monitor temperature? Why? Where does temperature change first? Last? Will you monitor glucose levels? Why? How often?

2. Should you give atropine prior to induction? Would you give atropine prior to an "awake" intubation? Why/why not? Would pancuronium do just as well?

3. How would you ensure temperature homeostasis? What is your choice of fluid management? Why? What if hyperalimentation is running? Would you discontinue and change over to a D_{20} solution? D_{10} solution? Not change? What are the effects of narcotic anesthetic techniques in this age group? Is MAC different in this age group? In what way? Is ketamine a choice?

4. What muscle relaxant would you choose? Why? Is there any specific advantage to cisatracurium?

Intraoperative Course [7, 8]

1. Direct arterial monitoring would be very helpful in this case, but technically difficult and associated with complications. Radial arterial cannulation should preferentially be done in the postductal left-sided location. Femoral arterial cannulation may be technically less difficult but circulation to the distal leg may be affected in a patient this small, even with a 22 g catheter. An alternative is a CVL through which blood products can be given and which also can be used for sampling. With a functioning oximeter, the need to measure arterial PaO_2 is lessened. In many cases, pre- and postductal oximeters are used. Temperature monitoring is very important given the ease with which hypothermia may occur and the problems hypothermia will cause. Rectal measurement gives a good indication of central temperature but care must be taken not to perforate the delicate rectal mucosa during insertion. An important part of intraoperative care of this infant will be frequent monitoring of serum glucose and electrolytes, platelet count, hemoglobin, pH, and blood gases. With the administration of either the existing hyperalimentation or D10, serum glucose will likely be maintained. A more complete discussion of glucose management is below in note 1 of "Additional Topics."

2. Atropine will help maintain a high infant heart rate during the induction and the case, but hypoxemia will still lead to bradycardia. Pancuronium also has a vagolytic effect on the heart rate but does not decrease oral secretions as does atropine.

3. Temperature maintenance begins prior to the start of the case. The OR temperature should be turned up prior to the arrival of the infant. Inspired gases can be humidified and warmed. When this is done, water "rainout" must be drained out of the circuit, and not into the infant's lungs. Additionally, the temperature of the inspired gases must be monitored and kept below 39°C to avoid burning the infant [9]. Maintenance glucose, as D10, at 100 mL/kg/day, must be given throughout the case, preferably through a separate IV, while blood products and other crystalloid are given through another IV. Any hyperalimentation already running should be continued at the same rate and once serum glucose is checked, the infusion rate can be carefully lowered. Opioid analgesics will decrease the stress response, help minimize postoperative catabolism, and in some cases high dose opioid analgesia has decreased mortality. MAC varies with age, although there is no data on the preterm weight newborn, particularly the low birth weight (LBW) or extremely low birth weight (ELBW) newborn.

4. Muscle relaxants are an important part of the anesthetic in cases such as these. Only rarely are the infants able to tolerate a MAC of the inhaled agents, so muscle relaxants are needed to assure immobility of the patient.

5. As the case progresses, the airway pressure suddenly rises, there is a diminution of breath sounds bilaterally, and the SpO$_2$ decreases steadily. What could be going on? What measures can you take to prevent this from occurring again?

Postoperative Course

1. When would you extubate? Why/why not? Is this baby at risk for postextubation croup? What factors are important for subglottic stenosis in the premature infant? Tracheomalacia?

2. How can you assess postoperative pain in the neonate? How would you manage pain in this patient? Why? Are there differences in pharmacokinetics of opioids in this age group? Why?

3. What are the long-term problems associated with necrotizing enterocolitis? Natural history of growth and development? Subsequent surgical problems? Nutritional status?

5. During the case, the infant is moved away from the anesthesiologist down the OR table and is difficult to reach or even see. A kink in the endotracheal tube can easily occur. The circuit is stiff with low compliance and may easily kink the softened warmed endotracheal tube. Other common causes of increased airway pressure needed for ventilation through this 2.5 mm endotracheal tube include mucous plugging, the development of a pneumothorax, or resistance to mechanical ventilation by the patient. Humidification of the inspired gases will help keep tracheal secretions from occluding the endotracheal tube, but has its own problems such as "rainout" of water into the ventilator tubing and excessive heating of the inspired gases.

Postoperative Course

1. Since the infant arrived intubated, requiring mechanical ventilation, was given opioids during the case, and now has an abdominal incision, extubation should not be done. The child would very likely hypoventilate or have apnea if extubated. If an infant is intubated with a tight fitting endotracheal tube, postextubation stridor or "croup" is a possibility, but not a certainly. Subglottic stenosis and/or tracheomalacia are complications of intubation to which newborns are subject. Although it is likely that the more trauma done to the trachea of a newborn the greater the chance of complications such as subglottic stenosis or tracheomalacia, any preterm newborn who has been intubated is at risk for them.

2. There are several scoring systems for the assessment of pain in the term and preterm newborn. The Neonatal Infant Pain Scale (NIPS) and the Crying, Requires oxygen, Increased vital signs, Expression Sleeplessness (CRIES), are composite measures of physiology and behavior, and among those most commonly used. Postoperative pain in this patient could be managed by systemic opioid administration [10]. Morphine and fentanyl both have prolonged elimination half lives in term and preterm newborns. There is evidence to support increased sensitivity to depression of respiratory drive in newborns but opioids can certainly be safely administered to newborns provided there is appropriate monitoring. Regional analgesia has been used in preterm newborns, but this patient still may have or develop bacteremia or coagulation abnormalities, two contraindications to regional analgesia.

3. Preterm newborns that have survived NEC may continue to have problems including malnutrition, intestinal obstruction, failure to thrive and residual hepatic disease resulting from TPN. Their nutritional status depends greatly on the amount of intestine damaged by NEC itself and the amount removed at surgery.

Additional Topics

1. Which infants are at risk for hypoglycemia? What threshold is used for the diagnosis of hypoglycemia in term infants? In preterm newborns? How would you treat hypoglycemia? What are the risks?

2. You need pressor support for a 2,000 g infant undergoing a diaphragmatic hernia repair. Which pressor will you choose? Why? Does it matter what the pH is? Why? In which ways do catecholamine receptors differ in the newborn from those of the adult? Is the stressed newborn any different? Can you use ephedrine? Phenylephrine?

3. How does continuous positive airway pressure (CPAP) work to improve pulmonary function in the premature infant? Which physics principle governs this? What is the role of surfactant?

Additional Topics

1. Hypoglycemia during general anesthesia can only be diagnosed by measurement of the serum glucose. Infants of diabetic mothers, SGA infants, infants with syndromes such as Beckwith–Wiedemann and nessidioblastosis are at increased risk. Treatment is with a "mini" bolus of 200–300 mg/kg over 90 s followed by an infusion of 6–10 mg/kg/min. The specific number at which hypoglycemia is diagnosed is the subject of much controversy. The diagnosis traditionally has had three criteria and is not applicable to the OR setting. The criteria are: the presence of clinical signs and symptoms (lethargy, pallor, cyanosis, jitteriness, apnea, seizures), a documented low serum glucose measurement, and resolution of the clinical signs and symptoms promptly after correction of the low glucose measurement. In the OR, a safe lower threshold for treatment is 60 mg%. This number is somewhat above the threshold recommended for newborns who are not under general anesthesia but, given the inability to suspect the diagnosis on clinical grounds, a higher threshold is needed. In contrast to earlier thinking, the absolute number used as the diagnostic criterion for hypoglycemia is not different for term or preterm newborns.

2. Dopamine use has been studied in term and preterm newborns. In the presence of normal pH, the dose range is similar to that used in older children and adults (2.5–20 mcg/kg/min). There is some indication that newborns respond to smaller doses than those commonly recommended. Acidosis significantly impairs the inotropic response to catecholamines. Epinephrine's potent inotropic and chronotropic effects are due to stimulation of alpha and beta receptors. Unless doses used are excessive, epinephrine can be safely used to support critically ill newborns. The usual range for infusion is 0.05–2 mcg/kg/min. Treatment of hypotension in critically ill newborns is best accomplished with direct-acting agents such as epinephrine.

3. Preterm newborns are deficient in surfactant [2]. This deficiency leads to increased surface tension in alveoli which then tend to collapse at end-exhalation, decreasing FRC. Recall the LaPlace equation which states that the pressure at the surface of a sphere is twice the surface tension divided by the radius of the bubble. Alveoli are not perfect spheres but the relationship still has applicability:

$$P(dyn / cm^2) = \frac{2T(dyn / cm)}{R(cm)}$$

On the basis of this relationship, pressure inside a small alveolus should be higher than that inside larger alveoli, leading to collapse of smaller alveoli and enlargement of larger alveoli. Surfactant promotes a decrease in surface tension even as the surface area of an alveolus is reduced, thus preventing collapse. The surface tension decreases to a greater extent than the radius, resulting in a diminishing transmural pressure gradient, stabilizing the smaller alveoli. Distending airway pressure helps to return the FRC to the volume it would be in a well newborn.

4. What factors are important in the etiology of retinopathy of prematurity?

5. How do you perform a leak test?

4. The major risk factor for the development of retinopathy of prematurity is, not surprisingly, prematurity itself. Gestational age and birth weight are the strongest predictors for the development of ROP. ROP, formerly called retrolental fibroplasia (RLF), was frequently seen in the 1940s–1950s when oxygen was routinely administered. It nearly disappeared in the 1970s when oxygen use was restricted, but with survival of smaller preterm newborns, the incidence is increasing. Annually, approximately 400 infants are blinded by ROP and 4,000 have serious retinal scars. In the OR, as in the NICU, the administration of supplemental oxygen should be done only when clinically indicated. Minimizing oxygen delivery to prevent the development of ROP should not put the infant at any risk of being exposed to hypoxemia.

5. The leak test is performed to determine whether or not the endotracheal tube size is appropriate to the child. Following intubation, the endotracheal tube is connected to the breathing circuit, the pop-off valve is closed and the fresh gas flow set at 2–4 L/min. As the pressure reading in the manometer rises, the anesthesiologist listens at the child's mouth or over the neck for the sound of a gas leak around the endotracheal tube. Ideally, the leak should be audible at approximately 15 cm H_2O. This degree of leak allows adequate positive pressure ventilation while not compromising blood flow to the tracheal mucosa.

Annotated References

1. Papageorgiopu A, Pelausa E, Kovacs L (2005) The extremely low-birth weight infant. Chapter 25. In: MacDonald MG, Mullett MM, Seshia MMK (eds) Avery's neonatology, 6th edn. Lippincott Williams & Wilkins, Philadelphia, pp 459–489
   This chapter reviews the epidemiology of low birth weight newborns as well as NICU management of these patients. Respiratory, cardiovascular, and fluid management are reviewed. The authors also discuss management of many of the common clinical problems that affect low birth weight newborns. Morbidity seen in low birth weight newborns is also included.

2. Whitsett JA, Rice WR, Warner BB et al. (2005) Acute respiratory disorders. Chapter 29. In: MacDonald MG, Mullett MM, Seshia MMK (eds) Avery's neonatology, 6th edn. Lippincott Williams & Wilkins, Philadelphia, pp 554–577
   The authors review in detail the embryology of lung development, the development of surfactant, the pathophysiology of respiratory distress in the preterm newborn and management of RDS.

3. Mancuso TJ (2008) Anesthesia for the preterm newborn. Chapter 33. In: Holzman RS, Mancuso TJ, Polaner DM (eds) A practical approach to pediatric anesthesia. Lippincott Williams & Wilkins, Philadelphia, pp 601–609

This chapter reviews the anesthetic considerations for preterm newborns including fluid and glucose administration, and discussion of the possible toxicity of various anesthetic agents in newborns.

References

1. Engle WA (2004) Age terminology during the perinatal period. Pediatrics 114:1362–1364
2. Whisett JA, Rice WR, Warner BB et al (2005) Acute respiratory disorders. In: MacDonald MG, Mullett MM, Seshia MMK (eds) Avery's neonatology, 6th edn. Lippincott Williams & Wilkins, Philadelphia, pp 557–562
3. Hill A (2005) Neurological and neuromuscular disorders. In: MacDonald MG, Mullett MM, Seshia MMK (eds) Avery's neonatology, 6th edn. Lippincott Williams & Wilkins, Philadelphia, pp 1396–1402
4. Flanagan M, Yeager SB, Weindling SN (2005) Cardiac disease. In: MacDonald MG, Mullett MM, Seshia MMK (eds) Avery's neonatology, 6th edn. Lippincott Williams & Wilkins, Philadelphia, pp 688–689
5. Levi M, Ten Cate H (1999) Disseminated intravascular coagulation. N Engl J Med 341:586–592
6. Blanchette V DYaCA (2005) Hemotology. In: MacDonald MG, Mullett, Seshia, MMK (eds) Avery's neonatology, 6th edn. Lippincott Williams and Wilkins, Philadelphia, pp 1193–1197
7. Mancuso T (2008) Anesthesia for the preterm newborn. In: Holzman RS, Mancuso TJ, Polaner DM (eds) A practical approach to pediatric anesthesia. Wolters Kluwer Lippincott Williams & Wilkins, Philadelphia, pp 601–609
8. Vitali S, Camerota AJ, Arnold JH (2005) Anesthesia and analgesia in the neonate. In: MacDonald MG, Mullet MD, Seshia MMK (eds) Avery's neonatology, 6th edn. Lippincott Williams and Wilkins, Philadelphia, pp 1557–1571
9. Bennett EJ, Patel KP, Grundy EM (1977) Neonatal temperature and surgery. Anesthesiology 46:303–304
10. Vitali S, Camerota AJ, Arnold JH (2005) Anesthesia and analgesia in the neonate. In: MacDonald MG, Mullet MD, Seshia MMK (eds) Avery's neonatology, 6th edn. Lippincott Williams and Wilkins, Philadelphia, pp 1561–1564

Chapter 2
Newborn Emergencies

A 14-h-old male, 2,400 g, born at 37 weeks gestational age, is scheduled emergently for repair of esophageal atresia with tracheoesophageal fistula. The newborn choked and gagged on the first glucose water feed. A contrast study confirmed the diagnosis. Vital signs are BP = 88/52 mmHg, RR = 44/min, P = 158 bpm, T = 37.2°C. His hemoglobin is 13.0 g/dL. An NG tube is in place. The infant is receiving nasal cannula oxygen at 300 mL/min.

R.S. Holzman et al., *Pediatric Anesthesiology Review: Clinical Cases for Self-Assessment,*
DOI 10.1007/978-1-4419-1617-4_2, © Springer Science+Business Media, LLC 2010

Preoperative Evaluation

1. Is this an emergency? What historical information might have helped anticipate the diagnosis? Are there other, safer, means to make the diagnosis than a contrast study?

2. What other evaluations of the newborn are needed prior to undertaking the induction of anesthesia? What conditions are likely or associated with EA/TEF?

3. Is a preoperative gastrostomy with local anesthesia indicated? Would the situation be different if the patient were preterm with RDS?

Preoperative Evaluation

1. While repair of the esophageal atresia (EA) with tracheo-esophageal fistula (TEF) may not be a true emergency, it is, at the least, very urgent. The longer the newborn is unrepaired the greater the risk for aspiration. Surgical correction should proceed very quickly but proper preparation can be accomplished in short order. The diagnosis can be suspected in cases of maternal polyhydraminos. In the delivery room, inability to pass a suction catheter into the stomach should raise the suspicion of EA. A contrast study is not needed to make the diagnosis. Aspiration of oral contrast is a significant risk. Plain X-rays may show the dilated, air-filled esophageal pouch. A film with a radiopaque catheter coiled in that pouch will confirm the diagnosis. If there is no gas in the abdomen, it is possible that the child has EA without TEF.

2. It is important to ascertain which type of TEF is present. Up to 80–90% of cases are esophageal atresia with a distal fistula between the posterior trachea near the carina and the stomach. The next most common, approximately 7%, is EA without TEF. Many other types and subtypes have been described. Up to 50% of patients with EA/TEF have other congenital anomalies. Cardiovascular anomalies make up one-third of the anomalies seen in these patients. The cardiac anomalies seen are, in order of occurrence, VSD, ASD, Tetralogy of Fallot, and coarctation of the aorta. Other organ systems involved in these patients are musculoskeletal (30%), gastrointestinal (20%), and GU (10%). Patients with EA/TEF may have the VATER syndrome which consists of vertebral defects or VSD, anal/arterial defects, TEF/EA, radial, or renal anomalies [2, 3].

3. In cases where the newborn is having severe respiratory compromise and positive pressure ventilation has been instituted, a ventilator breath may follow a path from the trachea through the fistula and distend the stomach. The abdomen can become very distended, further compromising ventilation. In these dire situations, an emergent gastrostomy may allow the abdominal pressure to be relieved enough for ventilation to continue [4]. Approximately 25% of newborns with EA/TEF are born preterm and in cases with respiratory distress, the situation is even more difficult since institution of positive pressure ventilation will require higher pressures. This will invariably also put gas into the stomach through the fistula.

Intraoperative Course

1. What monitors would you require for this case? Arterial line? Where? How will you assess intravascular volume? CVP catheter? How much information about preload would a foley catheter give you for this case?

2. What might be done to minimize the effect of the fistula at induction? Is IV or inhalation induction preferable? How should the airway be secured? Does the presence of the fistula alter the techniques for intubation? What should be done with the NG tube once intubation is accomplished?

Intraoperative Course

1. For otherwise well term newborns with EA/TEF, standard monitors, with the addition of "pre" (right hand) and "post" (left hand or either foot) ductal pulse oximeters and a foley catheter will often be sufficient. If there is pulmonary compromise, either from aspiration or because of prematurity, an arterial line is useful for frequent ABG determinations. A CVP catheter would not only give some information about intravascular volume but also be an excellent route for administration of resuscitation medications, should that be needed. If peripheral IV access is good in an otherwise well newborn with EA/TEF, the risk of placing a CVP line may not be justified. Urine output should mirror renal blood flow (GFR) but it is a secondary measure. In addition, the small volume produced may be difficult to accurately collect and measure. Nevertheless this monitor can provide useful information for these cases.

2. Avoidance of positive pressure ventilation is an important consideration in the anesthetic care of these patients. Positive pressure ventilation will force gas through the fistula into the stomach. IV access should be secured prior to any attempts at induction of anesthesia or intubation. Awake intubation is often done, followed by spontaneous ventilation with the infant breathing oxygen plus incremental doses of a potent vapor anesthetic. Alternatively, an inhalation induction can be done and when an adequate depth of anesthesia has been achieved and the airway anesthetized with a proper dose of topical anesthetic, laryngoscopy and intubation can be done. It has been commented that turning the bevel of the endotracheal tube anteriorly will decrease the chance of intubating the fistula but this is unproven. It also has been suggested that since the fistula is often relatively low in the trachea, a deliberate right main stem intubation should be done and the endotracheal tube then withdrawn to a position just above the carina, hopefully distal to the fistula. Great care is required while advancing the endotracheal tube in the trachea, however. The fistula may be quite large and the endotracheal tube may easily be placed into the fistula if it is advanced too far into the trachea [5]. An alternative that will allow positive pressure ventilation is performance of a rigid bronchoscopy following induction of anesthesia and placement of a Fogarty catheter through the fistula into the stomach. The balloon is then inflated and the catheter pulled taut, thus closing the fistula [6]. This technique allows positive pressure ventilation to proceed without distending the stomach. The surgeon will likely ask that the NG tube be advanced during the procedure to facilitate identification of the esophageal pouch.

3. Is controlled or spontaneous ventilation preferable for these cases? How would you determine whether or not a percutaneous gastrostomy is indicated prior to the definitive repair? Is a precordial stethoscope of particular importance for these cases?

4. After positioning and the start of the thoracotomy, breath sounds from the left axillary stethoscope markedly diminish and the SpO_2 decreases. What might be the cause? What would you do? Could the endotracheal tube have accidentally entered the fistula?

Postoperative Course

1. Is this patient a candidate for extubation at the conclusion of the surgery? If not, how should the newborn be ventilated? Should the NG tube be removed?

2. What options are there for postoperative analgesia? Does the presence of VATER syndrome affect your willingness to use regional analgesia? If the patient has no other anomalies, would regional analgesia be useful for this case? What drugs would you use?

3. Following extubation from minimal ventilator settings on postoperative day #1, the patient exhibits respiratory distress with inspiratory stridor. What might be the cause? What therapy would you begin? How would you decide whether or not to reintubate the child?

3. If the stomach distends after intubation, even with gentle assistance of respiratory efforts, and this distention is interfering with ventilation (leading to the use of higher ventilation pressures), percutaneous gastrostomy will allow some control of the situation. The usual position for surgery is left side down for a right thoracotomy. The surgeon retracts the right lung, leaving only the left lung for gas exchange. In this situation, a left axillary stethoscope will give the anesthesiologist immediate information about the adequacy of ventilation. The left bronchus is easily occluded by blood or secretions and may be kinked by the surgeon during the procedure; the anesthesiologist must be aware of these events as soon as they occur [7].

4. As mentioned above, secretions and/or blood may easily occlude the lumen of the trachea or right main bronchus. Additionally, the bronchus is often kinked by surgical retraction during the procedure. Even with occlusion of the fistula by a Fogarty catheter, there still may be room for the tip of the endotracheal tube, greatly decreasing or eliminating ventilation of the lungs [7].

Postoperative Course

1. For term infants who undergo a relatively uncomplicated repair, extubation is a possibility, but the intensive care nursery team who will care for the baby should be involved with the decision. The mode of ventilation, if extubation will be delayed, should be guided by the intraoperative course. It is often advisable to use a ventilator from the ICN for newborns in the OR since the anesthesia machine ventilators are not specifically designed for use in the newborn. The position of the NG tube is very important. It is generally left in a position such that the tip is just proximal to the esophageal anastomosis.

2. Postoperative analgesia can be provided by administration of local anesthetic and opioid into the epidural space [8]. If the patient has the VATER association, epidural catheter placement may be problematic but regional techniques should not be ruled out prior to review of an X-ray of the spine [9]. If regional analgesia is not undertaken, parenteral opioids can be used to provide analgesia. In either case, cardiorespiratory monitoring must be done [10].

3. Patients with EA/TEF may have significant tracheomalacia at the level of the dilated esophageal pouch. In utero, the dilated esophageal pouch may compress the developing trachea, leading to weakened cartilage. With vigorous inspiration this area of the trachea may partially collapse, and inspiratory stridor will result. It is unlikely that treatment of this problem with inhaled racemic epinephrine will be effective as it does with infectious croup, but if subglottic edema is part of the problem, a trial of this treatment should be undertaken. The infant should be reintubated if respiratory failure is imminent based on clinical and laboratory criteria. If reintubation is done, exquisite care must be taken with the NG tube and esophageal intubation must absolutely be avoided.

Additional Topics

1. What are the major preoperative considerations in evaluating a patient for congenital diaphragmatic hernia? What immediate interventions can be performed therapeutically? Sudden deterioration may indicate what? On which side?

2. What are the important differences between omphalocele and gastroschisis? What are the important anesthetic considerations during correction of these defects?

3. What are the considerations for anesthetic care during resection of a sacrococcygeal teratoma?

4. What are the anesthetic concerns for a child coming to the operating room for repair of pyloric stenosis?

Additional Topics

1. In the preoperative evaluation of newborns with congenital diaphragmatic hernia, the size of the hernia is important in predicting the severity of cardiorespiratory compromise and ultimate prognosis [11, 12]. Eighty percent of the defects are posterolateral, through the Foramen of Bochdalek, most commonly on the left. Twenty percent of newborns with CDH have associated cardiac defects, most often PDA [13]. Poor prognosis is associated with birth weight <1,000 g, gestational age <33 weeks, and an A-a gradient >500 mmHg [14]. Placement of a nasogastric tube may help ventilation by decompressing the stomach. Mechanical ventilation should be done with the lowest possible airway pressures [15]. Sudden deterioration may be due to the occurrence of a pneumothorax on the contralateral side from the hernia defect.

2. Omphalocele is herniation of intestine into the umbilical cord while gastroschisis is a defect in the abdominal wall. With omphalocele, a peritoneal sac covers the intestines (unless it is ruptured during delivery) but there is no covering in cases of gastroschisis. Infants with omphalocele are much more likely to have associated GI, cardiac, or craniofacial anomalies but only approximately 25% are preterm or low birth weight. In Beckwith–Wiedeman syndrome, omphalocele occurs in association with macroglossia, hypoglycemia, organomegaly, and gigantism. A much higher percentage of newborns with gastroschisis are born preterm. Two important anesthetic considerations for these conditions are fluid management and possible compromise of ventilation and/or circulation during replacement of the abdominal contents and attempted closure of the abdominal wall [16].

3. Sacrococcygeal teratomas can be quite large with an extensive blood supply. Their surgical excision can cause significant bleeding to the point that occlusion of the descending aorta may be needed as a temporary measure for hemostasis. The newborns' position may change from supine to prone more than once during the procedure [1].

4. Pyloric stenosis generally presents between 2 and 6 weeks of age with vomiting that is relentless and progressive but not bilious. The persistent vomiting may result in dehydration and hypochloremic metabolic alkalosis. Fluid replenishment and normalization of electrolytes should be accomplished prior to taking the child to the OR for a Ramstead pyloromyotomy. Suctioning of the stomach should precede induction of anesthesia. Several passes with an orogastric tube may be needed. Induction is by a rapid sequence technique. Rare occurrences of apnea in the postoperative period (possibly related to the still somewhat alkaline CSF) or hypoglycemia have been seen. These children generally do very well postoperatively, often taking PO's within hours of the end of the procedure. Analgesia can often be provided with PO/PR acetaminophen [17–20].

5. An infant, several hours old, is brought to the OR by the surgeon for respiratory distress with a diagnosis of infantile lobar emphysema. Is infantile lobar emphysema a surgical emergency? Why/why not? Should the patient undergo bronchoscopy first? Why/why not? What muscle relaxant would you choose? Why? A colleague of yours suggests the avoidance of nitrous oxide; do you agree?

6. A newborn is scheduled for exploratory abdominal surgery for obstruction. The abdomen is distended, meconium has not yet passed, and the intestines are palpable through the anterior abdominal wall. What is the most likely surgical diagnosis? What respiratory management concerns do you have? How will you approach securing the airway? Is it likely that this baby's sweat chlorides will be normal?

5. Congenital lobar emphysema is a relatively unusual cause of respiratory distress in the newborn and infant period. Presentation is usually within the first 6 months of life and includes tachypnea, tachycardia, and signs of respiratory distress [3]. The left upper lobe is the most commonly affected. Progressive air trapping leads to hyperinflation of the affected lobe. This lobe can then compress adjacent structures such as normal lung, vessels and even cause mediastinal shift. In infants who are rapidly worsening, this condition can certainly be a surgical emergency. Preoperative maneuvers such as chest tube placement or needle aspiration of the trapped air have not been successful in alleviating the respiratory distress in these children. Induction of anesthesia is a challenge. A slow inhalation induction with oxygen and sevoflurane or halothane, allowing the child to breath spontaneously, will minimize the possibility of increasing the size of the emphysematous lobe and worsening the situation [21]. If the infant hypoventilates, gentle positive pressure ventilation must be performed. If positive pressure ventilation must be delivered, consideration should be given to the use of high-frequency ventilation [22]. Intravenous ketamine has also been used to induce anesthesia in these cases. Caudally placed catheters have been used to provide analgesia for these procedures [23].

6. Meconium ileus results from obstruction of the distal small intestine by abnormal meconium [24]. This problem occurs almost exclusively in infants with cystic fibrosis; however, most infants with cystic fibrosis do not develop meconium ileus. This patient has cystic fibrosis until proven otherwise. The exocrine gland dysfunction in CF leads to pulmonary disease, pancreatic dysfunction, and abnormalities in sweat gland function that cause increased NaCl concentration in sweat. When a sweat chloride is measured at >60 mEq/L the diagnosis of CF is confirmed. The pulmonary compromise is due to thickened secretions and abnormal mucociliary clearance of those secretions. Small airways become obstructed and portions of lung become hyperinflated. There is an inconsistent response to bronchodilators. Induction of anesthesia in this newborn is complicated by full stomach considerations, the decreased FRC due to abdominal distention, and the possible pulmonary compromise due to cystic fibrosis. Once tracheal intubation is accomplished, the anesthesiologist should be prepared to suction the pulmonary secretions, possibly after lavage, to improve gas exchange and pulmonary mechanics.

Annotated References

1. Holzman, RS (2008) Gut development: surgical and anesthetic implications. In: Holzman RS, Mancuso TJ, Polaner DM (eds) Practical aspects of pediatric anesthesia. Wolters Kluwer Lippincott Williams and Wilkins, Philadelphia, pp 384–390

   This chapter reviews the development of the GI tract with discussion of the congenital anomalies that bring infants and children to the OR. Tracheoesophageal fistula is reviewed including the associated anomalies seen in other organ systems. Anesthetic goals and techniques are discussed including postoperative management.

2. Holzman, RS (2008) The body cavity and wall. In: Holzman RS, Mancuso TJ, Polaner DM (eds) Practical aspects of pediatric anesthesia. Wolters Kluwer Lippincott Williams and Wilkins, Philadelphia, pp 289–292

   This section reviews the embryology and pathophysiology seen in newborns with congenital diaphragamatic hernia. Anesthetic considerations are reviewed as well as peri-operative management issues.

3. Bishop, WP (2006) Pyloric stenosis. In: Kliegman RM, Marcdante KJ, Jenson HB, Behrman RE (eds) Nelson essentials of pediatrics, 5th edn. Philadelphia: Elsevier Inc, pp 599–600

   The author reviews the presentation, relevant diagnostic studies and medical management of infants with the diagnosis of pyloric stenosis. The central role of surgical correction is mentioned but anesthetic considerations per se are not included.

References

1. Seefelder C (2008) Abdominal tumors. In: Holzman RS, Mancuso TJ, Polaner DM (eds) Practical aspects of pediatric anesthesia. Wolters Kluwer Lippincott Williams and Wilkins, Philadelphia, pp 437–440
2. Kluth D, Steding G, Seidl W (1987) The embryology of foregut malformations. J Pediatr Surg 22:389–393
3. Kang BKB (2008) The foregut and chest. In: Holzman RS, Mancuso TJ, Polaner DM (eds) Practical aspects of pediatric anesthesia. Wolters Kluwer Lippincott Williams and Wilkins, Philadelphia, pp 391–392
4. Karl HW (1985) Control of life-threatening air leak after gastrostomy in an infant with respiratory distress syndrome and tracheoesophageal fistula. Anesthesiology 62:670–672
5. Koka B, Chacko SK (2006) Airway management of a newborn with trascheoesophageal fistula. In: Murphy M, Hung O (eds) Airway management and monitoring manual. McGraw-Hill, New York
6. Filston HC, Chitwood WR Jr, Schkolne B, Blackmon LR (1982) The Fogarty balloon catheter as an aid to management of the infant with esophageal atresia and tracheoesophageal fistula complicated by severe RDS or pneumonia. J Pediatr Surg 17:149–151

7. Andropoulos DB, Rowe RW, Betts JM (1998) Anaesthetic and surgical airway management during tracheo-oesophageal fistula repair. Paediatr Anaesth 8:313–319

8. Murrell D, Gibson PR, Cohen RC (1993) Continuous epidural analgesia in newborn infants undergoing major surgery. J Pediatr Surg 28:548–552; discussion 52–3

9. Valairucha S, Seefelder C, Houck CS (2002) Thoracic epidural catheters placed by the caudal route in infants: the importance of radiographic confirmation. Paediatr Anaesth 12:424–428

10. Tyler DC (1989) Respiratory effects of pain in a child after thoracotomy. Anesthesiology 70:873–874

11. Karamanoukian HL, Glick PL, Wilcox DT et al (1995) Pathophysiology of congenital diaphragmatic hernia. XI: Anatomic and biochemical characterization of the heart in the fetal lamb CDH model. J Pediatr Surg 30:925–928; discussion 9

12. Harrison MR, Keller RL, Hawgood SB et al (2003) A randomized trial of fetal endoscopic tracheal occlusion for severe fetal congenital diaphragmatic hernia. N Engl J Med 349:1916–1924

13. Schwartz SM, Vermilion RP, Hirschl RB (1994) Evaluation of left ventricular mass in children with left-sided congenital diaphragmatic hernia. J Pediatr 125:447–451

14. Reickert CA, Hirschl RB, Atkinson JB et al (1998) Congenital diaphragmatic hernia survival and use of extracorporeal life support at selected level III nurseries with multimodality support. Surgery 123:305–310

15. Karamanoukian HL, Glick PL, Zayek M et al (1994) Inhaled nitric oxide in congenital hypoplasia of the lungs due to diaphragmatic hernia or oligohydramnios. Pediatrics 94:715–718

16. Holzman R (2008) The Body Cavity and Wall. In: Holzman RS, Mancuso TJ, Polaner DM (eds) Practical aspects of pediatrics of anesthesia. Wolters Kluwer Lippincott Williamns and Wilkins, Philadelphia, pp 295–299

17. MacDonald NJ, Fitzpatrick GJ, Moore KP et al (1987) Anaesthesia for congenital hypertrophic pyloric stenosis. A review of 350 patients. Br J Anaesth 59:672–677

18. Davis PJ, Galinkin J, McGowan FX et al (2001) A randomized multicenter study of remifentanil compared with halothane in neonates and infants undergoing pyloromyotomy. I. Emergence and recovery profiles. Anesth Analg 93:1380–1386, table of contents

19. Cook-Sather SD, Tulloch HV, Liacouras CA, Schreiner MS (1997) Gastric fluid volume in infants for pyloromyotomy. Can J Anaesth 44:278–283

20. Campbell BT, McLean K, Barnhart DC et al (2002) A comparison of laparoscopic and open pyloromyotomy at a teaching hospital. J Pediatr Surg 37:1068–1071; discussion -71

21. Cote CJ (1978) The anesthetic management of congenital lobar emphysema. Anesthesiology 49:296–298

22. Goto H, Boozalis ST, Benson KT, Arakawa K (1987) High-frequency jet ventilation for resection of congenital lobar emphysema. Anesth Analg 66:684–686

23. Raghavendran S, Diwan R, Shah T, Vas L (2001) Continuous caudal epidural analgesia for congenital lobar emphysema: a report of three cases. Anesth Analg 93:348–350; 3rd contents page

24. Hartman GE, Boyajian MJ, Choi SS et al (2005) Surgical care of conditions presenting in the newborn. In: MacDonald MG, Mullet MD, Seshia MMK (eds) Avery's neonatology, 6th edn. Lippincott Williams & Wilkins, Philadelphia, pp 1119–1120

Chapter 3
Neuroanesthesia

An active 2-year-old, 12-kg boy is scheduled for a frontal craniotomy for a cranio-pharyngioma. HR = 100 bpm, BP = 110/60 mmHg, RR = 24/min, T = 37°C. A heart murmur is detected on preoperative examination.

R.S. Holzman et al., *Pediatric Anesthesiology Review: Clinical Cases for Self-Assessment,*
DOI 10.1007/978-1-4419-1617-4_3, © Springer Science+Business Media, LLC 2010

Preoperative Evaluation

1. What is the possible significance of a heart murmur? How should it be evaluated? Are any lab tests helpful? Which ones? Should this patient have a preoperative echocardiogram? Why? Should a cardiology consult be obtained? Why? A small atrial septal defect is diagnosed. Any significance?

2. What are the perioperative implications of this tumor? What is diabetes insipidus? What is antidiuretic hormone? Where is it made? How can diabetes insipidus be diagnosed preoperatively? How does the presence of diabetes insipidus affect your preoperative fluid management? How do you assess the need for perioperative steroids? What are the possible implications of inadequate steroid replacement? What other hormones can be affected? What are their anesthetic implications? What lab work would you require preoperatively? Explain.

Preoperative Evaluation

1. During routine random examinations, up to 30% of children will demonstrate an innocent murmur. There are several innocent murmurs of childhood, not associated with any cardiac pathology, with which a pediatric anesthesiologist should be familiar. The innocent murmur (Still's murmur) is characterized by a high-pitched, vibratory, short systolic murmur heard along the left mid-sternal border without radiation in children 2–7 years of age. An innocent venous hum resulting from turbulent flow in the jugular system may also be detected in the neck or upper chest. The hum can be changed or eliminated by position changes or light compression of the jugular veins in the neck. In some cases of increased cardiac output such as during febrile illnesses, murmurs of flow across normal semilunar valves are heard.

   The murmur of an ASD is similar to that appreciated in pulmonic stenosis. There is no murmur caused by the low velocity left to right flow across the ASD itself. A soft ejection-type (crescendo-decrescendo) murmur of relative pulmonic stenosis is heard at the upper left sternal border. This murmur results from the excessive flow across a normal pulmonary valve. The second heart sound is widely and persistently split as a result of this excessive flow. The most common type of ASD is the secundum type with the abnormal connection between the atria, a result of incomplete formation of the second atrial septum. PVR remains normal throughout childhood and CHF is quite infrequent. Adults with uncorrected ASDs do develop CHF and/or atrial flutter or pulmonary hypertension, so correction of the ASD is generally undertaken in early childhood. The significance of an ASD is that of the possibility of a paradoxical embolus in which air or clots in the venous system cross the ASD and lead to complications in the systemic arterial circulation.

2. Craniopharyngioma, a tumor of Rathke's pouch, may descend into the sella turcica and destroy part or all of hypothalamic and pituitary tissue as it enlarges, leading to hypopituitarism [1]. Preoperatively, the child should be evaluated for adrenal or thyroid dysfunction [2]. If ACTH secretion is impaired by the tumor, the production of glucocorticoids and androgens by the adrenal cortex will be below normal. If not evaluated preoperatively, adrenal insufficiency should be assumed and the patient treated accordingly. Diabetes insipidus is unlikely to be seen preoperatively. It is diagnosed by the presence of a large volume of dilute urine (Osm < 300 mOsm/mL) in the face of increasing serum osmolarity and increasing serum sodium. If replacement of urinary losses with dilute IV fluid such as D2.5W or D5, 0.2NS is insufficient, an infusion of aqueous vasopressin should be started. The preoperative lab tests ordered depend upon the clinical presentation but may include electrolytes, fasting glucose, thyroid function tests, and a CBC. Imaging studies ordered by the neurosurgeon should be reviewed as well.

Intraoperative Course

1. Would you premedicate this child? Why? Would you insert an intravenous catheter before he is asleep? Why? If not, or if the initial attempts are unsuccessful, what next? A colleague suggests intramuscular ketamine. Agree? Why? Is rectal methohexital or thiopental an option? Mask induction? Explain.

2. Would you insert an arterial catheter? Why? A central venous catheter? Why? If yes, where? Potential problems? Where do you want the tip to be? How do you confirm its position? What if multiple attempts are unsuccessful? Does the patient need a urinary catheter? Why? Would you use a precordial Doppler? Explain.

Intraoperative Course

1. The possibility of raised ICP should be considered when planning whether or not to administer a premedication. In a child such as the one presented who does not have intracranial hypertension, an inhalation induction is appropriate, with or without a premedication, depending upon the patient's (and the family's) level of anxiety. Placement of an IV for induction is also appropriate and would allow a more rapid induction without the possibility of airway compromise that some-times occurs during an inhalation induction and that would likely upset both the child and family. Ketamine is a potent cerebral vasodilator and also can cause sudden increases in ICP. Intramuscular midazolam is another possibility for a particularly anxious, uncooperative child who refuses oral premedication. Barbiturates have some advantages in neurosurgical patients, since this class of drugs does lower both cerebral blood flow (CBF) and the cerebral metabolic rate for oxygen ($CMRO_2$). Rectal administration of metholhexital in a dose of 25–30 mg/kg will induce a light sleep in most children despite the upset the route of administration causes at first. A small percentage of children, however, given that dose will develop airway obstruction.

2. An arterial catheter is appropriate for cases such as this in which large fluid shifts or blood losses are possible and/or frequent monitoring of serum ABGs or elec-trolytes is planned. The radial artery is the most convenient and commonly used site, although the posterior tibial and dorsalis pedis arteries in the foot are also acceptable sites. Complications of arterial cannulation include arterial occlusion, flushing of emboli through indwelling catheters, ischemia distal to a catheter and rarely, infection. A central venous catheter may be useful in this case as a mea-sure of preload. For neurosurgical procedures, cannulation of the femoral vein is an attractive option. A CVP catheter is not useful in treating venous air embo-lism (VAE) except as a route for administration of resuscitation medications, should that become necessary. Given the possibility of DI, a urinary catheter is an important monitor. VAE is a possible complication of pediatric neurosurgical procedures. A precordial Doppler is the most sensitive monitor of VAE, detect-ing even minute, clinically insignificant amounts of air. The precordial doppler is of limited use during electrocautery. Supplementing the doppler with another monitor of VAE such as the capnograph or end-tidal nitrogen monitoring is helpful since these monitors are not affected by electrocautery [3].

3. What agent would you use for induction? Why? Explain your choice of muscle relaxant, if you are using one. Explain your choice of agents for maintenance. Suppose the surgeon asked you to give mannitol. How much is appropriate? What is its expected effect? Are there potential problems with its administration?

4. During the craniotomy, the blood pressure decreases to 60/40 mmHg. Possible causes? End tidal CO_2 decreases as well. Causes? How can you differentiate hypovolemia from venous air embolism? Treatment? PEEP? How does the presence of the atrial septal defect influence your management? The hypotension persists. What is your next move? When are pressors indicated? Which would you choose? Why? Would you continue/restart the nitrous oxide? Explain.

3. Induction of anesthesia can be safely accomplished with either an inhalation or IV technique in this active 2-year old without evidence of raised ICP. Muscle relaxation should be part of the maintenance since any movement of the child once positioned would be dangerous. The goals of maintenance of anesthesia should include provision of a "slack brain" for the neurosurgeon and stable hemodynamics. The technique should allow for a rapid emergence at the conclusion of the procedure. Administration of opioid prior to pin placement and local anesthetic infiltration along the proposed incision will help minimize hemodynamic derangements. Mannitol administration may help reduce ICP and decrease the size of the brain, allowing better surgical exposure. Starting doses, in the range of 0.25–0.5 mg/kg IV, raise serum osmolality by approximately 10 mOsm. If given too rapidly, mannitol may cause transient hypotension. Repeated and large doses may increase serum osmolality to >320 mOsm, a dangerous level. Hypertonic (3%) saline has been used more recently in the treatment of raised ICP in patients with traumatic and nontraumatic cerebral edema and is an option to consider in the operating room.

4. Venous air embolism (VAE) is a distinct possibility in pediatric neurosurgical procedures. The incidence varies with the sensitivity of the detection device used, but up to 30–40% of children undergoing intracranial procedures have VAE. Maintenance of a generous circulating blood volume and the use of positive pressure ventilation help decrease the likelihood of a VAE. Once detected or suspected (unexplained hypotension) the anesthesiologist must alert the neurosurgeon who will flood the field, while the anesthesiologist ventilates with 100% oxygen and treats any hemodynamic instability. Vasoactive, inotropic agents may be needed to maintain the blood pressure at normal levels. Enhancing cardiac contractility may help to move any air from the right ventricle into the pulmonary circulation. The presence of an ASD in this patient is particularly troubling since air in the right atrium may cross to the left atrium and then travel to the cerebral or coronary circulation [4]. If hemodynamic instability persists, turning the patient to a left side down and head down position (Durant's Maneuver) may help move the air out of the right ventricular outflow tract and improve the hemodynamics. Hypovolemia may present similarly to VAE and if vigorous fluid administration is ongoing, the Doppler sounds may be difficult to interpret. In this situation, monitoring end-tidal nitrogen may help differentiate VAE from hypovolemia.

5. The urine output is 4 mL/kg/h. What is your differential diagnosis? Which lab tests might be helpful? The serum sodium is 155 mEq/L. Diagnosis? Treatment? Which intravenous fluids would you use? Why? Should they contain glucose? Why? How do you determine the rate of administration?

6. How much blood loss is acceptable prior to transfusion? Why? Are there alternatives? What are the risks?

7. The operation takes 10 hours. Would you extubate at the end? Pros/Cons? How would you minimize straining at extubation? Do you anticipate hypertension at the end of the case? Is this a problem? Why? Prevention/Treatment?

5. DI is a common complication of surgery for a craniopharyngioma [5–7]. It is caused by disruption of the ADH secreting cells. Diagnosis is made when the patient produces a large volume of dilute urine in the face of hypernatremia. The diagnosis is confirmed when the serum sodium is >145 mEq/L, the serum osmolality is >300 mOsm/L, the urine output is >4 mL/kg/h, and the urine osmolality is <300 mOsm/L. Treatment, outlined above, is directed at replenishing urine output and maintaining normal serum osmolality. Since the administration of water is not an option in the anesthetized patient, dilute IV fluids can be given to replenish the excessive water losses in the urine. If $D_{2.5}$ is used, hyperglycemia may result. If the serum osmolality remains high, an infusion of vasopressin offers the greatest flexibility in maintenance of fluid balance. An infusion of vasopressin, starting a 1 milliunit/kg/h, is begun and slowly increased until the urine output decreases to <2 mL/kg/h.

6. The lowest permissible hemoglobin depends upon the patient and the situation during the procedure. Measurement of an ABG or central venous blood gas (SvO_2) may give some information about the adequacy of oxygen delivery to the patient. Elevated serum lactate or lower than normal SvO_2 could indicate an imbalance between global oxygen delivery and oxygen consumption. The potential for continued bleeding is an important factor in deciding whether or not to administer blood/blood products. The risk of transmitting an infectious agent to a person via a transfusion varies from 1:100,000 for hepatitis A to 1:1–2,000,000 for HIV. Hemolytic transfusion reactions occur as often as 1:15–20,000 transfusions. Other results of transfusion include nonhemolytic transfusion reactions, urticaria or other allergic-type reactions, and possibly immunomodulation.

7. The usual criteria apply in considering whether or not to extubate this child. However, following neurosurgical procedures, it is important to assess neurological function and much easier to do so in an extubated, nonsedated patient. If opioids were a part of maintenance and the inhaled agents decreased as closure of the wound took place, straining and coughing prior to extubation should be minimal. Deep extubation is an option for this patient but experience with this technique is essential prior to undertaking it. Also, the anesthesiologist must be certain that the child has a very good mask airway while anesthetized prior to performing a deep extubation.

Postoperative Care

1. The urine output remains high postoperatively. How long do you anticipate this may persist? Treatment? What is vasopressin? Can you use it? How? Same for DDAVP? Dangers?

2. Eight hours postoperatively, the child has a seizure. Differential diagnosis? Treatment?

Additional Topics

1. What respiratory complications can you anticipate in the life of a child born with myelomeningocele? How does this happen with each problem? At what ages would you expect these various problems to present clinically?

2. A 3-year old showed up in the Pre Op Cl.inic scheduled for the removal of an orbital dermoid. He has four cafe-au-lait spots on his trunk and buttocks. He has had headaches recently, and his pediatrician noticed his blood pressure was elevated (135/105 mmHg). Want more? His Mom has noticed some "flushing" spells recently. What do you think may be going on? There is a family history of neurofibromatosis. Are there any associated endocrinopathies?

Postoperative Care

1. DI may persist for several days following surgery for craniopharyngioma and may even be permanent [5]. Management using an IV infusion of vasopressin offers greater flexibility but once longer-term therapy is indicated, the route of administration should be switched to intermittent IV then intranasal. Oral desmopressin is available in addition to the intranasal form. The usual starting dose is ten times the intranasal dose.

2. Other postoperative complications seen after this procedure include hyperthermia and seizures. Retraction of the frontal lobes during this lengthy procedure may be responsible for this postoperative problem. On occasion anticonvulsants are begun intraoperatively and continued postoperatively. Hyperthermia may result from damage to the hypothalamic thermoregulatory mechanisms.

Additional Topics

1. Myelodysplasia is an abnormality of fusion of the neural groove during the first month of gestation. The resulting sac-like herniation of the meninges is called meningocele, and if neural elements are contained within the sac, then it is called myelomeningocele. There are often accompanying abnormalities such as hydrocephalus, tethered cord, and Arnold-Chiari type II malformations present in these children. At birth, fluid losses through the defect may lead to dehydration. Intraoperatively, during the initial repair, high third space fluid losses are an important consideration. Since the majority of myelomeningocles are in the lumbar region, as the child grows older, the resulting urinary insufficiency leads to electrolyte abnormalities [8]. In addition, as they age, various bladder augmentations and other procedures are often done on these children leading to additional difficulties with electrolytes. The paralysis at and below the level of the lesion leads to the development of thoraco-lumbar scoliosis. As the scoliosis worsens, pulmonary function is impaired [9–11].

2. Neurofibromatosis is differentiated into two forms, NF-1 (90%) and NF-2 (10%). This patient has NF-1. This disease can affect nearly every organ system. The tumors characteristic of the condition are overgrowths of Schwann Cells and endoneurium. Clinically, café-au-lait spots, axillary or inguinal freckling, neurofibromas, bone lesions, and optic gliomas are seen. Precocious sexual development is seen as a result of invasion of the glioma into the hypothalamus. CNS tumors account for significant morbidity in these children. In addition, the incidence of pheochromocytoma, rhabdomyosarcoma, Wilms tumor, and leukemia is higher than in the general population.

3. What is the Glasgow Coma Scale? What is the maximum total score you can get? How many points do you get for being brain dead?

4. A patient with cerebral palsy and spasticity needs to have his heel cords (Achilles tendons) lengthened. Is he likely to have swallowing problems? How will you evaluate him for the potential to reflux and aspirate? Should he receive a rapid sequence induction? With which intravenous agents? Your choice of muscle relaxant? What if he has "no veins?"

3. The Glasgow Coma scale is used to assess cortical and brainstem function.

Activity	Best response	Score
Eye opening	Spontaneous	4
	To verbal stim	3
	To pain	2
	None	1
Verbal	Oriented	5
	Confused	4
	Inappropriate words	3
	Nonspecific sounds	2
	None	1
Motor	Follows commands	6
	Localizes pain	5
	Withdraws from pain	4
	Flexion to pain	3
	Extension to pain	2
	None	1

4. Cerebral palsy is a static encephalopathy that has a changing clinical presentation over time. It is a disorder of posture and movement often associated with seizures, resulting from a lesion in the developing brain. Children with CP often have surgical procedures as treatment for contractures, scoliosis, gastroesophageal reflux, and other problems [12]. If a rapid sequence induction is planned, succinylcholine may be used. Its use in children with CP has been studied, and serum potassium increases as it does in patients without CP given succinylcholine [13]. If there is no IV access, IM administration of Ketamine, glycopyrrolate, and succinylcholine is an option.

Annotated References

1. Bendo AA, Kass IS, Hartung J, Cottrell JE. (2006) Anesthesia for neurosurgery. In: Barash PG, Cullen PG, Stoelting RK (eds) Clinical anesthesia, 5th edn, Lippincott Williams and Wilkins Philadelphia, Pa. Chapter 27, pp 773–774
   Sections of this chapter review, among other topics, the clinical presentation, monitoring and management of venous air embolism in neurosurgical patients, the pathophysiology of intracranial pressure, specific issues regarding pituitary tumors, and management of patients with head injury.

2. Levine DA, (2006) Cerebral Palsy. In: Kliegman RM, Marcdante KJ, Jenson HB, Behrman RE (eds) Nelson essentials of pediatrics, 5th edn. Elsevier Saunders, Philadelphia, Section II, pp 57–58

This section reviews briefly the diagnosis and subtypes of cerebral palsy. Risk factors for the development of this condition are also discussed.

References

1. Karavitaki N, Wass JA (2008) Craniopharyngiomas. Endocrinol Metab Clin North Am 37:173–193, ix–x
2. Muller HL (2008) Childhood craniopharyngioma. Recent advances in diagnosis, treatment and follow-up. Horm Res 69:193–202
3. Culp WC, Jr, Culp WC (2007) Gas embolisms revisited. Anesthesiology 107:850–851; author reply 3–4
4. Buompadre MC, Arroyo HA (2008) Accidental cerebral venous gas embolism in a young patient with congenital heart disease. J Child Neurol 23:121–123
5. Dusick JR, Fatemi N, Mattozo C et al (2008) Pituitary function after endonasal surgery for nonadenomatous parasellar tumors: Rathke's cleft cysts, craniopharyngiomas, and meningiomas. Surg Neurol 70(5):482–490
6. Wisoff JH (2008) Craniopharyngioma. J Neurosurg Pediatrics 1:124–125; discussion 5
7. Sigounas DG, Sharpless JL, Cheng DM et al (2008) Predictors and incidence of central diabetes insipidus after endoscopic pituitary surgery. Neurosurgery 62:71–78; discussion 8–9
8. Woodhouse CR (2008) Myelomeningocele: neglected aspects. Pediatr Nephrol 23(8):1223–1231
9. Sherman MS, Kaplan JM, Effgen S et al (1997) Pulmonary dysfunction and reduced exercise capacity in patients with myelomeningocele. J Pediatr 131:413–418
10. Swaminathan S, Paton JY, Ward SL et al (1989) Abnormal control of ventilation in adolescents with myelodysplasia. J Pediatr 115:898–903
11. Kirk VG, Morielli A, Gozal D et al (2000) Treatment of sleep-disordered breathing in children with myelomeningocele. Pediatr Pulmonol 30:445–452
12. de Veer AJ, Bos JT, Niezen-de Boer RC et al (2008) Symptoms of gastroesophageal reflux disease in severely mentally retarded people: a systematic review. BMC Gastroenterol 8:23
13. Dierdorf SF, McNiece WL, Rao CC et al (1985) Effect of succinylcholine on plasma potassium in children with cerebral palsy. Anesthesiology 62:88–90

Chapter 4
Central Nervous System/Orthopedics

A 12-year-old, 50-kg girl with myelomeningocele and T10 paraplegia has a 90°
thoracic curve and is scheduled for a posterior spinal fusion with instrumentation. She
has a functioning ventriculoperitoneal shunt and is allergic to penicillin, vancomycin,
milk, nuts, and bananas. She self-catheterizes, and is incontinent of feces. Her hematocrit is 32%, and she has six units of designated donor blood available.

R.S. Holzman et al., *Pediatric Anesthesiology Review: Clinical Cases for Self-Assessment,*
DOI 10.1007/978-1-4419-1617-4_4, © Springer Science+Business Media, LLC 2010

Preoperative Evaluation

1. Of what anesthetic significance is scoliosis? What are the implications of the 90°
   curve? Why?

2. What would you like to evaluate further? Why?

   (a) With what specific tests will you evaluate the respiratory system? Why?
   (b) With what specific tests will you evaluate the cardiovascular system? Why?
   (c) Are there other organ systems that you are concerned about in this patient?
       Why/Why not?

Preoperative Evaluation

1. Scoliosis surgery usually involves extensive surgical tissue trauma in the prone position and considerable blood loss. Extensive bone dissection may promote air entrainment and air embolism, along with fat embolism and the potential for spinal cord ischemia. As the spinal curvature increases above 65° it produces rotational spine deformity, narrowing of the chest cavity, and maldistribution of ventilation and perfusion matching. Progression of spine rotation deformity potentially predisposes to spinal cord ischemia during the surgical correction. The restriction of lung volumes has its greatest effect on the reduction of the vital capacity. The vital capacity is further diminished by 60% after thoracic surgery on the first postoperative day and gradually recovers over the following 7 days. Further ventilatory compromise can occur from splinting of muscles due to inadequate pain control after surgery and diminished central respiratory drive from opioid analgesics. Therefore, all patients with advanced scoliosis curvature will require postoperative ventilatory support.

2. I would like to assess baseline pulmonary function prior to surgery and anesthesia to explain to the patient the need and risks for postoperative ventilatory support. I will order pulmonary function tests (PFT) and a room air arterial blood gas. PFT will assess the degree of restrictive and obstructive dysfunction. It is effort-dependent and can be useful in a cooperative patient. ABG assesses oxygenation and ventilation by quantitating the abnormalities of gas exchange.

   I will evaluate the cardiovascular system by requesting an electrocardiogram to evaluate conduction and rhythm abnormalities. Echocardiography can assess structural abnormalities and performance of the myocardium. A cardiac MRI may be needed if the chest wall is severely deformed and an adequate echo window cannot be obtained. The reason for evaluation of the cardiovascular system is that a longstanding severe scoliosis can increase pulmonary vascular resistance and right ventricular strain and dysfunction by several mechanisms: reduced alveolar vasculature, increased alveolar capillary pressure by compression from deformed ribs, and chronic hypoxemia and hypercarbia.

   Other system disorders that are involved in this disease include chronic urinary tract obstruction, infection, and possible renal insufficiency.

3. Of what significance is the myelomeningocele for preoperative evaluation of the patient? Why?

   (a) Are there any other associated anatomic abnormalities that influence the anesthetic plan?

   (b) Which anesthetic agents would you select?

   (c) Does the patient need a sleep study?

   (d) How would you evaluate the functioning of the ventriculoperitoneal shunt?

3. Preoperative evaluation of a child with myelomeningocele should consider possible autonomic nervous system dysfunction, symptoms of ventriculoperitoneal (VP) shunt malfunction (onset of new symptoms such as headaches, for example), control of seizures, extent of neurological deficit, lower extremity contractures, and a history of latex allergy.

   (a) The presence of contractures of the lower extremities and overweight (due to nonambulation) requires extra care to avoid pressure injury. The VP shunt requires care to avoid shunt compression and avoidance of insertion of a central line on the ipsilateral side. Brainstem compression may occur by hyperextension of the cervical spine if a Chiari malformation is present and uncorrected.

   (b) I will select the combination of an inhaled anesthetic such as sevoflurane and nitrous oxide and intravenous opioids. In general, there is a decreased requirement for a neuromuscular blockade agent due to the reduced muscle mass in the lower extremities. There are reduced analgesic and anesthetic requirements for the lower extremities and perineal surgery because of impaired sensation. Standard doses of opioids and other CNS depressants may cause excessive sedation and respiratory depression postoperatively due to a right shift of the carbon dioxide response curve. Brain stem compression by the Chiari malformation produces a rightward shift of the carbon dioxide response curve, thereby increasing susceptibility to the respiratory depressant effects of the anesthetic technique.

   (c) This patient does not need a sleep study because she has no history of obstructive sleep apnea or difficulties.

   (d) Malfunction of the VP shunt produces variably severe signs and symptoms of increased intracranial pressure such as unexplained abdominal pain, nausea, and vomiting, decline in school performance, decreased mental status, and persistent or morning headaches. Head and neck radiographs may be helpful to visualize a shunt catheter disconnection and migration. Measurement of CSF pressure at the ventricular reservoir, if the pressure is high, may indicate obstruction to peritoneal drainage. Definitive diagnosis can be made by checking the ventricular drainage on MRI with a contrast injection.

Intraoperative Management

1. Intraoperative monitoring:

   (a) How will you monitor this patient?

   (b) Is an arterial line necessary? Why/why not?

   (c) Where would you place a central venous line?
   (d) Is this likely to cause any problems with her ventriculoperitoneal shunt?

   (e) What if she had a ventriculoatrial shunt?

   (f) When would you consider a pulmonary artery catheter?

   (g) Will end-tidal CO_2 sampling be accurate in this patient? Why/why not?

   (h) Is it likely that somatosensory evoked potentials will be used to monitor this patient? Why/why not?

2. Induction of anesthesia:

   (a) Having had numerous prior procedures, the patient is terrified of needles and requests a mask induction. Your response?

   (b) Why? How do you justify it to the patient?

Intraoperative Management

1. Intraoperative monitoring:

   (a) I will monitor the patient with standard ASA monitoring guidelines including ECG, end-tidal carbon dioxide, inspired oxygen concentration, end-tidal anesthetic concentration, temperature, and urine output.

   (b) I will use an intra-arterial blood pressure monitor to observe changes in blood pressure from excessive blood loss, rapid fluid shift, latex anaphylaxis, and potential autonomic instability as well as obtain samples for lab studies such as arterial blood gas analysis, hematocrit, electrolytes, calcium, and magnesium.

   (c & d) I will place the central venous line into the internal jugular vein because of direct access to the superior vena cava. I will place the central venous line on the contralateral side of the VP shunt to avoid entanglement or puncture with the catheter.

   (e) If the patient has a venticulo-atrial (VA) shunt then I will definitely avoid catheterization of the internal jugular vein because the additional catheter may further narrow the internal jugular vein lumen, impede cerebral venous drainage, and provide a conduit for potential contamination of the shunt catheter. A subclavian, femoral, or axillary vein catheter are safer alternatives in this case.

   (f) I would consider a pulmonary artery catheter if there was preoperative evidence of severe pulmonary hypertension and/or ventricular dysfunction to monitor pulmonary artery pressure and cardiac output as a guide to fluid and inotropic therapy.

   (g) The measurement of the $ETCO_2$ in this patient may not be accurate because of the ventilation–perfusion mismatch and increased respiratory dead space.

   (h) I do not think lower extremity SSEP monitoring is useful in this patient because of the severe sensory and motor impairment.

2. Induction of anesthesia:

   (a) I will induce this patient with an inhalation agent via mask provided that she does not have significant gastroesophageal reflux and venous access cannot be readily established; however, these patients are known to have difficult IV access.

   (b) I will justify the need for IV induction if the patient has GERD and explain to her and the family that the potential for aspiration pneumonitis overrides the fear of needles. The fear of needles can be minimized by providing oral anxiolytic premedication and a topical anesthetic.

Anesthetic Maintenance

1. What anesthetic agents would you use for maintenance? Why?

2. Should you anticipate any particular sensitivity to opioids?

3. Would the use of somatosensory evoked potentials affect your answer? Why/ why not?

Intraoperative Events

1. Forty-five minutes after the start of surgery the patient becomes progressively difficult to ventilate, with peak inspiratory pressures increasing from 25 to 45 cm. H_2O, blood pressure falling from 100/64 to 64/34, oxygen saturation decreasing to 92 from 99%, and wheezing noted. You also note hives on the forearms.

   (a) Your considerations? Why?
   (b) What is your differential diagnosis?
   (c) Specific therapeutic interventions? Why?

   (d) Would diphenhydramine help? Why/why not?

Anesthetic Maintenance

1. I will use a balanced anesthetic technique consisting of an opioid supplemented with a low dose of volatile agent to maintain an adequate depth of anesthesia, hemodynamic stability and minimize the suppression of SSEP recordings.

2. Yes, as discussed above, the presence of an uncorrected Chiari malformation type II and III may compress the brainstem and suppress the CO_2-response function. Hence the patient can be sensitive to opioid-induced respiratory depression.

3. Yes, volatile agents even in low concentrations can suppress the SSEP to a greater extent in the presence of mild sensory impairment, compared with total intravenous anesthesia (TIVA). A low dose volatile agent <MAC of 0.5% usually produces clinically acceptable suppression of neural membrane potentials in patients with normal sensibility. If the SSEP recordings are unsatisfactory in the presence of a low ET dose of inhaled agent then I would proceed with a TIVA technique.

Intraoperative Events

1. (a & b) These are manifestations of a possible allergic reaction, most likely owing to latex anaphylaxis in this particular patient. I will check with the surgical team and nursing staff that latex containing material is not used during the surgery. Other possible causes are a drug or blood product-induced anaphylaxis/anaphylactoid reaction, pneumothorax, and occlusion of the endotracheal tube with secretions and kinking, or endobronchial intubation.

   (c) I will immediately notify the surgeon and nursing staff, discontinue volatile agents and provide 100% oxygen, stop any ongoing antibiotic infusion, auscultate the lungs for pneumothorax and endobronchial intubation, and suction the endotracheal tube to check for possible occlusion. If these causes are excluded then I will administer IV epinephrine 10–20 mcg in incremental boluses to stabilize hemodynamics and relieve the bronchospasm. I will also call for help.

   (d) Diphenhydramine is useful in the treatment of allergic reactions but is not the first line of treatment. It blocks central and peripheral H_1 receptors and antagonizes the effect of histamine released from mast cells during immune-mediated allergic reactions.

2. The patient loses 750 mL of blood during the first 1½ h of the procedure.

    (a) At what point would you begin transfusion?

    (b) Even with autologous blood? Why/why not?

    (c) Is there a role for hetastarch in this case?
    (d) Is there a disadvantage to using it? Why?

    (e) What other efforts can you direct to blood conservation?

Postoperative Course

1. As the patient begins pulling at the endotracheal tube at the end of the case, you loosen the tape, and she vomits. With retching, you can hear air flow in the pharynx, and the patient phonates.

    (a) Your considerations?
    (b) What therapeutic interventions will you make? Why?

2. The patient is extubated and in the PACU for an hour. She appears more difficult to arouse than before, although her heart rate is slow (60) and she appears comfortable. As you wake her, she mumbles about the "worst headache she's ever had."

    (a) Your considerations?
    (b) How would you evaluate the patient?

    (c) How would you intervene in this patient, specifically?

2. (a) I will start blood transfusion right away because of the loss of 750 mL of blood amounts to 20% of patient's total blood volume and it will decrease the Hct from 32 to 25%. If blood loss continues at this rate it will significantly impair oxygen carrying and delivery capacity and expose the patient to hypoxemia.

   (b) I will use the autologous blood first. As the procedure continues the blood loss will increase and expose the patient to hemodynamic instability and the risk of spinal cord ischemia and generalized hypoxemia.

   (c & d) Hetastarch can be useful to replace volume loss provided that the patient's Hct is above 25%. There is a limited experience with the use of hetastarch in children and it has the potential to cause platelet dysfunction when used at an infusion rate greater than 15 mL/kg in a 70 kg adult.

   (e) Intraoperative blood conservation can be achieved by salvaging red blood cells with use of "Cell Saver®" or similar technologies. Other measures such as acute hemodilution and deliberate hypotension are associated with potentially high risks for spinal cord ischemia due to reduced oxygen carrying capacity. A preoperative strategy that can be helpful to conserve blood is autologous blood donation.

Postoperative Course

1. (a & b) The endotracheal tube dislodged out of the glottis. I will remove the endotracheal tube and suction the secretions and vomitus and assist ventilation with 100% oxygen via a face mask.

2. (a & b) I will examine the patient for increased intracranial pressure which can occur from VP shunt malfunction as a result of kinking or disconnection. Other differential diagnoses are opioid-induced hypercarbia and headache and cerebral hypoperfusion due to hypotension, low Hct. Excessive neck rotation and flexion/extension intraoperatively may impede internal jugular vein drainage particularly from compression by the VP shunt catheter and internal jugular vein central line, leading to increased CSF pressure and cerebral edema.

   (c) I will provide 100% oxygen and assist ventilation via mask. If the patient remains sedated, develops hypertension and bradycardia, and the headache persists or progresses, I would consider reintubation and hyperventilation. If the condition does not improve, I would consider measuring VP shunt reservoir pressure and tapping the shunt. If there was no improvement, I would consider an emergency MRI to assess cerebral edema and/or compression of the posterior fossa contents.

General References

1. Geiger F, Parsch D, Carstens C (1999) Complications of scoliosis surgery in children with myelomeningocele. Eur Spine J 8:22–26
2. Lubicky JP, Spadaro JA, Yuan HA, Fredrickson BE, Henderson N (1989) Variability of somatosensory cortical evoked potential monitoring during spinal surgery. Spine 14:790–798
3. Mazon A, Nieto A, Pamies R, Felix R, Linana JJ, Lanuza A, Caballero L, Estornell F, Garcia-Ibarra F, Alvarez-Garijo JA (2005) Influence of the type of operations on the development of latex sensitization in children with myelomeningocele. J Pediatr Surg 40:688–692
4. Rendeli C, Nucera E, Ausili E, Tabacco F, Roncallo C, Pollastrini E, Scorzoni M, Schiavino D, Caldarelli M, Pietrini D, Patriarca G (2006) Latex sensitisation and allergy in children with myelomeningocele. Childs Nerv Syst 22:28–32
5. Ronchi CF, Antunes LC, Fioretto JR (2008) Respiratory muscular strength decrease in children with myelomeningocele. Spine 33:E73–E75
6. Suarez Delgado JM, Hernandez Soto R, Vilches Martin MJ, Romero RR, Vaz Calderon MA, Garcia Perla JL (1998) Anaesthetic considerations for myelomeningocele in neonates. Paediatr Anaesth 8:363–364

Chapter 5
Otolaryngology

A 3-year old previously healthy boy riding a tricycle on the sidewalk falls over the handlebar when the tricycle hits a pothole. He sustains an anterior neck injury and presents to the emergency room with stridor, aphonia, and a puffy neck. The ORL surgeons want to bring him to the OR urgently. He had eaten 2 h previously (full meal). Admission vital signs: BP 120/85, HR 130, RR 45/min, Hematocrit 35.

R.S. Holzman et al., *Pediatric Anesthesiology Review: Clinical Cases for Self-Assessment,*   199
DOI 10.1007/978-1-4419-1617-4_5, © Springer Science+Business Media, LLC 2010

Preoperative Evaluation

1. Why could this patient have stridor?

    (a) Is it important to differentiate inspiratory, expiratory, and biphasic stridor?
    (b) How will it influence your anesthetic management?
    (c) Why is he aphonic?
    (d) Is this of significance to your anesthetic plan?

2. What is the etiology of the puffy neck?

    (a) How would you go about evaluating it?
    (b) Of what importance is it to your plan?

3. What other injuries would you be concerned about?

    (a) How critical is it to rule out these other injuries?
    (b) Is this an urgent situation? An emergent situation? A life-threatening situation? Why?
    (c) Does this patient need a chest tube?
    (d) Does this patient need to be intubated in the emergency room? Why or why not?

Preoperative Evaluation

1. Stridor is the result of turbulent airflow produced by partial obstruction or narrowing of the airway, at the supraglottic, glottic, and infraglottic spaces, or combinations. Inspiratory stridor is characteristic of obstruction at the supraglottic or glottic larynx while expiratory stridor is characteristic of airway collapse in the infraglottic area. Biphasic stridor may reflect obstruction in both locations or tracheomalacia. The physical examination findings aid in anticipating the possible level of obstruction to be encountered as well as influencing the anesthetic technique, particularly with regard to controlled vs. spontaneous ventilation. He is likely aphonic because of acute vocal cord dysfunction such as vocal cord paralysis or impaired adduction ability of the vocal cords such as might occur from arytenoid dislocation.

2. The puffy neck may be due to soft tissue swelling from subcutaneous hematoma and tissue dissection or subcutaneous emphysema as a result of airway disruption; physical diagnosis and chest X-ray will confirm the diagnosis. Both will influence the anesthetic plan, particularly if the cause is subcutaneous emphysema from airway disruption, because positive pressure ventilation will make the problem worse.

3. Associated injuries could include head injury, facial injury, neck injury with cervical spine trauma, closed chest injury such as pulmonary or cardiac contusion, and blunt abdominal trauma. These associated injuries should be rapidly ruled out with physical examination and radiological studies including CT scan of the chest and abdomen if needed because the occult manifestations of these injuries such as elevated intracranial pressure, impairments of ventilation and gas exchange, and cardiac performance as well as occult bleeding may all worsen under anesthesia; other surgical services may have to be consulted. The airway situation is nevertheless a critical situation and examination of the airway for disruption must move along quickly because of the potentially life-threatening nature of the problem. If the patient has a minor pneumothorax, a chest tube prior to induction of anesthesia may not be necessary. Intubation in the emergency room in the absence of an anatomic airway diagnosis is hazardous because of the possibility of further disruption of the airway and worsening of the pneumothorax and subcutaneous emphysema.

Intraoperative Management

1. Does this patient need an arterial line? Why or why not?

   (a) Should he be monitored for myocardial ischemia? How would you do this? Which leads are most sensitive in a pediatric patient?
   (b) Does this patient need a precordial doppler? Why or why not? Where would you place it?
   (c) Would a TEE be more sensitive? Specific? Would you place one?

2. Should an NG tube be placed prior to induction?

   (a) What are the hazards of a full stomach in this setting?
   (b) Would you consider a rapid sequence induction?
   (c) Fiberoptic trans-nasal intubation?
   (d) Awake oral intubation? Why/why not?
   (e) What are the risks, advantages, and potential disadvantages of each?
   (f) Should cricoid pressure be used?
   (g) What are the risks of cricoid pressure in this setting?

Intraoperative Management

1. If the patient is not hemodynamically compromised in his current state and gas exchange is acceptable, then placement of an arterial line is not as important as moving along expeditiously with the surgery. Significant compromise of vital signs and gas exchange might warrant placement by additional personnel while the primary procedure, examination of the airway, is ongoing, or if it is anticipated that the patient will need airway support in the intensive care unit postoperatively. If there is physical or radiological evidence to support chest and myocardial contusion then monitoring for ischemia and arrhythmias should include two lead simultaneous monitoring such as II and V5. A precordial Doppler probe is not necessary for the anticipated procedure and a TEE is likely to interfere with the surgeon examining the airway. If there are questions of myocardial function then a transthoracic echo probe could be utilized.

2. There are several risks to placing an NG tube. First of all, if the trauma included a facial fracture there is always the possibility of a deep LeForte fracture, like a LeForte III, extending to the skull base; therefore, the NG tube could worsen that damage. Furthermore, there can be significant pharyngeal and laryngeal soft tissue damage from blind placement of the NG tube, and if the pathology is in the supraglottic or glottic larynx, the attempts at tube placement in this child may worsen such damage. These risks must obviously be weighed against the "full stomach" considerations inasmuch as the airway will not be "protected" prior to or during the examination. A rapid sequence induction of anesthesia, while one alternative, exposes the patient to the risk of nondiagnostic airway instrumentation with a laryngoscope and endotracheal tube. If the examination is to be complete and include the entire laryngeal apparatus, the endotracheal tube will have to be removed by the endoscopist anyway. The use of cricoid pressure, while justifiable for "full stomach" reasons, may likewise cause further damage if laryngeal structures are already damaged or disrupted, so it should be used with caution, if at all, and then only after consultation with the surgeon

3. Assume spontaneous inhalation induction, without cricoid pressure.

   (a) Stridor worsens with deepening of the anesthetic; continuous positive air-
       way pressure (CPAP) makes the stridor worse. What is the differential
       diagnosis?
   (b) Would a muscle relaxant help at this point? Succinylcholine?
   (c) Stridor worsens to the point where little gas exchange is occurring and the
       patient's saturations are in the low 90s. More CPAP seems to make it worse.
   (d) Would an emergency tracheostomy help? What about transtracheal jet ven-
       tilation? What are the hazards of each?
   (e) Laryngoscopy during light anesthesia reveals arytenoid dislocation with
       prolapse of the left arytenoid cartilage and fold into the laryngeal inlet.
       Then the patient develops laryngospasm. What would you do next?

4. Assume intubation is performed through the laryngeal inlet in this setting. Should
   the patient continue breathing spontaneously or be relaxed?

   (a) What are the hazards? Advantages?
   (b) Patient stops breathing spontaneously…you begin positive pressure ventila-
       tion; subcutaneous emphysema worsens, and profound hypotension occurs.
       Your differential? Treatment?.

Perioperative Care

1. After the arytenoid is reduced and the larynx fracture is repaired, when would
   you extubate the patient? What criteria would you use?

   (a) Should a tracheostomy be performed? What are the advantages?
       Disadvantages?
   (b) Should the patient remain intubated postop?
   (c) Breathing spontaneously, or mechanically ventilated? What are the advan-
       tages and disadvantages of both in this patient?

3. CPAP usually makes stridor better because it tends to pneumatically stent soft tissue obstruction, such as pharyngeal wall collapse during the induction of anesthesia. It may worsen upper airway obstruction if the cause is noncompliant solid tissue such as laryngeal tumor or arytenoid dislocation with prolapse into the larynx during inspiration. For these lesions, a muscle relaxant will not help and may actually worsen the airway obstruction because of relaxation of contiguous muscles and loss of adjacent airway support. The difficulty at this point is knowing what to do next, because all decisions now have to be based on the anatomy involved. I would proceed with a direct laryngoscopy and, while visualizing the larynx, use topical lidocaine (2%, with a volume limited to approximately 5 mg/kg) to spray the supraglottic larynx, vocal cords, and infraglottic structures. The endoscopist should have a rigid bronchoscope immediately available. Based on the anatomy identified, I would reapply the mask and wait for the topical to take effect while holding gentle positive pressure and maintaining spontaneous breathing, then have the endoscopist complete the balance of the airway exam prior to intubation either with the bronchoscope or an endotracheal tube and repositioning the dislocated arytenoid cartilage.

4. Even if the problem identified is the arytenoid cartilage dislocation, there is still an air leak causing the subcutaneous emphysema, so spontaneous respiration without the use of nitrous oxide should continue. If the patient stops breathing, then the gentlest positive pressure ventilation should be utilized, realizing that this strategy will probably worsen the subcutaneous emphysema and pneumothorax. In this circumstance, the patient may very well need a prophylactic chest tube. Other strategies that can be pursued include stimulating respiratory drive with the use of carbon dioxide through the breathing circuit or doxapram to shift the CO_2 response curve [1].

Perioperative Course

1. Because of the smaller airway diameter in children, airway edema impairs respiration much more than in adults. I would plan to keep the patient intubated for several days postoperatively. The strategy for extubation should be based on the recovery from airway edema following surgery; therefore, the development of an airway "leak" with positive pressure ventilation has been one criterion used. I would favor extubating in the operating room after the surgeon examines the airway. A tracheostomy may be required if several such attempts fail. Spontaneous breathing may continue, but distal airway collapse with prolonged spontaneous breathing through an endotracheal tube may occur, so pressure support ventilation is a better strategy if contemplated for any longer than a few hours.

2. You are called to the PACU 2 h postop because the patient has not moved his arms or legs since awakening.

    (a) Your differential diagnosis?

    (b) How would you evaluate?

    (c) Is there anything diagnostically or therapeutically to be done at this point?

3. You see the patient 3 days postop in the ICU; he has developed a high fever, looks septic, and has radiographic signs of a mediastinitis…why?

Additional Questions

1. What is the CHARGE Association?

    (a) Of what importance is choanal atresia in the first week of life?

    (b) What special considerations are there for the surgical correction?

    (c) Are there specific anesthetic implications?

2. Of course, you should make sure that the patient is able to hear you, understand your question, and is strong enough to follow your command, i.e., recovered reasonably well from the effects of general anesthesia with neuromuscular blockade. Assuming all this is true and you do not have to administer reversal agents such as naloxone, flumazenil, or neostigmine, then the most worrisome possibility is impairment at the level of the cervical or thoracic spinal cord such as hematoma or spinal cord trauma or ischemia. If the patient is clearly capable of following commands but cannot do so because of obvious motor impairment, immediate diagnostic evaluation by MRI is warranted with the possibility of further spinal cord exploration and decompression surgically if needed. Throughout this time, attention to the adequacy of ventilation and oxygenation is critical because of secondary edema and inflammation possibly extending the effect of the initial lesion.

3. An esophageal perforation as a result of the shock wave could have occurred at the time of the initial injury. This may be treated medically with antibiotics, may require drainage in the operating room, and/or continued support in the ICU with intubation.

Additional Questions

1. The CHARGE association is an acronym that stands for colobomas of the eye, heart disease, atresia of the choanae, retarded growth, genital anomalies, and ear anomalies. Because these anomalies occur early in embryological development, there can be varying stages of severity for each, along with impairments of development of other contiguous structures such as the branchial arches and occipital somites. It is therefore not uncommon to have a short neck, short mandible, small mouth, clefting of the lip or palate, a range of cardiac anomaly severity, and failure to thrive. In the newborn period, severe respiratory distress may occur which cannot be relieved by a nasal airway. Likewise, nasogastric intubation for decompression or feeding may not be possible.

2. A 12-year-old boy presents with a growth in the nasopharynx and is scheduled for biopsy.

   (a) What concerns do you have?
   (b) Of what significance is the diagnosis of juvenile nasal angiofibroma?
   (c) What implications does it have for anesthetic management?
   (d) Is it important to know about the extent of this tumor prior to anesthesia? Why?
   (e) What implications does it have for management?
   (f) The patient will first be scheduled for coil embolization under anesthesia in the interventional radiology suite. How will your anesthetic management be influenced for this procedure?
   (g) How should the CO_2 be controlled?
   (h) Is there an optimal choice of anesthetic agents?
   (i) Should the patient be managed with controlled hypotension? Why/why not?

3. A 15-year old is scheduled for incision and drainage of a peritonsillar abscess; she has trismus and is frightened.

   (a) What are your considerations for anesthetic induction?
   (b) Should this patient undergo an awake intubation?
   (c) Rapid sequence induction?
   (d) Should she receive a muscle relaxant?
   (e) What about an awake trans-nasal fiberoptic intubation?
   (f) How is this situation different from a Ludwig's Angina patient?

2. Most childhood tumors in the nasopharynx are benign, but can have significant consequences nevertheless. Encephaloceles, dermoids, and benign teratomas can occur as congenital remnants, in which case they present at an early age with airway obstruction, or more insidiously in older patients. The juvenile nasal angiofibroma is the most aggressive of these benign tumors presenting in early adolescence, usually in boys. They extend locally into the surrounding nasopharyngeal tissue and cranially through the skull base. They are typically evaluated radiologically by CT scan, magnetic resonance angiography (MRA), and/or angiogram and at the same time, embolized to reduce the vascularity for subsequent surgical resection. Because transit time in vascular areas is related to volume, pressure, and pH, all three can be positively influenced by the anesthetic technique. For placement of embolization devices, increased volume, normal to slightly higher than normal blood pressure, and moderate controlled hypercarbia may facilitate coil placement. For the surgical procedure, this physiology should be reversed, so that bleeding may be decreased through the use of controlled hypotension, volume reduction, and positive pressure-controlled hyperventilation

3. This is a very typical presentation – an older pediatric patient with a sore throat, difficulty swallowing, often sick for a few days, and occasionally, voice changes with difficulty talking. She may even have some mild respiratory distress. Although the majority will have been treated successfully with antibiotics, those coming to surgery have usually failed such therapy. Most patients will have had CT scans of their upper airway preoperatively, and therefore the extent of the peritonsillar abscess is easy to evaluate. Trismus is difficult to evaluate with regard to predicting the ease of direct laryngoscopy and endotracheal intubation. It is typically relieved following induction with a hypnotic agent and the use of a muscle relaxant unless the inflammation and edema have been progressive over several days. Assuming that the clinical exam and radiological evaluation do not suggest anatomic difficulties with a rapid sequence induction of anesthesia, direct laryngoscopy, and intubation of the trachea, this would be the optimal choice. Secondary choices include topical anesthesia, sedation, and an awake "look" or placement of an endotracheal tube; however, the risks of patient discomfort, coughing, and potential disruption of the abscess may outweigh the benefit. An alternative would be the maintenance of spontaneous ventilation either following intravenous induction with a hypnotic agent or mask induction with a volatile agent. A transnasal fiberoptic intubation would be very hazardous because the peritonsillar abscess often extends into the upper pole of the tonsillar bed, right at the junction of the soft palate, and instrumentation of the soft tissue in the area could be a significant risk for abscess disruption.

4. A 5-year-old Haitian girl who speaks only French is scheduled for partial reduction glossectomy for cystic hygroma.

   (a) How will you evaluate her?
   (b) Her tongue protrudes 7 in. beyond her mouth, and the distal 3 in. are dessicated and macerated. How will you begin your induction sequence?
   (c) Is it likely that you will be successful at orally intubating her?
   (d) Nasally intubating her?
   (e) How would you preoxygenate?
   (f) What are your postoperative considerations?

5. Differentiate epiglottitis, croup, and bacterial tracheitis.

   (a) What difference does it make to your anesthetic management to consider these as different entities?

4. There are several important features here; first of all, the inability to provide positive pressure ventilation or even supplemental oxygenation by mask is most influential on the anesthetic plan. Second, the patient does not speak English and therefore will have a more difficult time cooperating with an anesthetic plan that involves sedation, topicalization, and awake intubation. Her ability to cooperate must be carefully assessed with the aid of a translator in the presence of the parents who can help to explain what the anesthesiologist will be doing. An IV should be established first to provide sedation to the point of arouseable somnolence. A variety of medications can be used for this purpose, but a combination of midazolam and fentanyl would probably be my choice. Topical anesthesia can be provided by lidocaine (a 2% concentration in this age group should be enough) to the level of the laryngeal inlet. Depending on the choice made, direct laryngoscopy or fiberoptic laryngoscopy (transnasal or transoral) can be accomplished. Supplemental oxygen can be delivered by an assistant while asking the patient to take deep breaths. Postoperatively, depending on the duration and extent of the surgery, she may have swelling that would make nasal reintubation more comfortable for the patient and more secure for her ICU stay.

5. Epiglottitis refers to the acute bacterial infection of the supraglottic larynx that had historically been caused by Hemophilus influenza type B. The typical clinical appearance is the sudden onset of fever and airway distress in the absence of a URI in a toxic-appearing young child (typically 2–5 years old). They are often sitting, rather than recumbent, because they can breathe more easily. Radiographically, they typically have a thumb sign of the epiglottis. Croup, or laryngotracheobronchitis, is typically more gradual in its onset, preceded by several days of URI-like symptoms, and usually caused by URI-related organisms such as parainfluenza. Many patients have a typical "barking" cough with or without stridor while others can have significant upper airway obstruction. Biphasic stridor supports the diagnosis of laryngotracheobronchitis. The age group is somewhat younger, usually 6 months–3 years of age. Radiographically, a "steeple" sign is present in the subglottis. Bacterial tracheitis may present with fever, stridor, voice change with a brassy quality, and a toxic appearance. The trachea usually has purulent debris, crusting, ulceration, and membranes that may require removal. A range of gram positive and gram negative organisms are often the culprits. These patients often need to be supported with endotracheal intubation and perioperative intensive care. It is important to differentiate the disorders because airway support is often necessary for epiglottitis and bacterial tracheitis while airway instrumentation and endotracheal intubation should usually be avoided for croup.

6. How does a laryngeal cleft occur embryologically?

   (a) What are the implications for airway management?
   (b) Should these patients receive a tracheostomy in the newborn period? Why/
       why not?

7. What are your considerations for using jet ventilation as part of your management of the airway during laser surgery for juvenile laryngeal papillomatosis?

8. You are called into a colleague's room because the laser aperture was accidentally left open and the laser fired on a polyvinylchloride endotracheal tube that
   remained in place just prior to extubation and after the suspension laryngoscope
   was placed; the patient has flames and smoke in the tube and singed lips. Your
   colleague's sleeve has caught fire, and he is preoccupied with that. What do you
   do next?

6. Failure of complete separation of the primitive foregut into the trachea and esophagus can result in varying degrees of residual communication between the two. It can be as subtle as a small communication between the arytenoid cartilages indicating incomplete formation of the interarytenoid muscle or complete communication at the cranial portion of the larynx and upper third of the trachea, making them functionally one tube. These infants have an abundance of pharyngeal secretions, recurrent aspiration pneumonias, choking episodes, and respiratory distress, typically associated with attempts at feeding. A significant portion also have tracheoesophageal fistulas. A tracheostomy may be ineffective in establishing an airway because of the tendency for the tracheostomy tube to pass through the posterior wall of the trachea into the esophagus. It is usually better to attempt a primary closure of the mucosa separating the trachea and esophagus through suspension laryngoscopy while maintaining endotracheal intubation. The alternative, open repair and separation of the trachea and esophagus, is often fraught with hazards of perioperative tissue breakdown and formation of fistulous communications [2].

7. Jet ventilation [3] accomplishes several things that intubation with a metal tube or foil-wrapped tube cannot. First of all, it provides unimpaired access to the airway and complete visualization for the surgeon. Second, it decreases the risk of fire by not having any combustible material within the airway at all. The hazards are several: there is a risk of barotrauma and dissection of tracheal, pretracheal, or pharyngeal tissue if the driving pressure of the jet is too high, and for that reason, a pressure/compliance curve is an optimal strategy, where the amount of driving pressure is just enough to ventilate the patient, assessed by using chest wall movement and/or breath sounds as an endpoint for adequate ventilation. The airway is unsecured, and therefore, debris and smoke can be "jetted" into the unprotected airway, so efforts at ventilation should be made in concert with the surgeon's laser resection.

8. The colleague will probably be adequately cared for by the OR personnel, who likely know how to handle this straightforward situation. The airway situation is more complicated because it is less frequently encountered. Working in conjunction with the surgeon, ventilation of the lungs has to be discontinued and all anesthetic gases including oxygen have to be discontinued as well. The flames should be extinguished with saline, and the endotracheal tube removed. All of these steps should take place virtually simultaneously. At that point, the patient's lungs should be ventilated by mask, and the surgeon should prepare to evaluate the trachea endoscopically for damage and burns. Depending on the degree of burn and damage, endotracheal intubation and perioperative mechanical ventilation may be required.

Specific References

1. Yost C (2006) A new look at the respiratory stimulant doxapram. CNS Drug Rev 12:236–249
2. Fernández A (2003) Anaesthetic management in a case of a type IV laryngotracheo-oesopha-geal cleft. Paediatr Anaesth 13:270–273
3. Sosis M (1997) Anesthesia for airway laser surgery. In: Sosis M (ed) Anesthesia equipment manual. Lippincott-Raven, Philadelphia, pp 279–291

General References

4. Holzman R (1994) Pediatric critical incidents. In: Gaba D, Howard S, Fish K (eds) Crisis man-agement in anesthesiology. Churchill-Livingstone, New York, pp 267–290
5. Holzman R (1998) Prevention and treatment of life-threatening pediatric anesthesia emergen-cies. Semin Anesth Perioperat Med Pain 17:154–163
6. Holzman R (2000) Anesthesia in the child and adolescent. In: Wetmore R, Muntz H, McGill T (eds) Pediatric otolaryngology: principles and practice pathways. Thieme Medical Publishers, New York, pp 31–47

Chapter 6
Head and Neck

A 1-year-old, 9-kg boy is scheduled for repair of orbital hypertelorism for Apert's syndrome. He appears congested but afebrile, with a blood pressure of 92/55 mmHg, pulse 120 bpm, respiration 32/min, and temperature 37°C. Hematocrit is 33%. He is on no medications, and his parents report that he is terribly afraid of doctors after coming to the craniofacial clinic so often. He has never had any previous surgery.

R.S. Holzman et al., *Pediatric Anesthesiology Review: Clinical Cases for Self-Assessment,*
DOI 10.1007/978-1-4419-1617-4_6, © Springer Science+Business Media, LLC 2010

Preoperative Evaluation

1. Will this patient have a difficult airway? In what way?

   (a) What can you do to figure this out ahead of time?
   (b) Should a fiberoptic bronchoscope be ready?
   (c) How does Apert's syndrome develop?
   (d) Does this patient have proptosis?

2. Is this a plastic surgery or neurosurgery operation? Why?

3. What difficulties, if any, would you anticipate with access for this patient? Why?

Preoperative Evaluation

1. That depends on what you mean by a difficult airway. The midface is hypoplastic, the eyes appear to be proptotic, although that is more a reflection of the hypoplastic midface and orbits but normal size eyes. The hypoplastic skull base contributes to abnormal development of the sphenoid, frontal, and maxillary sinuses, which in turn often lead to an appearance of chronic congestion, simply because sinus and nasal drainage is impaired. The branchial arches, however, are typically not affected, so that mandibular development proceeds normally. The combination often results in chronic upper airway congestion, moderately difficult fit for a mask, but relatively easy laryngoscopy and intubation [1]. Originally thought to be due to premature closure of the coronal suture, the defect is more complicated because abnormal fibroblastic growth occurs in various areas of the membranous and cartilaginous neurocranium (skull base), accounting for the abnormal shape of the head as well as the midface hypoplasia [2].

2. This again depends on how you look at it. The morphological defect is craniofacial, the etiology of which are fibroblast abnormalities in the deep and superficial cranium and their contiguous structures. The surgical approach is a bifrontal craniotomy with multiple osteotomies and (hopefully) preservation of an intact dura. There can, however, be neurosurgical consequences if there is a dural puncture, or even with the prolonged reconstructive surgery, dural exposure, and large blood loss and fluid shifting that occurs. Many of the patients have elevated intracranial pressure as a result of their cranial dysmorphism as well as CNS developmental abnormalities such as agenesis of the corpus callosum. Early intervention with ventricular shunting is common.

3. Polysyndactyly of the hands and feet is common, and therefore, intravenous access may be difficult.

Intraoperative Course

1. What monitors will you choose? Why?

   (a) Does this patient need an arterial line? Why?
   (b) What are the risks of central line placement in this patient? Would you insert one? Why?
   (c) How would you precisely localize the placement of a central line for air aspiration? Are there any other ways?
   (d) Does this patient need a precordial doppler? Why?
   (e) Would a transesophageal echo be better? Why/why not?

2. What are your considerations for anesthetic induction? Why?

   (a) Your colleague stops by and suggests an awake intubation? What do you think?
   (b) You select an intramuscular preinduction technique in the preop holding area with ketamine because of the extreme separation anxiety, and the patient obstructs within 30 s in the mother's arms and begins to turn blue. What do you do next?
   (c) Will an oral airway help?
   (d) Is this patient a difficult intubation?
   (e) Should you continue with the case?

Intraoperative Course

1. Because of the typical age of repair, the insidious blood loss, and multiple osteo-tomies in the cranial vault and other bones above the level of the right atrium, secure IV access anticipating large volume transfusion, intra-arterial access for volume assessment, blood sampling and postoperative care as well as monitoring for venous air embolism is essential for these cases. At least two relatively large bore (for age) IVs should be established, as well as an arterial line and a precordial Doppler. Central venous access should be considered if adequate peripheral vein access could not be found. If the intention is to potentially use the central line for air evacuation following venous air embolism, then a multiorificed catheter would be more effective; however, early detection prior to any cardiovascular compro-mise is more important than central venous access to treat the consequences of venous air embolism. Precise localization of the tip of the catheter can be accom-plished by (1) chest X-ray confirmation (2) use of a saline-filled catheter as an intracardiac electrode and confirmation with large biphasic P waves on ECG (3) use of transesophageal echocardiography (TEE). A precordial Doppler should still be used because of its sensitivity and noninvasive nature. A TEE, while also sensi-tive and specific, is more invasive and requires more attention for interpretation.

2. Considerations for anesthetic induction include the patient and family's emo-tional state – the patient is fearful because of multiple visits to the clinic as well as "stranger anxiety" typical for this age, the parents are fearful as well because they know this is a big operation with significant morbidity. There is also the larger context of the uncertainties of the family with a chronically ill, syndromic child. While there may be advantages to a parent present induction in the operat-ing room such as decreased crying and decreased aerophagia, thereby lowering the risk of intragastric air and regurgitation, these advantages may be outweighed by the relatively minimal chance that this infant will be consoled by a parent's presence, the likely difficulty with the mask fit because of the midface hypopla-sia and the presence of impaired secretion elimination because of the sinus abnormalities with the strong possibility of airway irritability, laryngospasm, or bronchospasm on induction. If intramuscular ketamine were selected to be administered in the preop holding area, it would not be surprising that the crying from the pain of the injection along with the increased salivation and impaired drainage from the underlying anatomic abnormality as well as the effect of ket-amine would result in breath-holding and laryngospasm. The patient would become cyanotic rapidly because of his age. Positive pressure ventilation could be attempted if he was apneic, or CPAP applied if he was making respiratory efforts, but a mask fit might be difficult under this circumstance, which might lead to the requirement for muscle relaxation (succinylcholine plus atropine IM, laryngoscopy, and endotracheal intubation in the holding area). An oral airway might help, but if the obstruction is at the level of the vocal cords, it might not. Assuming that intubation solved the previous airway issues, then it would be reasonable to proceed with the case

3. What will be your primary anesthetic technique? Why?

    (a) Will you use nitrous oxide? Why/why not?
    (b) What is your choice of muscle relaxant, if any? Why?

4. During surgery, the patient suddenly develops a drop in blood pressure, brady-cardia, and a drop in end-tidal CO_2.

    (a) What is your differential diagnosis?
    (b) How can you go about narrowing the possibilities?
    (c) What would you do? Why?
    (d) Blood pressure is 60/40 with a heart rate of 60; how would you manage his depth of anesthesia? Why?

Postoperative Course

1. Would you leave this patient intubated? Why/why not?

    (a) What criteria will you use to decide about extubation? Why?
    (b) At the end of the procedure, during planned extubation, the desaturation recurs while the patient is struggling, bearing down, and breath-holding. Your management? Why?

2. You are called urgently to the ICU 6 h postop; the patient has pulled out all of his IVs and A-line.

    (a) Where will you attempt his vascular access? Why? (remember he has polysyndactyly)

3. A balanced technique with fentanyl/air/oxygen and isoflurane would be my choice. Nitrous oxide should be avoided because of the risk of venous air embolism and also because body cavities will be opened and subsequently closed. Muscle relaxation can be accomplished with pancuronium because the procedure will be long in duration and pancuronium acts favorably as far as preservation of heart rate and blood pressure in infants. It is also less expensive than other nondepolarizing neuromuscular blocking agents.

4. Decreased blood pressure and a drop in end-tidal CO_2 suggest a decrease in perfusion and blood volume delivery to the systemic as well as pulmonary circulation. The accompanying bradycardia, however, is ominous for inadequate myocardial perfusion/cardiac ischemia and a process more immediately threatening than acute volume depletion, so included in the diagnosis must be significant venous air embolism. The Doppler will help to confirm the diagnosis with a characteristic "chirping" and whooshing sound; if a central venous line is present, air may be aspirated from it, simultaneous with asking the surgeons to flood the operative field, turning off the volatile agent in the setting of the hypotension and bradycardia, the administration of atropine and/or epinephrine with volume, and changing the patient position, if possible, to head-down or head-down and left lateral decubitus, to trap the entrained air into the apex of the right ventricle and not cause an air lock in the pulmonary circulation. CPR might actually be therapeutic with regard to breaking up larger air pockets into smaller ones until the intravascular air clears the pulmonary circulation.

Postoperative Course

1. There are good reasons for extubating as well as good reasons for leaving the patient intubated. It will be easier for assessment of neurological status if the patient can be extubated and it will result in less tracheal trauma. On the other hand, the airway will probably be more stable in this patient with a congenitally abnormal face, for whom a mask fit would be difficult and postoperative supplemental oxygen would be hard to administer. The patient could be kept sedated to minimize movement and coughing. Much would also depend on the volume received intraoperatively; a significant amount of facial puffiness might suggest tracheal edema that would require the overnight availability of an anesthesiologist.

2. This situation makes the patient very vulnerable and an IV should be quickly restarted. The difficulty is that with polysyndactyly, there is usually poor venous access. Nevertheless, alternate sites may have to be chosen, such as femoral or subclavian; internal jugular would probably prove to be more difficult because of the positioning of the head and neck required. Arterial access may be easier to establish in the extremities, but the femoral artery or axillary artery should be kept in mind as alternate sites.

Additional Questions

1. What is Goldenhar's syndrome?

   (a) How does it develop?
   (b) What are the anesthetic considerations?
   (c) Are there particularly significant associated anomalies?
   (d) Do these patients tend to get easier to take care of over time?

2. A 5-year old was hit by a car while riding his bike, and sustained an over-the-handlebar fall into the pavement, suffering a LeForte I fracture, mandibular fracture, a Colle's fracture, and various bumps and bruises. He comes to the operating room in a soft collar in preparation for oral surgery to repair his facial trauma.

   (a) Your considerations for anesthetic induction? Maintenance?
   (b) What are your considerations for anesthetic emergence?
   (c) How will you wake him up? (wired, blood in stomach, antiemetic, coughing, extubate?)

Additional Questions

1. Goldenhar's syndrome is the eponym for hemifacial microsomia, an anomaly characterized by variable hypoplasia of the mandibular division of the first branchial arch, including the mandibular ramus, body and temporomandibular joint, hypoplasia of soft tissue components of the face and jaw, and hypoplasia of the facial nerve [3]. The more severe forms are typically very difficult intubations because of the inability for the jaw to move, and breathing through a natural airway (and therefore support through a mask airway) may be difficult because of a small pharynx. Because this anomaly occurs early in embryological life during branchial arch formation, anomalies of other contiguous areas are not uncommon, including fusion of occipital somites that can give rise to the Klippel–Feil anomaly of cervical vertebral fusion, cardiac defects such as atrial and ventricular septal defects, and cleft palate. Anomalies of the first branchial cleft such as low set, misshapen ears, and sensorineural hearing loss are common as well.

2. You have to be concerned as much about what you do not see as what you do see; the fact that he has multiple facial fractures and therefore the potential for airway trauma or difficult laryngoscopy and intubation may be the tip of the iceberg; he may also have chest and cardiac contusions, blunt abdominal trauma, closed head injury, and a period of unconsciousness and altered sensorium with or without concussion. All of these are less obvious in physical exam and therefore must be suspected and inquired about during the history, with any additional appropriate laboratory tests. Assuming that these other issues have been ruled out, then the amount of bleeding, soft tissue injury with swelling, bony injury, and trismus will affect the ease of induction, mask fit, and intubation. A 5-year old will not likely tolerate an awake laryngoscopy and intubation, so a decision will need to be made about the amount of trismus present that is likely to be relieved with the induction of anesthesia (and therefore facilitate intubation) vs. the amount of soft tissue swelling and/or bony injury that may make laryngoscopy and exposure difficult. Radiological evaluation may be very helpful in this regard, especially if stridor is present. It is important to discuss the extent of the repair, as it is likely that a nasal intubation will be necessary if internal maxillary fixation is to be applied. Emergence considerations are important as well; coughing, bucking, and valsalva maneuvers should be avoided and in general, a smooth wake up is best. It may be well advised to keep the patient intubated for several days until soft tissue swelling decreases and an air leak is reestablished. Extubation may be accomplished in the intensive care unit or in the operating room

3. What is the developmental history of a cleft lip and palate?

    (a) What associated anomalies should you expect?
    (b) Are there other associations of cleft palate with craniofacial deformities?
    (c) How can you assess the potential for intubation difficulty?
    (d) Would you use a muscle relaxant as part of your anesthetic technique?
    (e) Narcotics?
    (f) Why does a cleft palate develop with Pierre–Robin syndrome?

4. A 9-month old is scheduled for exploration of the posterior triangle of the neck for a large right-sided cystic hygroma that is half the size of his face.

    (a) What are your anesthetic considerations?
    (b) Are these patients difficult to intubate? Under what circumstances?
    (c) Why does the surgeon want to do a posterior triangle exploration?
    (d) He asks you to leave the right arm free of IVs in case he has to do an axillary exploration…why would he ask that?

5. You are evaluating a patient with the Klippel–Feil syndrome.

    (a) What are your anesthetic considerations?
    (b) How does this syndrome happen?
    (c) Are there other congenital anomalies associated with it?

3. Typical cleft lip formation occurs along a line joining the primary and secondary palates through the middle of the ipsilateral ala. Clefting of the primary and/or secondary palate may also occur in continuity with a cleft lip. Clefting of the soft palate may also occur, because palatal fusion occurs progressively from anterior to posterior portions of the palate. There may be associated anomalies of structures or organ systems that are developing at the same time as the midface and palate, such as the heart and occipital somites. A cleft palate may also occur in association with glossoptosis (Pierre–Robin Sequence), in which case it is more properly considered a deformation by interference with the progressive midline fusion of the maxillary shelves. A paramedian palatal cleft can occur with branchial arch abnormalities such as hemifacial microsomia (Goldenhar's syndrome) [3]. It is important to carefully evaluate any association with branchial arch abnormalities because of the potential for difficult laryngoscopy and intubation. The use of any specific anesthetic technique should be directed to the desired end-point of the surgery as well as any anticipated difficulty with extubation. These patients will occasionally have significant obstructive or mixed sleep apnea; attention to perioperative monitoring for apnea and hypoxia is probably more important than any particular anesthetic technique.

4. "Cystic hygromas," more properly known as lymphangiomas, typically present in this area of the head and neck as lobular, multiloculated collections of cysts and lymphatic vessels filled with clear or serous fluid. There are a variety of often bewildering and challenging presentations because while most arise in the posterior triangle of the neck in continuity with the fascia of the collis longi muscle, they may extend into the axilla, the anterior triangle of the neck, and intraorally. In addition, bleeding may occur into the cysts, forming clot and therefore hard, extrinsically compressive masses to the oral cavity and therefore the airway. The airway may therefore be difficult to visualize in these patients and each should be looked at individually for the potential for difficult mask fit, visualization, and tracheal intubation.

5. The Klippel–Feil syndrome is the result of varying degrees of fusion of occipital somites resulting in fused cervical vertebrae. It is often associated with other vertebral anomalies such as hemivertebrae, spondylolisthesis or scoliosis, congenital heart disease, and branchial arch abnormalities, again because these structures develop at about the same stage of embryological life. Often a clinical tip to cervical vertebral anomalies is a low-set ear, neck webbing, and a low hairline at the neck. Laryngoscopy and visualization of the airway may be difficult and fiberoptic intubation is frequently necessary.

Specific References

1. Nargozian C (2004) The airway in patients with craniofacial abnormalities. Paediatr Anaesth 14:53–59
2. Holzman R (1998) Anatomy and embryology of the pediatric airway. In: R J (ed) The difficult pediatric airway. W.B. Saunders Co. Ltd, Philadelphia, pp 707–727
3. Holzman R (1992) The child with Goldenhar syndrome for cleft lip repair. In: Linda S (ed) Common problems in pediatric anesthesia. Mosby Year Book, St. Louis, pp 99–106

Chapter 7
Ophthalmology

A 2-year-old, 8.5-kg girl is scheduled for bilateral rectus recession. She was born at 34 weeks, required some supplemental oxygen for a few days but not intubation or mechanical ventilation, and went home with an apnea monitor for a month that "never alarmed" according to the parents. Her vital signs are blood pressure of 92/55, P 120, R 32, and T 37°C. Hematocrit is 32. She is on phospholine iodide for treatment of her variable strabismus. She has never had any previous surgery.

R.S. Holzman et al., *Pediatric Anesthesiology Review: Clinical Cases for Self-Assessment,*
DOI 10.1007/978-1-4419-1617-4_7, © Springer Science+Business Media, LLC 2010

Preoperative Evaluation

1. What are the problems with the medication this patient is on? Why?

   (a) Are there medications you would avoid?
   (b) Would you avoid succinylcholine anyway?
   (c) Are there any medications you would advise the surgeon to avoid?

2. Of what significance is the early history of prematurity? Why?

   (a) Do you still anticipate problems?
   (b) Should this patient have a retinal exam preoperatively for ROP? Why/Why not?
   (c) Is the concentration of inspired oxygen a concern in your anesthetic plan?
   (d) Should this patient receive narcotics?

3. Is this patient at greater risk for the development of malignant hyperthermia? Why/Why not?

   (a) How can you further determine this?
   (b) Should the patient have a muscle biopsy?
   (c) Would you use a clean technique? Why/Why not?

Preoperative Evaluation

1. As an anticholinesterase, echothiophate iodide (phospholine iodide) is used to nonspecifically increase the contractile state of extraocular muscles in an effort to "medically" rebalance the squint. An anticholinesterase administered in this manner may also delay the metabolism of ester local anesthetics and prolong the effect of depolarizing neuromuscular blocking agents. It may shorten the duration of nondepolarizing agents, resulting in an increased dose administered to achieve a desired effect. It will also increase intraocular pressure in patients with closed angle glaucoma. The duration of its effect in chronically treated patients may last for weeks. Its main purpose currently is to produce miosis and reduce the intraocular pressure of patients with open angle glaucoma [1].

2. She is quite small for her age, so the first thing to be concerned about is failure to thrive; an average 2-year old should weigh about 12 kg. If she is simply small for her age and has been consistently at the lower end of the growth curve, then reassurance from the pediatrician along with an adequate nutritional history would probably suffice, but it is very possible that with poor intake, she may be anemic, immunodeficient, and have other issues that require further medical consultation. She may have retinopathy of prematurity, which has been associated with a history of supplemental oxygen therapy in prematures and many other neonatal factors as well; however, the index of suspicion for severe retinopathy is probably low, because the treatment was of short duration. Nevertheless, it would be reasonable for the ophthalmologist to do a quick exam just to answer the question about the appearance of the fundus so that it can be documented, and it is likely that with this history an exam would have been done anyway. It would not dissuade me from delivering a routine anesthetic consisting of an F_iO_2 of 0.3–0.4 following 100% oxygen prior to intubation. Likewise, I would not be concerned about a significant risk of respiratory depression with judicious amounts of opioids, with this history of 2 years of age in an otherwise asymptomatic ex-34 weeker.

3. Malignant hyperthermia has been associated in the past with strabisms, principally through case reports in the ophthalmology literature, although a higher than background rate (fourfold higher) association with masseter muscle spasm has been described in strabismus patients who underwent anesthetic induction with halothane and succinylcholine. The association between masseter muscle spasm and the subsequent development of malignant hyperthermia remains unclear. I would proceed, therefore, with a routine inhalation induction but nevertheless try to avoid succinylcholine for the more typical reason of its higher incidence of masseter muscle spasm and other possible adverse effects such as rhabdomyolysis or hyperkalemia in children. In addition, many ophthalmologists prefer not to have the sustained extraocular muscle contracture, produced as a side effect of succinylcholine, influence their measurements for the procedure.

Intraoperative Course

1. What monitors will you choose? Why?

    (a) Does this patient need an end-tidal CO_2 monitor? Why/Why not?
    (b) Would you use an agent analyzer? How would agent analysis be of specific help?

2. What are your considerations for anesthetic induction? Why?

    (a) Your colleague stops by and suggests pretreating with an anticholinergic? What do you think? Should this patient have been premedicated with an anticholinergic an hour earlier?
    (b) Is intravenous administration during induction more or less effective for prevention of the oculocardiac reflex? Why/Why not?

Intraoperative Course

1. Monitors should include all routine noninvasive monitors, end-tidal CO_2 monitoring as well as specific agent analysis. An agent analyzer identifies the specific agent utilized, and in addition, will identify combined agents if, for example, sevoflurane is used for induction of anesthesia but changed over to isoflurane for maintenance.

2. My principal consideration for this child, who is certainly small for her age but in reasonable health according to her vital signs and hematocrit, is her separation/preoperative anxiety. This can be dealt with by anxiolytic premedication with or without a parent-present induction. The premedication is more likely to be anxiolytic than the presence of the parent, although there is much variation. Moreover, many parents wish to be present for a variety of reasons beyond "reassurance," such as curiosity and education, and these may be very reasonable because ultimately satisfying these needs will inform future decisions, and may be helpful for siblings as well. However, parents should not feel compelled to go into the operating room or participate in the parent-present induction if they do not wish to do so. Many in the past have felt that an anticholinergic premedication in the setting of strabismus surgery is required to decrease the incidence of the oculocardiac reflex. When working with experienced surgeons, the bradycardia of the oculocardiac reflex is most rapidly treated by asking the surgeon to stop the traction on the extraocular muscle. If an anticholinergic is needed to treat the bradycardia, it can be administered intravenously at that time. Most patients, however, do not experience the bradycardia of the oculocardiac reflex in the hands of a skilled surgeon, so their routine exposure to an anticholinergic is not necessary.

3. Is a muscle relaxant necessary for this case? Why?

    (a) What is your choice of muscle relaxant? Why?

    (b) Will you use nitrous oxide? Why/why not?

    (c) Should this patient routinely receive antiemetics? What is your choice? Why?

    (d) What are the disadvantages of metoclopramide in a child compared with an adult?

    (e) Is total intravenous anesthesia with propofol a real advantage?

    (f) Would ondansetron be of any greater benefit?

    (g) How does ondansetron work?

3. A muscle relaxant is not necessary for this case, as long as the patient is well anesthetized and motionless. Movement under the microscope will be magnified, and there is the possibility of significant compromise of the surgical procedure and injury to the patient. Surgeons often have a preference for operating with or without the administration of a neuromuscular blocking agent and will often make that part of their preoperative discussion with the anesthesiologist. The most important thing, however, is consistency of anesthetic technique with regard to the surgeons' caliper measurements for muscle resection and recession. The choice of muscle relaxant will depend on the anticipated length of the surgery (i.e., the number of muscles). Pancuronium, with its associated tachycardia, may be a very reasonable choice for this particular procedure. Neuromuscular blockade should be monitored carefully because of the echothiophate treatment. I would use nitrous oxide as part of the anesthetic technique, with only a minor concern about its possible contribution to perioperative nausea and vomiting (PONV), which is likely to occur in any event with this patient because of the association of PONV with strabismus surgery. Prophylactic antiemetic administration is very reasonable given the high association of strabismus surgery with PONV. For years, droperidol was routinely administered to strabismus surgery patients, but now there is concern about its effect on cardiac conduction and its possible contribution to Torsades, an extremely rare event which nevertheless resulted in a "Black Box" warning from the FDA which effectively stopped the use of droperidol as an antiemetic. Other antiemetics include ondansetron, a selective 5-HT3-receptor antagonist which blocks serotonin, both peripherally on vagus nerve terminals and centrally in the chemoreceptor trigger zone. Metoclopramide can also be used, but is associated with a higher incidence of tardive dyskinesia in children than in adults, although these are typically in larger dose ranges than those administered by anesthesiologists. Propofol-based TIVA may have some advantages in that it has an antiemetic effect and would also allow avoidance of the use of potent inhalation anesthetic agents. Its antiemetic effect, however, may be of questionable duration into the postoperative period, so a more sustainable strategy might involve the use of ondansetron, dexamethasone, and possibly metoclopramide.

4. During surgery, the patient suddenly develops a drop in heart rate from 110 to 54 beats/min.

    (a) What is your differential diagnosis?

    (b) How can you go about treating? What would you do? Why?

    (c) Why does this happen?

    (d) What is the specific pathway of this reflex?

    (e) Does greater anesthetic depth block this reflex?

    (f) What is a traction test? What is a duction test?

    (g) Blood pressure is cycling continuously on the automated blood pressure cuff and there is no reading; the heart rate is 24 beats/min and the surgeon has backed way off; how would you proceed? Why?

Postoperative Course

1. What are the advantages of a deep extubation?

    (a) Would you choose this method? Why/why not?

    (b) What are the risks of a Valsalva maneuver in this patient?

    (c) What if she had just undergone an open globe procedure?

4. The most likely cause of this bradycardia is the oculocardiac reflex, mediated in its afferent limb by the long and short ciliary nerves, synapsing in the ciliary ganglion and traveling through the ophthalmic division of the trigeminal nerve. The efferent limb travels from the motor nucleus of the vagus nerve through the peripheral portion of the vagus nerve and terminates in the heart. Other causes include hypoxia, hypertension, elevated intracranial pressure, and other noxious stimuli mediated through the vagus. Direct myocardial depression from the inhalation anesthetic, specifically through its antichronotropic effects, or cardiac effects of other drugs, such as opioids, should also be included in the differential diagnosis. The first maneuver would be to make the surgeon aware of the heart rate and request that he or she discontinue their procedure; the patient may then be observed for a relatively rapid return to a normal heart rate. If this does not occur, then an anticholinergic should be promptly administered IV. An increase in anesthetic depth may block this bradycardia, but it may also contribute, because of the antichronotropic effect, to a worsening of the bradycardia. When traction is applied to the extraocular muscles it will eventually produce a bradycardic response followed by a recovery tachycardia upon release of the traction. Fatigue of the oculocardiac reflex typically occurs with subsequent manipulation; this is generally referred to as a *traction test*. A *forced duction test* is a maneuver used to evaluate mechanical restriction to ocular movement. The sclera is grasped with a forceps and the eye is moved into each field of gaze. This allows the surgeon to differentiate between a paretic muscle and a muscle with restricted movement. Many surgeons prefer that neuromuscular blockade be used during a forced duction test to eliminate the variability in muscle tone with the changing depth of anesthesia. This test is most useful for those undergoing repeat strabismus surgery or in those with paralysis or prior trauma causing a mechanical restriction.

Postoperative Course

1. A deep extubation, when well conducted, will allow for a motionless emergence without bearing down or "bucking" on the endotracheal tube with resultant strain and an increase in mean arterial and central venous pressure as well as head and neck venous pressure. There is, in addition, some evidence that suggests higher oxygen saturations through emergence following deep extubation in children [2]. The Valsalva maneuver would increase venous pressure in the head and neck and influence the accumulation of edema in the surgically resected tissue; however, this is less of a problem in extraocular surgery than with intraocular surgery, such as an open globe. Most pediatric patients, however, will cry after these procedures, testing the closure of the globe anyway.

2. You are called urgently to the PACU 15 min postop because the patient has been screaming, banging her head against the siderails, not making any sense, and is inconsolable. She is scratching at her eyes.

   (a) What is your differential diagnosis?
   (b) Should you sedate her?
   (c) Get a blood gas?
   (d) Give her physostigmine?

Additional Questions

1. A 5-year old just fell from the Jungle Gym at MacDonald's with a Big Mac in his mouth, and landed on a rock causing an open eye injury. The ophthalmologist wants to go to the operating room right away because the eye is salvageable and the surgery should be accomplished as quickly as possible. The child is crying in the emergency room when you see him. He is otherwise healthy, hematocrit 36%. What anesthetic plan and counseling will you give to the parents?

2. Emergence delirium can occur for a variety of reasons; the most common in this situation would be the delirium associated with emerging from a sevoflurane anesthetic (the etiology of which remains unclear) and the central nervous system effects of anticholinergic syndrome, resulting from the administration of anticholinergics during surgery or as part of the reversal of neuromuscular blockade, particularly if atropine was used (tertiary ammonium molecule which can cross the blood–brain barrier). There is a lower chance of this syndrome with the use of glycopyrrolate, a quarternary ammonium molecule which is much less likely to cause CNS effects because it is a polar molecule. Hypoxia, respiratory distress, and pain should be considered in the differential diagnosis as well. Sedation may work if the patient is having a difficult time adjusting to the emergence and is at risk for self-injury, although ideally she should simply be protected from hurting herself until the delirium (if that is what it is to be determined) passes. A blood gas is unlikely to help in further delineating hypoxia beyond the reading of a pulse oximeter probe. The administration of Antilirium (physostigmine), a centrally acting anticholinesterase, may be useful diagnostically, but its synergy with echothiophate should prompt concern.

Additional Topics

1. This is one of the "classical" controversies in pediatric anesthesia, balancing the risk of the full stomach and aspiration of gastric contents with the risk of extrusion of a portion of the vitreous. It is also important not to forget that, in dealing with the whole patient, there may be other associated injuries, in this case, the possibility of loss of consciousness or orbital fracture. Assuming these other possibilities are ruled out and it is decided to proceed to the operating room as quickly as possible to obtain the best possible result, my priority would be a calm, anxiolytic induction of anesthesia. If an IV is in place, this would probably entail sedation with an intravenous anxiolytic such as midazolam. If an IV is not in place, then I would choose an oral premed with midazolam. It is tempting to consider a rapid sequence induction of anesthesia with cricoid pressure and succinylcholine; however, succinylcholine has been associated with an elevation of intraocular pressure, even with the administration of intravenous barbiturates and/or "precurarization." A good alternative would be to use the priming method with a nondepolarizing neuromuscular blocking agent, with the administration of one-tenth of the intubating dose, waiting for 2–3 min for a partial depletion of acetylcholine quanta at the neuromuscular junction, and then intravenous induction (with thiopental or propofol) followed by an intubating dose of the nondepolarizing neuromuscular blocking agent. The onset of adequate relaxation for tracheal intubation usually follows within 90 s, during which time gentle ventilation with positive pressure up to 10–12 cm H_2O and cricoid pressure may be delivered. Although part of the counseling for the parents should include the seriousness of the situation with regard to balancing the aspiration considerations against eye salvage, practically speaking, if the patient has already been crying, he may suffer no more risk with anesthetic induction than he already has prior to surgery [3].

2. A 1-month old is scheduled for congenital cataract aspiration. Following anesthetic induction with halothane/nitrous oxide/oxygen, the surgeon places a needle into the anterior chamber and begins to instill a saline–epinephrine solution, which the nurse quickly realizes was not the 1:200,000 dilution he asked for but 1:1,000. Should you stop the halothane technique? Should you intubate and change to a nitrous-narcotic technique? Should you mask with sevoflurane? What are the comparative advantages and disadvantages? What would you do? Why?

3. What happens to intraocular pressure with a vigorous Valsalva maneuver? (Describe the pathway, specifically, and how it affects the aqueous humor.) Is it rational to use a muscle relaxant if a patient performs a Valsalva maneuver? Are there any relaxants to be avoided? Why? What about a barbiturate?

4. What are the systemic effects of the following antiglaucoma drugs that are of significance to the anesthesiologist?

   (a) Timolol
   (b) Acetazolamide
   (c) Pilocarpine

2. The volume of this solution of saline and epinephrine in this space will be very small, so very little of the 5 mcg/mL of epinephrine will be given. Moreover, the epinephrine will produce local vasoconstriction, further reducing its own uptake. In addition, the area is not well vascularized (probably less so in the patient with congenital cataracts); therefore, the rate of absorption of this small amount will likely be slow. In addition, infants are much more tolerant of higher plasma levels of epinephrine than are adults. Therefore, although there is some theoretical concern about the administration of exogenous epinephrine in the setting of an alkane anesthetic such as halothane, which has the potential for sensitizing the myocardium to arrhythmias, practically speaking, this is unlikely to be a significant concern. On the other hand, even a small amount of 1:000 epinephrine (1,000 mcg/mL) is a considerable toxic dose and preparation should be made immediately for the administrative of medications to counteract the massive adrenergic effect this dose may have.

3. The effect of the Valsalva maneuver is as follows: it raises the central venous pressure, it impedes drainage of the aqueous humor through the canal of Schlemm into the episcleral venous system, it increases intraocular blood volume, and therefore increases intraocular pressure. The administration of a nondepolarizing muscle relaxant may be necessary to immobilize a patient if a Valsalva maneuver occurs during an alteration of the depth of anesthesia. If succinylcholine is chosen, it may actually elevate intraocular pressure as a result of its tonic effect on extraocular muscles. It may be more efficacious to administer thiopental or propofol intravenously to acutely lower the intraocular pressure.

4. *Timolol* (or betaxolol), both beta blockers, lower intraocular pressure and treat glaucoma by decreasing production of aqueous humor. There are some systemic effects to be considered, especially for timolol, such as negative chronotropy and a more prominent beta-2 effect which has been associated with a small incidence of asthma. Betaxolol may be better in this regard because of its more selective beta 1 effect.

   Acetazolamide is a carbonic anhydrase inhibitor and is also used to decrease the secretion of aqueous humor through its effect of inhibiting the sodium pump in the ciliary body. It may, however, cause a metabolic acidosis due to its systemic effect that can be treated by the administration of bicarbonate. Longer-duration treatment may lead to hypokalemia and nephrolithiasis.

   Pilocarpine is a cholinomimetic used for glaucoma. It causes miosis and therefore increases the size of the canals of Schlemm, promoting outflow of the aqueous humor.

5. An ex-premie is scheduled for an examination under anesthesia and cryotherapy for retinal detachment. What exactly is cryotherapy? What is the difference between that and a scleral buckle procedure? How will you anesthetize him? Where will you measure his oxygen saturation? Should you anticipate any other problems specific to his ex-premature state? What if he had a to-and-fro, machinery-like murmur? How about Tetralogy of Fallot, s/p a Blalock–Taussig shunt?

5. Cryotherapy is used when retinopathy of prematurity has lead to cicatrix forma- tion in the retina and impending retinal detachment and loss of vision. Cryotherapy is used to produce a chorioretinal scar, sealing a retinal break as a result of the accumulation of subretinal fluid with subsequent detachment. Cryotherapy may be used as part of a sequence including a scleral buckling procedure for reattach- ment of the retina to the pigment epithelium. In scleral buckling, the sclera is physically indented to bring the retinal tear closer to the pigment epithelium. External drainage of the subretinal fluid may be necessary as well. The anes- thetic required is a general endotracheal anesthetic. Special consideration has to be given to the use of nitrous oxide; if chosen as part of the anesthetic technique, the air in the posterior chamber may actually increase in volume if nitrous oxide is continued once the eye is closed; therefore, nitrous oxide should be discontin- ued approximately 20 min prior to sealing the chamber. Alternatively, nitrous oxide can be avoided as part of the anesthetic technique. Oxygen saturation can be measured in any extremity or the earlobe and should provide an accurate reflection of retinal saturation. While there may be theoretical concerns about oxygen treatment in the setting of established retinopathy of prematurity, the patient already has very significant injury from multifactorial causes, and the entire patient has to be considered. Patients with coexisting conditions such as cardiac lesions may require additional considerations for oxygen monitoring.

A to-and-fro, machinery-like murmur describes the findings of a patent ductus arteriosus. To the extent that the ductus may have a left to right shunt or right to left shunt, oxygen saturation should probably be measured preductally, i.e., in the right hand or earlobe and not in the left hand or in the feet. The patient with a Blalock– Taussig shunt will probably have a right subclavian to pulmonary artery anastomo- sis, and therefore the accuracy of the pulse oximeter reading in the right hand may be called into question. Earlobe saturation measurement may therefore be more accurate as far as cerebral (and therefore ophthalmic) oxygen concentrations.

Specific References

1. Wallace D, Steinkuller P (1998) Ocular medications in children. Clin Pediatr 37:645–652
2. Patel R (1991) Emergence airway complications in children: a comparison of tracheal extubation in awake and deeply anesthetized patients. Anesth Analg 73:266–270
3. Seidel J (2006) Anesthetic management of preschool children with penetrating eye injuries: postal survey of pediatric anesthetists and review of the available evidence. Paediatr Anaesth 16:769–776

General Reference

4. Gayer S (2006) Anesthesia for pediatric ocular surgery. Ophthalmol Clin North Am 19:269–278

Chapter 8
Respiratory System

A 3-year-old male, 15 kg, is scheduled for functional endoscopic sinus surgery, bilateral myringotomy and tubes, and nasal ciliary biopsy. Vital signs are BP 90/60 mmHg, P 125 bpm, as palpated by his PMI in the right precordium, and T 37.2°C. His hemoglobin is 13.0 g/dL. He has a productive cough, mild expiratory wheezing, does not have a runny nose, and is completing a 14-day course of ampicillin. He uses a beclomethasone inhaler twice daily.

R.S. Holzman et al., *Pediatric Anesthesiology Review: Clinical Cases for Self-Assessment,*
DOI 10.1007/978-1-4419-1617-4_8, © Springer Science+Business Media, LLC 2010

Preoperative Evaluation

1. Why is this patient wheezing?

    (a) How would you like to further evaluate the wheezing? Why?
    (b) How will it affect anesthetic management?

2. What are the implications of dextrocardia for this patient?

3. Is this patient adequately treated with his current medication regimen?

    (a) What would you add? Why?
    (b) Any specific implications for anesthetic management?
    (c) Are there significant neuroendocrine effects to be expected from the use of beclomethasone through the inhalation route?

4. Should this patient be premedicated? With what? Why?

    (a) What about a parent-accompanied induction?

Preoperative Evaluation

1. Wheezing, in the setting of asthma or other diseases with bronchoreactivity, is a result of airway narrowing due to inflammation and the accumulation of airway secretions. In chronic conditions, the inflammatory response, particularly in children, may result in tracheo- or bronchomalacia, worsening the wheezing because of the loss of integrity of the cartilaginous matrix of the airways and airway collapse with increased work of breathing. The increased work of breathing is worth mentioning as well because it contributes to the symptomatology of wheezing by producing more turbulent flow and worsens the underlying metabolic condition of the patient because the harder they work to breath, the less efficient their breathing becomes. They therefore have to work harder and utilize more calories to breathe, worsening their failure to thrive.

   The evaluation of wheezing is initially clinical, with attention to the respiratory rate, utilization of accessory muscles of respiration such as intercostal muscles, neck muscles, and gross movement of the entire rib cage. In addition, intercostal retractions may be seen. Tachypnea is the first sign of respiratory distress unless the patient is already exhausted. The wheezing may be inspiratory, expiratory, or biphasic, and this will lead to a further refined diagnosis of supraglottic, infraglottic, or mixed airway obstruction. A careful history and the patient's responsiveness to bronchodilators will provide further information as to the etiology of the wheezing. There may be cardiovascular consequences as well, including pulmonary hypertension and right heart failure. Anesthetic management should be directed to optimal preinduction medical management through sympathomimetics and anticholinergics, with additional steroids as needed.

2. The dextrocardia may be an isolated finding, but is more likely related to Kartagener's syndrome, which is characterized by ciliary dysmotility and abnormal PMN leukocyte motility. Patients develop chronic otitis media, sinusitis, recurrent respiratory infections, and bronchiectasis. Sterility in males is due to abnormal spermatozoa motility. Situs inversus or dextrocardia is associated with the syndrome.

3. Single drug medical management is probably inadequate; beclomethasone is good for chronic treatment but not adequate for acute exacerbations. Sympathomimetic and, in particular, anticholinergic therapy may be required for the unstable preoperative patient. An albuterol inhaler and ipratropium may be appropriate additional medications for achieving this purpose. The beclomethasone can have systemic effects, although these may not be clinically significant.

4. Premedication may be helpful for several reasons; it will lessen anxiety (for the parent as well as the child) and will also decrease the secretion of endogenous catecholamines and lower the risk of induction laryngospasm. In addition, lower anxiety will decrease crying and aerophagia, which may increase the chance of aspiration. A benzodiazepine alone should not shift the CO_2 response curve and cause significant respiratory depression. A more complete "preinduction" premed such as a benzodiazepine + ketamine + and anticholinergic orally will serve several purposes: amnesia, anxiolysis, bronchodilation, and drying of secretions.

Intraoperative Course

1. How will you set up the ECG monitor? Why?

    (a) Would an arterial line be a good idea Why/Why not?
    (b) Would you place it preinduction? Why?
    (c) Is a sidestream capnometer more accurate than a mainstream capnometer for this case?
    (d) What about transcutaneous CO_2 analysis?

2. Should you give an anticholinergic prior to induction? Why/why not?

    (a) Is this patient at risk for inspissation of secretions?
    (b) How deeply should the patient be anesthetized for intubation?
    (c) How will you know when he is deep?
    (d) Should intravenous induction agents be avoided? Why/why not?
    (e) What about a rapid-sequence intravenous induction?
    (f) Is propofol better than thiopental for induction?

Intraoperative Course

1. The ECG monitor should be configured for dextrocardia with a mirror image of the usual lead placement. An arterial line is probably not necessary for this type of surgery, which should be relatively short, without a large blood loss. On the other hand, if the patient's respiratory status deteriorates as the case proceeds, one should have a low threshold for arterial line placement in this patient with known reactive airways. Sidestream and mainstream capnography differ because the sidestream capnograph aspirates a bulk sample of respiratory gases continuously while the mainstream capnograph detects respiratory gas moieties by an infrared beam transmitted through the gases in the endotracheal tube without bulk gas sampling. The main disadvantage of the mainstream capnometer in children is that the detector is bulky relative to the diameter of the endotracheal tube; particularly under the drapes in a warm patient, there is a tendency for the mainstream capnometer to kink the endotracheal tube. The aspiration side channel in the sidestream capnometer is much lighter and does not kink the tube. Transcutaneous CO_2 analysis can be helpful when skin blood flow can be relied upon; in cold patients and low cardiac output states, it becomes less reliable. General anesthetics can also alter skin blood flow, but children preserve their cutaneous blood flow better than adults, and therefore, in the warm child, transcutaneous CO_2 analysis is relatively reliable.

2. It is worthwhile administering an anticholinergic prior to induction; however, it is important to be aware of the dose administered. The most logical choice is a reasonable dose of glycopyrrolate intravenously (if an IV is present) or inhalation administration of ipratropium bromide. Inspissation of secretions is not a significant concern, because anticholinergics change the volume of elaborated secretions but not their water content [1–3]. In general, patients should be deeply anesthetized as well as adequately treated with sympathomimetics, anticholinergics, and steroids, in order to additionally attenuate their bronchoreactivity. The usual clinical signs should be followed for depth, such as heart rate, blood pressure, and abdominal muscle tone. The eye signs, particularly pupillary dilatation, may be less reliable because of the administration of the sympathomimetics and anticholinergics both causing mydriasis. Intravenous induction agents do not need to be avoided as long as you remember that they are primarily hypnotics and anesthetic depth is more influenced by the volatile agents and narcotics. Ketamine may also act synergistically for depth of anesthesia and sympathomimetic effects. A traditional rapid sequence induction may be associated with more bronchoreactivity because the patient is relatively light and succinylcholine has been associated with the initiation of bronchospasm when it is biotransformed to its monocholine moieties. The choice of intravenous induction agent makes relatively less difference as long as an adequate depth of general anesthesia is achieved by one of the above strategies.

3. What is your choice for anesthetic maintenance? Why?

   (a) How would the use of sevoflurane for maintenance compare to isoflurane?
   (b) Would desflurane be a good choice after induction and during maintenance?
   (c) Is MAC different in this age group? In what way?
   (d) Is ketamine a choice? Why/why not?
   (e) A colleague suggests that he would avoid nitrous oxide in this patient? Do you agree?
   (f) The surgeon would like to apply 4% cocaine to the nose and mucosa of the maxillary antrum for topical analgesia and vasoconstriction? Do you agree?
   (g) How much will you tell him he can use?

4. What muscle relaxant would you choose? Why?

   (a) Is there any specific advantage to cis-atracurium or vecuronium over rocuronium or pancuronium?

5. What are the advantages of allowing this patient to breath spontaneously through-out the entire case? Would you do it? Why/Why not?

   (a) What breathing system would you choose? Why?
   (b) Does it matter which breathing system you use if the patient is breathing spontaneously as opposed to through a circle absorption system?

6. Shortly following the application of 4% cocaine, the patient's blood pressure is noted to be 180/110, with a heart rate of 220 bpm. As the surgeon begins, it increases to 210/120 with a heart rate of 230.

   (a) Why?
   (b) What else could it be? What can you do?
   (c) Should you attempt to slow the heart rate? Why?
   (d) What can you do to slow the heart rate?

3. A balanced anesthetic with a significant component of deep inhalation anesthesia with a volatile agent would probably be best. The opioids are excellent for providing analgesia and rapid attenuation of surgical stress while the potent volatile agents are excellent bronchodilators because of their effect on airway smooth muscle. At equi-MAC concentrations, the volatile agents are almost all equally efficacious at bronchodilatation, although there still seems to be some advantage to halothane, which is mitigated by the fact that it is an alkane anesthetic that sensitizes the heart to endogenous catecholamines. It also has more profound anti-inotropic and anti-chronotropic effects on the heart, which are of concern in pediatric practice. Ethrane is a reasonable choice although it is a little pungent, and desflurane is even more pungent. It has also been associated with laryngospasm during induction of anesthesia in children. Ketamine may be a reasonable choice because of the reasons outlined above. Avoiding nitrous oxide allows you to use a higher F_iO_2 and may also be important if the pulmonary vascular resistance is elevated and pulmonary hypertension is present. Cocaine is an excellent topical vasoconstrictor but it is unnecessary to use a 4% concentration in this age patient; 1–2% would be enough for topical analgesia and vasoconstriction, up to 3 mg/kg.

4 A variety of muscle relaxants can be chosen as long as their histamine release and potential for allergic reaction is minimal. Curare and atracurium (mixed *cis* and *trans* enantiomers) were associated with histamine release, but pancuronium, vecuronium, and *cis*-atracurium should release minimal histamine. There has been some concern recently with allergic reactions to rocuronium, and mivacurium has also been associated with a greater amount of histamine release when administered rapidly.

5. There may be an advantage to spontaneous breathing due to less turbulent airflow distal to an area of obstruction, according to the Hagen–Poiseuille equation. For the majority of patients, muscle relaxation with positive pressure ventilation will provide optimal operating conditions and maximize patient safety because of less chance for movement. For severely obstructed patients, the spontaneous breathing strategy may become necessary. I would choose a circle absorption system for the economy of fresh gas flow. An alternative would be a variation of the Mapleson circuits, either a D (Jackson Rees modification of Ayre's T) or an A (Magill system, optimal for spontaneous breathing). However, both of these Mapleson systems require a much higher fresh gas flow, with its attendant loss of temperature and wastefulness of volatile agent, than a circle absorption system, which can have fresh gas flows lowered to within very low flow or closed circuit range.

6. The direct effect of absorbed cocaine is the etiology of these findings. There are two options – if the cocaine is packed in the nose and is continuing to be delivered, the packing should be removed and suction applied to remove any trace quantities pooled at the mucosal level. Medications that act directly as antihypertensives can be administered if these expectant measures are ineffective, such as sodium nitroprusside (Nipride) in doses ranging from 0.5 to 10 mcg/kg/min and esmolol or propranolol, also in small divided doses and titrated to effect.

7. Sudden increase in peak airway pressure and desaturation (bronchospasm): the patient desaturates to 87% over 30 s, and diffuse biphasic wheezing develops with a rise in peak inspiratory pressure to 55 cm H_2O.

   (a) What would you do first?
   (b) And next? Why?
   (c) Where could the problem be?
   (d) If this is truly bronchospasm, what could you do anesthetically to fix it?

Postoperative Course

1. When would you extubate? Why?

   (a) Would you extubate deep?
   (b) Is this patient at risk for postextubation croup?
   (c) For postextubation laryngospasm?
   (d) Tracheomalacia?

2. What are the risks to this patient of reversal of neuromuscular blockade? Why?

   (a) What are the alternatives?
   (b) Would you not use a reversal agent?
   (c) Is neostigmine better/worse than pyridostigmine or edrophonium?

7. There should be a logical and rapid progression through a differential diagnosis of mechanical obstruction at the level of the breathing circuit and endotracheal tube and then to the level of the patient's trachea and major conducting airways. Such obstruction can be due to a kinked tube or a tube obstructed with secretions or a mucus plug, or the airway obstructed with a mucus plug. If there is no obvious kink in the endotracheal tube then a suction catheter can be passed through the endotracheal tube until you are convinced that the tube is clear. If mechanical obstruction is ruled out then diffuse inspiratory and expiratory wheezing can be accounted for by bronchospasm. Albuterol can be delivered via the endotracheal tube but it may be more efficacious if the bronchospasm is severe to deliver dilute epinephrine (i.e., 0.1 mcg/kg) intravenously to see if the bronchospasm will break. Anesthetically, the patient should probably be deepened with the volatile agent; ketamine and intravenous glycopyrrolate may also be effective.

Postoperative Course

1. Arguments can be made for deep and awake extubation. I would extubate awake because there is a better assessment of oxygenation, ventilation, and other airway needs, even though some studies have shown a higher saturation with deep extubation [4]. Postextubation croup is probably more related to subglottic irritation from the intubation as well as a loose basement membrane. Postextubation laryngospasm is a much more likely possibility in any child with irritable airways.

2. Neuromuscular blockade and controlled ventilation often result in less efficient respiratory mechanics because of the cephalad migration of the diaphragm, decrease in FRC, and decreased efficiency of alveolar airflow because of positive pressure ventilation. The reversal of neuromuscular blockade with an anticholinesterase and anticholinergic may result in bronchospasm and increased salivation.

Additional Questions

1. What are the anesthetic induction considerations in the patient with pulmonary sequestration? What immediate interventions can be performed therapeutically for deterioration during induction?

2. Is infantile lobar emphysema a surgical emergency? Why/why not? Should the patient be bronchoscoped first? Why/why not? What muscle relaxant would you choose? Why? A colleague of yours suggests the avoidance of nitrous oxide; do you agree?

Additional Questions

1. Pulmonary sequestration is the result of early isolation of pulmonary tissue from the developing lung bud. Sequestration may occur as intralobar or extralobar, depending on whether the abnormal tissue is located within the pleura or outside of it. The abnormal tissue may have cystic and solid areas with mixtures of air, rudimentary air sacs, and bronchi and chronically inflamed areas. Deterioration during the induction of anesthesia may be a result of communication of the sequestration with the respiratory or gastrointestinal tract, resulting in respiratory distress or GI symptoms. Spontaneous breathing may be more optimal in this regard until the communication can be identified, isolated, and ligated along with the blood supply to the sequestration. Extralobar sequestration, although extrapleural, generally presents at an earlier age with recurrent infections. Arteriovenous malformations are also commonly associated.

2. It may or may not be, depending on the timing and severity of presentation. A deficiency of bronchial cartilage, bronchial stenosis, or extrinsic vascular compression from the pulmonary artery may result in congenital lobar emphysema, characterized by overinflation and air trapping in the affected lobe with compression atelectasis of adjacent parenchyma and possible mediastinal displacement. Males are affected more often than females. There is progressive respiratory distress in the newborn period or in early infancy. Rapid deterioration requires urgent surgery, and when accompanied by a mediastinal shift, increased intrathoracic pressure, impaired venous return, and decreased cardiac output may result. The diagnosis is made by chest X-ray when bronchovascular marking is present in a hyperlucent area of lung. Bronchoscopy should be considered in the older infant if there is a possibility of intraluminal obstruction causing lobar emphysema. Surgical excision in the neonate, however, may be an emergent procedure if the lobe is expanding rapidly. Vigorous positive pressure should be avoided during anesthetic induction and spontaneous ventilation should be preserved. Nitrous oxide should be avoided, as should muscle relaxants.

3. A frightened 8-year old with a large anterior mediastinal mass presents for supra-clavicular lymph node biopsy, and his parents want to know whether he can be asleep for the procedure? What does the answer depend on? Why? Under what circumstances would you want a perfusion team present?

3. An anterior mediastinal mass may or may not cause symptoms depending on its encroachment on the tracheobronchial tree and the right heart and pulmonary circulation. Physical diagnosis is not always helpful with regard to the severity of the chest disease, because even patients with more than 50% airway narrowing may only be symptomatic with orthopnea; the superior vena caval syndrome is relatively rare in pediatric patients [5–7]. Pulmonary function tests may be helpful in demonstrating inspiratory and expiratory compromise. At 8 years of age, a MAC plus good local anesthesia by the surgeon is a very acceptable plan. The patient should also be placed in Semi-Fowler's position for optimal comfort for ventilation and gas exchange. Premedication with oral benzodiazepines may be a very rational plan and will lessen the patient's anxiety and improve the chances for a successful operating room course. For patients whose risks increase because of greater than 50% airway encroachment or significant tumor impingement on the pulmonary circulation or the right ventricle, it is not a bad idea to have a rigid bronchoscope available. In the highest risk situations, when the patient has had episodes of syncopy which may be related to a drop in pulmonary blood flow as a result of right heart obstruction, it may be worthwhile to have both groins prepped and draped and have a perfusion team standing by to cannulate and go on to cardiopulmonary bypass immediately.

4. A 14-year-old girl is admitted for evaluation of dysphagia, chest pain and a weight loss of 7 kg over 3–4 weeks. At 5 years of age she received an allogenic bone marrow transplant for aplastic anemia which was complicated by the chronic sclerodermoid form of severe graft-vs-host disease with generalized skin involvement, muscle wasting and restrictive lung disease requiring supplemental oxygen (0.5 L/min) and nocturnal biphasic intermittent positive airway pressure (BIPAP) ventilation. She is afebrile, with a heart rate of 110–140 beats per minute and a respiratory rate of 18–24 breaths per minute. Her room air oxygen saturation is 91%, increasing to 98% with 0.5 L/min of oxygen. The rigid chest wall shows almost no expansion during inspiration. Pulmonary function tests are:

FVC = 17% of predicted
FEV_1 = 18% of predicted
FEV_1/FVC = 96% of predicted
TLC = 64%
RV = 194%
RV/TLC = 78%
ABG: (0.5 L/min O_2) pH = 7.27, pCO_2 = 95 mm Hg, pO_2 = 183 mm Hg

Her ECG is unremarkable apart from a sinus tachycardia. Her echocardiogram ruled out right ventricular dysfunction but is suspicious for elevated right ventricular pressure. Her barium swallow demonstrated a web at the cervical esophagus with mild distal narrowing. She is coming to the OR for an endoscopic esophageal dilatation which the gastroenterologists feel should take about 1/2 hour to 45 minutes.

Assuming she is currently optimally prepared and this is her usual baseline state, what are your plans for intraoperative anesthetic technique and postanesthetic care? What are the likely complications and pitfalls?

4. Because of the severe restrictive ventilatory defect and the esophageal obstruction, I would begin the induction of anesthesia in the sitting position while continuing spontaneous ventilation. The patient has severe CO_2 retention and I would expect a severe decrease in the minute ventilation response to hypercarbia, so it might be worthwhile to consider a respiratory analeptic to shift the CO_2 response curve, such as doxapram [8]. It would probably be necessary to use a small amount of continuous positive airway pressure to maintain the FRC. As the patient lost consciousness, she could be placed in a more supine position, cricoid pressure applied, and the trachea could be intubated at that point. She is indeed a "full stomach," but, in my opinion, the risks of rapid sequence induction and commitment to positive pressure ventilation are outweight by the advantages of spontaneous breathing with a careful and slow induction of anesthesia with the preservation of spontaneous breathing. Positive pressure may cause interventricular septal shifting that will significantly decrease her stroke volume and cardiac output, so I would be concerned about delivering positive pressure ventilation and committing her to controlled ventilation if it could be avoided. Even a small amount of controlled ventilation may be enough, particularly in this patient, to drive her CO_2 below apneic threshold, the CO_2 required for spontaneous breathing. She has a severe restrictive ventilatory defect with incipient changes in the pulmonary circulation and right heart. She has a "cuirass" type of pulmonary physiology which prevents deep breaths either during spontaneous ventilation and most importantly during controlled ventilation [9]. Because of the progressive vascular sclerosis that is characteristic of graft vs. host disease, placement of peripheral arterial catheters may carry significant risk of ongoing vascular obstruction, even after the arterial catheter is removed. Notwithstanding her history (and anticipated complication) of elevated pulmonary vascular resistance and right heart problems, these are well understood and changes intraoperatively can be interpreted in light of these findings and supporting evidence from noninvasive monitors such as $ETCO_2$ and pulse oximetry [10].

References

1. Kaliner M, Shelhamer J, Borson B, Nadel J, Patow C, Marom Z (1986) Human respiratory mucus. Am Rev Respir Dis 134:612–621
2. Tamaoki J, Chiyotani A, Tagaya E, Sakai N, Konno K (1994) Effect of long term treatment with oxitropium bromide on airway secretion in chronic bronchitis and diffuse panbronchiolitis. Thorax 49:545–548
3. Taylor R, Pavia D, Agnew J, Lopez-Vidriero M, Newman S, Lennard-Jones T, Clarke S (1986) Effect of four weeks' high dose ipratropium bromide treatment on lung mucociliary clearance. Thorax 41:295–300
4. Patel R, Hannallah R, Norden J, Casey W, Verghese S (1991) Emergence airway complications in children: a comparison of tracheal extubation in awake and deeply anesthetized patients. Anesth Analg 73:266–270
5. Pullerits J, Holzman R (1989) Anesthesia for mediastinal masses. Can J Anaesth 36:681–688

 6. Shamberger R, Holzman R, Griscom N, Tarbell N, Weinstein H (1991) CT quantitation of tracheal cross-sectional area as a guide to the surgical and anesthetic management of children with anterior mediastinal masses. J Pediatr Surg 26:138–142
 7. Shamberger R, Holzman R, Griscom N, Tarbell N, Weinstein H, Wohl M (1995) Prospective evaluation by computed tomography and pulmonary function tests of children with mediastinal masses. Surgery 118:468–471
 8. Hirshberg A, Dupper R (1994) Use of doxapram hydrochloride injection as an alternative to intubation to treat chronic obstructive pulmonary disease patients with hypercapnia. Ann Emerg Med 24:701–703
 9. Patrick J, Meyer-Witting M, Reynolds F, Spencer G (1990) Perioperative care in restrictive respiratory disease. Anesthesia 45:390–395
10. Schure A, Holzman R (2000) Anesthesia in a child with severe restrictive pulmonary dysfunction caused by chronic graft-versus-host disease. J Clin Anesth 12:482–486

Chapter 9
Cardiac I

A 3-year-old male with a diagnosis of tetralogy of Fallot and a right Blalock–Taussig shunt (created at 1 month of age) presents with a history of gradually decreasing exercise tolerance and increasing frequency of hypercyanotic episodes. He had a hematocrit of 69% 2 months previously. He is scheduled for complete repair of his lesion.

R.S. Holzman et al., *Pediatric Anesthesiology Review: Clinical Cases for Self-Assessment*, DOI 10.1007/978-1-4419-1617-4_9, © Springer Science+Business Media, LLC 2010

Preoperative Evaluation

1. What is the tetralogy of Fallot? Is it really four lesions? What is the principal anatomic lesion?

2. What are the reasons that this child would have received a palliative shunt for his first surgical procedure rather than a definitive repair? Are there any long-term consequences to a Blalock–Taussig shunt of importance to you as an anesthesiologist?

3. The patient is extremely apprehensive and very scared of needles. How will you gain his confidence so that you can perform a physical exam? How will you assess him for volume status and dehydration? Would you expect his hematocrit to be any different today than it was 2 months ago? What do you expect his oxygen saturation to be? Any additional lab studies you would like to see? Any additional diagnostic cardiac information you would like to have? What would you expect to find on echocardiogram?

4. He has a Tet spell in the examining room...how do you manage it? What is a Tet spell, physiologically and anatomically? Why do you choose the maneuvers you choose? Would it be any different in the preoperative holding area? How about in the operating room during induction?

Preoperative Evaluation

1. The primary lesion in tetralogy of Fallot is a conoventricular malalignment ventricular septal defect (VSD). As a result of this lesion there is anterior and superior displacement of the aorta and "crowding" of the pulmonary outflow tract. This lesion produces aortic override (50% or more of the aorta over the VSD), hypoplasia of the pulmonary outflow tract (pulmonic stenosis), and dynamic right ventricular outflow tract (RVOT) obstruction due to anterior deviation of the conal septum and muscle bundles in the RVOT. Right ventricular hypertrophy (RVH) occurs secondary to fixed and dynamic RVOT, *not* as a primary manifestation of the lesion.

2. A palliative shunt is typically done in institutions not versed in infant cardiac surgery utilizing cardiopulmonary bypass (CPB). The long-term adverse consequences of such a shunt would be: (1) poor growth of the native pulmonary arteries due to preferential blood flow to one lung, stenosis at the anastamosis site, or chronic low pulmonary blood flow. In the worst case scenario, the branch pulmonary arteries might become discontinuous. (2) progression of RVH as placement of a shunt does not address RVOT obstruction and thereby does not remove the stimulus for continued hypertrophy.

3. Volume status would be assessed in this child as in any child of similar age. The erythrocytosis associated with cyanosis is progressive; however, hematocrits above 70% are rare. A baseline oxygen saturation of 60–70% with desaturation episodes into the 40–50% range would be expected. A platelet count would be useful as erythrocytosis is associated with thrombocytopenia. A PT and PTT would be useful as chronic cyanosis is associated with poorly defined coagulation abnormalities. It would be necessary to know the status of the pulmonary vasculature. Specifically, it is necessary to know whether the pulmonary arteries are continuous and of normal size. The echocardiogram will demonstrate severe RVH and there will be bidirectional flow across the VSD. It is possible that the flow across the VSD could be entirely right to left with all pulmonary blood flow supplied by the Blalock–Taussig (BT) shunt.

4. A "tet spell" is simply an exacerbation of the *dynamic* component of RVOT obstruction that results in increased right to left shunting across the VSD. It will be precipitated by physiologic perturbations that reduce the caliber of the RVOT: (1) reduced venous return, (2) increases in shortening and thickening of the free wall and septum of the RV. Treatment is directed at these causes. Alternatively treatment can be directed toward increasing systemic vascular resistance (SVR) which will reduce right to left shunting at the VSD *but does nothing to treat the underlying cause of the "tet spell."* The only difference between the holding area and the operating room is the extent of monitoring, qualified personnel, and drug choices available.

Intraoperative Course

1. Are there any specific drugs would you like to have ready in the OR, besides the "usuals?"

2. What kind of monitoring will you select? Place prior to or postinduction? Any specific considerations for placement of the monitors? Invasive lines? ECG?

3. How will you induce anesthesia? Maintenance? Fluid management strategy? Any particular considerations for the Blalock–Taussig shunt?

Treatment Modalities:

- **Improved venous return**

  - Volume infusion – at least 10–15 mL/kg
  - Sedation – reduces tachypnea (morphine is used most frequently). Administration of an alpha agonist (phenylephrine) – reduces venous unstressed volume and improves venous return

- **Relaxation of the RVOT**

  - Sedation
  - Negative inotropes – beta blockers (esmolol), anesthetic agents (halothane). Heart rate reduction may also increase the caliber of the RVOT by increasing RV end-diastolic and end-systolic volumes.

- **Increasing SVR**

  - Administration of an alpha agonist (phenylephrine)

  - Aortic or femoral artery compression   manual compression of the abdominal aorta, hip flexion

Intraoperative Course

1. Phenylephrine, infusions of dopamine, epinephrine, milrinone, and tranexamic acid.

2. ECG (5 lead including V_5), pulse oximeter $\times 2$ (upper and lower), BP $\times 2$ (upper and lower, arterial line, and BP cuff), and CVP. ECG, pulse oximeter, and BP cuff prior to induction. Right arm may not be a reliable source of central BP measurement given the presence of a right Blalock–Taussig shunt (BTS).

3. Induction and maintenance of anesthesia could be accomplished with any agent or combination of agents that preserve myocardial contractility and pulmonary blood flow. Maintenance of pulmonary blood flow via the BTS is dependent on maintenance of systemic BP and a normal or low pulmonary vascular resistance (PVR). Appropriate PVR can be obtained with a high FiO_2 and pH of 7.45 or above. pH can best be maintained in this range with a mild respiratory alkalosis ($PaCO_2$ of 30–35 mm Hg in the absence of a metabolic acidosis). The ventilatory settings to accomplish this should be achieved with the lowest mean airway pressures possible to avoid mechanical impairment of pulmonary blood flow. This usually is accomplished with a tidal volume of 10–12 mL/kg, an I:E ratio of 1:3, and a rate of 10–15 bpm.

4. What are your considerations as regards the hemodilution associated with cardiopulmonary bypass?

5. Do you expect any coagulation problems? Would you use any particular pharmacological management strategy in this regard?

6. What are your considerations as regards weaning from cardiopulmonary bypass?

7. What are your transport considerations from the OR to the intensive care unit?

Postoperative Course

1. What is the postpump syndrome? Is there a cardiac component? A pulmonary component? A psychological component?

4. Hemodilution is an expected consequence of CPB. In this instance, the high hematocrit will likely lead the perfusionist to prime with a little or no blood to attain a target hematocrit of 25–35%. The prime will most likely be a crystalloid or colloid solution. The danger to this patient will be a dilutional thrombocytopenia and factor deficiency secondary to the reduced plasma volume associated with erythrocytosis. This could be countered by adding FFP rather than a crystalloid or colloid solution.

5. The clotting abnormalities have been previously delineated. Use of a lysine analog antifibrinolytic agent such as transexamic acid (TXA) or epsilon-aminocaproic acid (EACA) is warranted. The serine protease inhibitor aprotinin is currently unavailable for use.

6. The major CPB weaning issues are:

   • Reduced RV systolic function as a consequence of less than optimal preservation of the hypertrophied RV and the ventriculotomy that may be necessary to close the VSD/augment the RVOT.
   • Reduced RV diastolic function for the reasons outlined above.
   • Residual volume load on the RV from either pulmonary insufficiency (from a transannular patch) or a residual VSD. A residual VSD will be very poorly tolerated as it presents an acute volume load to a chronically pressure overloaded RV.
   • Right to left shunting at the atrial level if the foramen ovale has been left open as a pop-off valve.
   • Atrial arrhythmias, particularly junctional ectopic tachycardia (JET) if the VSD was closed across the tricuspid valve.

7. Transport to the ICU with continuous BP, pulse oximetry, ECG. Blood or colloid for volume infusion. Hemodynamic stability while the patient is being ventilated with the transport bag should be obtained prior to leaving the OR.

Postoperative Course

1. Postpump syndrome is now known to be the consequence of the systemic inflammatory response syndrome (SIRS). SIRS is characterized by tissue and endothelial injury leading to enhanced capillary permeability (capillary leak syndrome) and transmigration of leukocytes into interstitial fluid with subsequent activation of sequestered leukocytes, elaboration of chemoattractants, and amplification of the inflammatory process. The spectrum of SIRS induced responses ranges from tissue edema to end-organ dysfunction and failure. The magnitude of this response is enhanced in neonates/infants and small children due in part to the high circuit surface area to blood volume ratio as compared with adults.

2. What arrhythmias will you tell the nursing staff in the ICU to anticipate? Why?

2. JET (junctional ectopic tachycardia) is the most likely. The substrate for this arrhythmia is injury to myocardium in and around the AV node occurring as consequence of surgical retraction of the tricuspid annulus. JET typically manifests with a junctional rate only slightly faster than the sinus node rate and is the only narrow complex tachycardia in which the atrial rate is less than the ventricular rate (A:V ratio < 1:1). Much less commonly (10%), there may be retrograde activation of the atrium with inverted p waves noted and an A:V ratio of 1:1. In either case, there is loss of AV synchrony (loss of atrial kick). At a HR < 160–170 bpm this arrhythmia may be well tolerated. It is unlikely to be tolerated in the presence of restrictive diastolic function at any rate. JET with HR > 170 bpm is associated with hemodynamic instability and increased postoperative mortality.

Neither cardioversion nor adenosine is effective. Treatment of JET is atrial pacing at a rate slightly faster than the junctional rate reinitiating A–V synchrony. This therapy is effective unless the junctional rate is very fast (>160–170 bpm) at which point atrial pacing at a faster rate is unlikely to improve hemodynamics because the reinitiation of A–V synchrony is offset by the reduction in diastolic filling time present at these rates.

References

1. DiNardo JA (2008) Anesthesia for congenital heart disease. In: DiNardo JA, Zvara DA (eds) Anesthesia for cardiac surgery, 3rd edn. Blackwell Publishing, Oxford, pp 167–251
2. Kussman BD, DiNardo JA (2008) The cardiovascular system. In: Holzman RS, Mancuso TJ, Polander DM (eds) A practical approach to pediatric anesthesia. Lippincott Williams and Wilkins, Philadelphia, pp 306–374
3. DiNardo JA (2008) Tetralogy of Fallot. In: Yao F-SF (ed) Yao and Artusio's anesthesiology problem-oriented patient management, 6th edn. Lippincott Williams and Wilkins, Philadelphia, pp 403–425

Chapter 10
Cardiac II

A 4-year-old boy presents for pectus excavatum repair. He has a Holmes heart type of double-inlet left ventricle (single ventricle, great vessel concordance, hypoplastic pulmonary outlet chamber), tolerates exercise well, and has an Hct of 45%. He has a Glenn shunt. His pectus excavatum is so severe, however, that the cardiac surgeons would like it repaired prior to sternotomy and cardiac surgery.

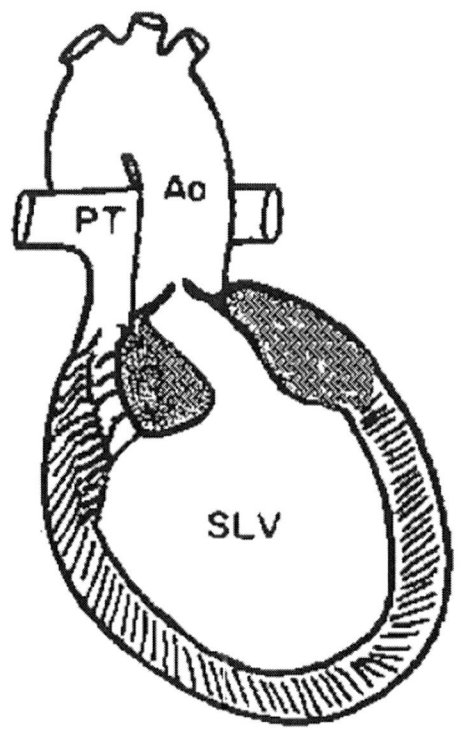

R.S. Holzman et al., *Pediatric Anesthesiology Review: Clinical Cases for Self-Assessment,*   269
DOI 10.1007/978-1-4419-1617-4_10, © Springer Science+Business Media, LLC 2010

Preoperative Evaluation

1. What is the difference between a single inlet and a double inlet ventricle? Why would it matter? What are the morphologic components of any ventricle? Is it important to your anesthetic management to understand the outlet component? Is there a difference whether or not the outlet component is concordant or discordant with the ventricular morphology? Why?

2. What is a Glenn shunt? How does it differ from a Fontan procedure? In what way are the differences relevant for anesthesia? Are there any specific differences with regard to anesthesia for venous to pulmonary artery shunts compared with systemic arterial to pulmonary artery shunts such as the Blalock–Taussig shunt (BTS) or Waterston shunt? When would it matter?

Preoperative Evaluation

1. A double inlet ventricle is one in which both AV valves drain into one ventricle resulting in complete mixing of systemic and pulmonary venous blood. Subsequent delivery of this mixed blood to the systemic and pulmonary circulations then occurs in parallel (not series) from one ventricle. These two features are the basis of single ventricle physiology. The morphological components of a ventricle are the inlet, the body, and the outlet. A "ventricle" which is composed of only an outlet portion is called a bulboventricular foramen (BVF). Transposition of the Great Vessels (TGV) refers specifically to the anatomic circumstance wherein there is concordance of the atrioventicular connections associated with discordance of the ventriculoarterial connections. Corrected transposition (C-TGV) refers specifically to the anatomic circumstance wherein there is discordance of the atrioventricular connections associated with discordance of the ventriculoarterial connections. In the case of single ventricle physiology, concordance or discordance of the ventriculoarterial connections becomes academic as systemic and arterial flow are derived from one ventricle. The relevant issue is whether the outflow to either circulation from the single ventricle is obstructed. In the case described here there is potential for subpulmonary obstruction at the level of the communication to the BVF and pulmonary outflow tract.

2. A classic Glenn shunt is an end-to-end anastamosis of the superior vena cava (SVC) to the right pulmonary artery (RPA) in which the RPA is separated from the main PA. Thus all pulmonary blood flow is derived from the SVC to RPA. A bidirectional Glenn (superior cavopulmonary anastomosis) is currently the procedure of choice. It involves an end to side anastamosis of the SVC to the right pulmonary artery in which the RPA is in continuity with the main PA and LPA. Thus all pulmonary blood flow is derived from the SVC to RPA *and* LPA. All IVC blood is delivered to a common atrium (mixing with pulmonary venous blood) following a Glenn shunt. These shunts are not dependant on systemic arterial pressure to provide pulmonary blood flow, as is the case with systemic to pulmonary artery shunt such as the BTS or Waterston.

   The Fontan procedure creates continuity between the IVC and the SVC and the pulmonary artery. Following a Glenn shunt, Fontan physiology would be created by surgically creating continuity between the IVC and the pulmonary artery. Following a Fontan all systemic venous blood is delivered to the pulmonary circulation.

3. Of what significance are the exercise history and the hematocrit? What if he was simply short of breath with exertion, but had a hematocrit of 45%? What if the hematocrit was 57% and he was also short of breath? Does this patient need to come into the hospital the night before surgery for intravenous hydration? Why/why not? What would your choice of fluid be? Full maintenance rate, 1/2 maintenance? Why?

4. Should this patient receive a premedication prior to coming to the operating room? What if he was extremely apprehensive? What would be the potential advantage? If the patient became profoundly sedated and difficult to arouse to anything except vigorous shaking, would that be a problem? Why?

3. The hematocrit is consistent with adequate pulmonary blood flow and systemic oxygen delivery as there is no compensatory erythrocytosis. The good exercise tolerance is consistent with preserved ventricular function, systemic oxygen delivery, and chronotropic reserve. In patients with a palliated congenital heart lesion, loss of chronotropic reserve may be a component of impaired exercise tolerance. A hematocrit of 57% and shortness of breath would warrant further evaluation, specifically, an echocardiogram to evaluate ventricular function, AV valve regurgitation, and patency of the Glenn pathway. Cardiac catheterization would be necessary to rule out decompressing venous collaterals from the Glenn pathway to the IVC or directly to the pulmonary venous system. These collaterals would diminish pulmonary blood flow and increase right to left shunting (systemic venous blood to the common atrium). In addition, cardiac catheterization would delineate the extent of pulmonary arteriovenous malformations (AVMs); these are a source of intrapulmonary right to left shunting (systemic venous blood delivered directly to the pulmonary veins). These AVMs develop in patients with Glenn shunts due to a lack of hepatic venous blood being delivered to the lungs. The hormonal factor present in hepatic venous blood that promotes this process has not been identified. A similar phenomenon occurs in cirrhotic patients, not as a result of deprivation of the pulmonary bed of hepatic venous blood, but as a result of severely impaired hepatic synthetic function. This patient should be admitted the night before surgery and given full maintenance fluids. This is necessary to prevent dehydration in the setting of pre-existing erythrocytosis.

4. The decision to premedicate should be individualized to the patient's preoperative physiological status. Over-sedation of this patient would likely cause pulmonary venous desaturation as a result of hypoventilation and development of pulmonary V/Q mismatch and shunt. This patient is no more at risk for development of this than a normal patient; however, the consequence in terms of systemic arterial saturation is more severe given that this patient's arterial saturation is a weighted average of the volume and saturation of pulmonary venous blood and the volume and saturation of systemic venous (in this case IVC) blood.

Intraoperative Course

1. Other than routine noninvasive monitors, does this patient need any invasive monitoring? Why/why not? Would a central line be helpful? Why? How about a pulmonary artery catheter? Would you go to the cardiac catheterization lab before surgery to place one? What if the cardiac surgeons do not want you to place an arterial line because of his upcoming cardiac repair? Does his ECG need to be configured in any particular way for a morphological left ventricle? Is it just as accurate to place leads on his lateral chest? Should they be placed on his back for the pectus repair? What would this show you that would be different from normal lead placement?

2. How would you induce anesthesia for this patient? What would be important in your decision? Is an inhalation anesthetic better than high dose fentanyl? Is ketamine an acceptable choice if the patient is screaming and crying uncontrollably in the preop area? Why/why not? Would you be worried about the patient under this circumstance?

3. The patient is given an intramuscular injection of ketamine/midazolam and glycopyrrolate in the midst of crying in the preoperative holding area, and over the course of 30 s remains as blue as he was when he was crying; but now he is not crying, and is still blue. Your management? Is oxygen likely to help? What else would you do? What effect would manipulating resistance in the pulmonary and systemic circulation have? How can you do this in the holding area?

4. The parents have agreed to you placing a thoracic epidural for intraoperative care and postoperative pain management. What are your considerations for placement of a thoracic epidural in a 4-year old? When would you place it? What technique would you use? Any specific considerations for this patient? Is volume loading required? How would you administer a test dose? How accurate is it? What effect is a thoracic epidural likely to have on pulmonary vascular resistance? Is this a particular consideration for this patient? What if the principal impedance to pulmonary blood flow is at the level of the pulmonic infundibulum; how would this affect your use of an epidural intraoperatively?

Intraoperative Course

1. A central line via the right internal jugular vein would end up in the RPA if a classic Glenn was present and in the MPA if a bidirectional Glenn was present. In either case the transduced pressure would be the mean PA pressure. The difference between the MPA pressure and the mean common atrial pressure would be the transpulmonary gradient (TPG). Placement of a pulmonary artery catheter would allow measurement of the MPA and the common atrial pressure indirectly via a PAOP. However, placement of such a catheter would be highly impractical as it would require fluoroscopy and a trip to the cardiac catheterization laboratory and would provide little additional information. An arterial line would be a necessity and the appropriate site could be negotiated. Standard ECG lead placement would reveal qRS forces directed leftward and anterior and would be consistent with left ventricular hypertrophy (LVH).

2. The major anesthetic goal here would be avoidance of elevated PVR, and in the case of a classic Glenn shunt, dynamic obstruction to pulmonary blood flow into the BVF. In the case of a bidirectional Glenn, dynamic pulmonary outflow obstruction would be irrelevant. An inhalation induction in this patient would be prolonged given the reduced Qp:Qs. The only disadvantage to this is that a longer period of airway management (along with the risk of aspiration, laryngospasm, etc.) as compared with an intravenous induction would be necessary. Ketamine administration is acceptable as long as it is not accompanied by hypercarbia and/or hypoxia.

3. Oxygen by mask followed by initiation of positive pressure ventilation with oxygen if necessary. There is no danger of overcirculation in this patient (i.e., PVR reduced to the point where Qp:Qs is so high that systemic perfusion is impaired) given that Glenn physiology is present.

4. Hypovolemia will exacerbate dynamic subpulmonary outflow obstruction. Aggressive prehydration prior to initiation of thoracic epidural blockade would be necessary.

Postoperative Management

1. What criteria will you use to extubate? Is this patient likely to have an increased dead space to tidal volume (Vd/Vt) ratio? Why? Is he likely to have impaired efficiency of oxygenation (significant shunt)? What about his ventilatory mechanics – how might they be affected by his underlying problems? How will you then decide? If his saturation is 95% on 100% FiO_2, should he be extubated? Why/Why not?

2. One of your colleagues suggests that the patient should be given furosemide (Lasix®) so he will have less lung water and it will be easier for him to breathe. Do you agree? Why/why not?

   Of what significance is volume depletion in this patient? Are there any specific implications for his shunt? What are they? How might they manifest themselves?

Postoperative Management

1. V_d/V_t will be increased in a patient with a Glenn shunt due to an increase in Zone 1 lung. This is the direct result of low pulmonary artery pressure (i.e., SVC pressure).

2. Lasix will reduce lung water and work of breathing if interstitial lung water is present. This would be best determined by physical exam and CXR. Volume depletion could in theory contribute to shunt thrombosis and a drastic reduction in pulmonary blood flow.

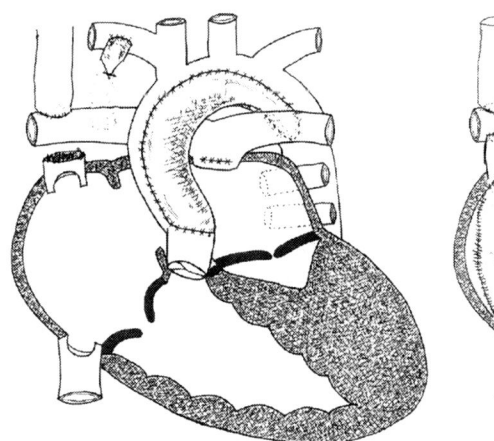

Bidirectional Glenn

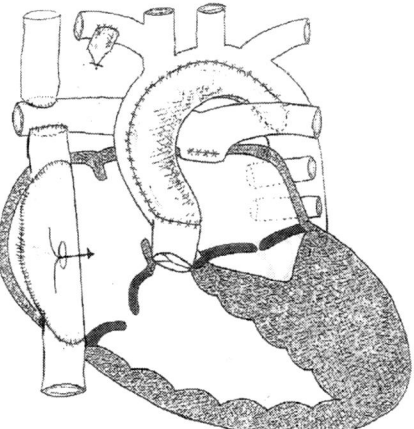

Fenestrated Fontan

Additional Questions

1. What differences are there in the architecture of the immature and adult myocardium, and what physiological implications does this have? How would it affect your anesthetic management? What would the length-tension curve look like compared with an adult myocardium?

2. Why should systemic to pulmonary artery shunts be clamped or ligated as soon as bypass begins? Of what importance is this to your anesthetic management?

3. A 12-month-old child with trisomy 21 presents for reduction of macroglossia. On examination you hear a murmur. Would you be prepared to continue with this case? Are there any cardiac abnormalities you would expect? What implications are there for anesthetic management?

4. A 14-year-old male presents for posterior spinal fusion. He has a history of a univentricular heart and has been palliated with a Fontan procedure, s/p fenestration. Describe briefly the Fontan operation. What is the function of the fenestration? Does it require a separate procedure to close? What are the anesthetic goals in a patient of this sort undergoing a spinal fusion?

5. A 3-year-old female presents for bilateral ureteral reimplantation. She has tetralogy of Fallot, a functioning right Blalock–Taussig shunt, and a resting oxygen saturation of 87% on room air and a hematocrit of 69%. What are your thoughts? What are you going to tell the parents? What are you going to tell the surgeon? What are the risks of erythropheresis? Is erythropheresis effective? How would you perform it?

Additional Questions

1. The architecture of the immature myocardium is characterized by reduced contractile elements and smaller myocytes than adults. In addition, the fetal myocardium has a decreased sarcoplasmic reticulum and a poorly developed or absent T-tubule system as compared with adults. This results in a greater dependence on transsarcolemmal calcium influx for generation of contractile function and a greater susceptibility to the negative inotropic properties of anesthetic agents. The fetal tension-length curve is characterized by greater resting tension (impaired diastolic relaxation) and lower developed active tension (impaired systolic function and a propensity to develop afterload mismatch).

2. All systemic to pulmonary artery communications whether anatomical or surgical need to be controlled prior to initiation of CPB to prevent recirculation of CPB pump flow into the pulmonary circulation. In the presence of uncontrolled communications, some portion of CPB flow will go to the lungs and the left atrium. This will produce systemic hypoperfusion and distention of the nonbeating, unvented heart.

3. The most likely defect in this patient would be an endocardial cushion defect comprised of a primum atrial septal defect (ASD), an inlet ventricular septal defect (VSD), and a common AV valve. This is associated with a large left to right physiologic shunt (high Qp:Qs) and high pulmonary artery pressures. Eventually, this child would be at risk for development of elevated PVR due to pulmonary vascular occlusive disease with a gradual decrease in left to right shunting.

4. The Fontan procedure creates continuity between the IVC, the SVC, and the pulmonary artery. Following a Glenn shunt, Fontan physiology would be created by surgically creating continuity between the IVC and the pulmonary artery. Following a Fontan, all systemic venous blood is delivered to the pulmonary circulation. A fenestrated Fontan involves placing a 4 mm hole in the baffle of the tunnel connecting the SVC and IVC to the pulmonary artery. When the transpulmonary gradient (TPG) is high, transpulmonary blood flow and delivery of blood to the systemic atrium is low, resulting in a low cardiac output syndrome. In this circumstance, the fenestration permits systemic cardiac output to be maintained at the expense of systemic oxygen saturation by allowing a small right to left shunt at the atrial level with delivery of venous blood to the systemic atrium. These fenestrations are closed in the cardiac catheterization laboratory following hemodynamic evaluation with temporary balloon occlusion.

5. This child has outgrown her shunt and has erythrocytosis in response to chronic hypoxemia. Erythropheresis is effective in reversing the coagulation abnormalities associated with erythrocytosis and in reducing the risk of cerebrovascular accident. It is generally performed using either isotonic crystalloid solution or FFP. Systemic air embolism is a risk of this procedure.

6. A child with Wolff–Parkinson–White (WPW) syndrome is anesthetized for ablation of the re-entrant tract. Prior to commencing the procedure the patient's heart rate increases to 285. ST depression is evident. The cardiologist says not to worry – if the patient stays in the rhythm it will speed up the EPS mapping. What do you think? What would you do? What would you tell the cardiologist?

7. A 13-day-old child with Transposition of the Great Arteries/intact ventricular septum arrives in the hospital on Friday afternoon and is booked for repair on Saturday morning. The child is receiving Prostaglandin E1, is not intubated, and appears comfortable with a saturation of 89% on room air. When you question the cardiologist regarding the cost-effectiveness of operating on a weekend how do you defend your position? What is the likely concern of the cardiologist? Discuss involution of the ventricular mass of the physiological right ventricle postnatally. What is this due to? How rapidly does it occur, i.e., when does it become physiologically significant?

6. The patient needs to be either chemically or electrically cardioverted. This is an unstable rhythm that will likely deteriorate to ventricular fibrillation (VF).

7. The exact time frame of involution of LV mass is unknown but clinical experience suggests that the LV remains prepared to accommodate systemic afterload for 2–4 weeks following ductal closure in Transposition of the Great Arteries with Intact Ventricular Septum (TGA/IVS). The gradual postnatal decrease in pulmonary artery pressure following ductal closure and the subsequent reduction in LV afterload are responsible for this involution. The continued administration of PGE_1 places the child at risk for apnea and an ongoing volume requirement with accumulation of interstitial edema.

8. A 5-year-old male, S/P truncus arteriosus repair as a newborn, regularly followed by his cardiologist, but full details not available because he recently moved to the area, presents to the ER with an acute abdomen. The general surgeon suspects acute appendicitis and wants to proceed with surgery as soon as possible. What is a truncus arteriosus? What problems may develop as a result of the repair? How can you assess these clinically? What preoperative investigations are indicated?

8. Truncus arteriosus: The truncal valve (common aortic and pulmonary valve) may have more than three leaflets and may be dysplastic, with both stenosis and regurgitation. Definitive repair for truncus arteriosus involves: (1) VSD closure such that the truncal valve becomes the neoaortic valve and (2) creation of RV to PA continuity with a valved conduit. The most likely sequelae following repair of truncus arteriosus are conduit stenosis/insufficiency and truncal valve (neoaortic valve) insufficiency. Conduit dysfunction with significant RV dysfunction will be obvious on physical exam (enlarged liver, systemic venous hypertension, pleural effusions). Significant truncal valve dysfunction will have similar physical findings to aortic insufficiency or stenosis. A preoperative echocardiogram is warranted.

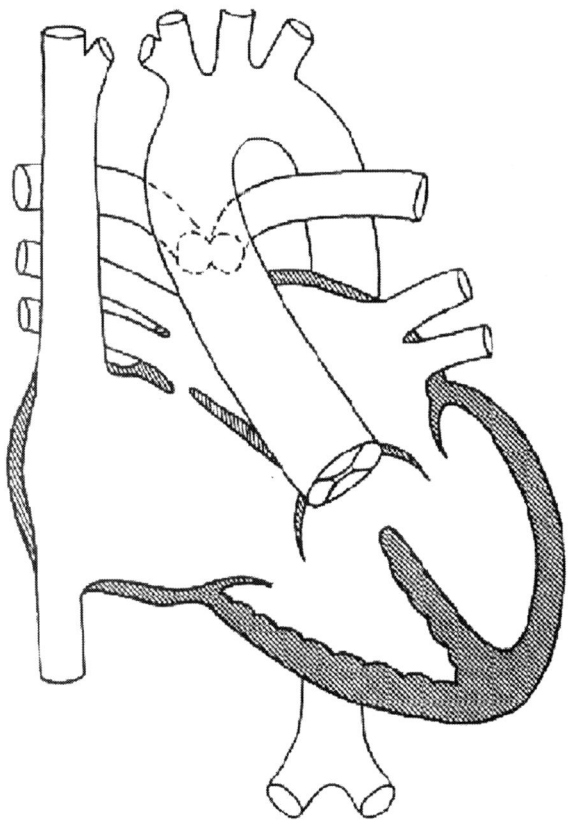

9. A 2-month-old with aortic stenosis/mitral stenosis, S/P stage one palliation (Norwood) with failure to thrive, is referred for placement of a gastrostomy tube. What is a Norwood operation? What do you understand by the term "parallel circulation?" What problems may arise after the Norwood operation? How can you assess these clinically? What investigations are indicated? How would you induce this patient? What monitoring would you use? What postoperative management would you recommend?

9. Single ventricle physiology is used to describe the situation wherein complete mixing of pulmonary venous and systemic venous blood occurs at the atrial or ventricular level and one ventricle then distributes output to both the systemic and pulmonary beds. As a result of this physiology the:

- Ventricular output is the sum of pulmonary blood flow (Q_p) and systemic blood flow (Q_s).
- Distribution of systemic and pulmonary blood flow is dependent on the relative resistances to flow (both intra and extra-cardiac) into the two parallel circuits.
- Oxygen saturations are the same in the aorta and the pulmonary artery.
- This physiology can exist in patients with one well-developed ventricle and one hypoplastic ventricle as well as in patients with two well-formed ventricles.
- Problems following the Norwood procedure include: RV dysfunction with TR, residual aortic arch obstruction, and inadequate pulmonary blood flow secondary to shunt stenosis or patient growth.

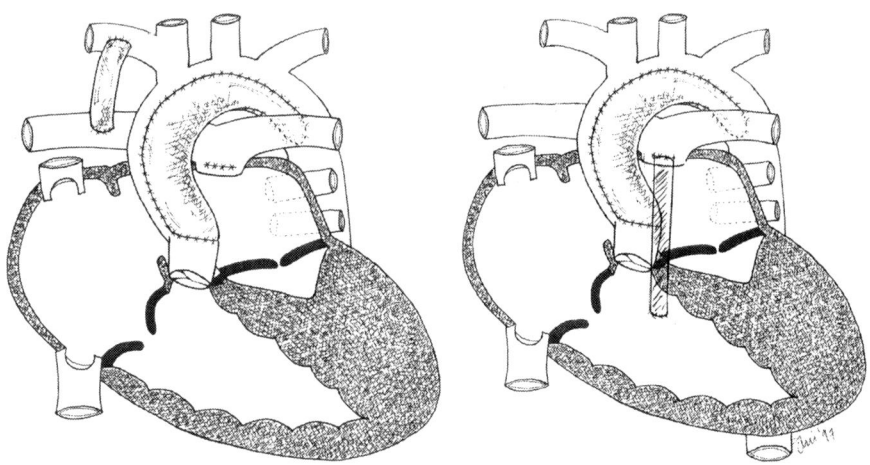

Norwood with BT shunt   Norwood with RV–PA conduit (Sano)

10. A 3-month-old with Shone's syndrome, S/P coarctation repair, has progressive inspiratory and expiratory stridor. He is in the emergency room with significant retraction and respiratory distress. He nevertheless has improved after a single dose of racemic epinephrine and now is monitored in the ICU. Saturation is 98% in humidified head box oxygen with soft biphasic stridor, but he is still tachypneic and is scheduled for direct laryngoscopy and bronchoscopy. What is Shone's syndrome? What is the etiology of the pulmonary hypertension? Describe your clinical evaluation. What might you find on the CXR? How would you induce this patient? Is an inhalational induction safe? Is it indicated for this procedure? What is the effect of airway obstruction on pulmonary artery pressure and cardiac output? How would you maintain anesthesia in this patient particularly as the ORL service wants to perform a functional examination to rule out tracheomalacia?

11. A 10-year-old with coarctation of the aorta is scheduled for repair by thoraco-tomy. Describe your clinical assessment of this patient. What preoperative investigations are important? How will they affect surgical management? Would you perform one lung anesthesia? What is the smallest double-lumen endotracheal tube available? What is the smallest patient you would consider a candidate for a double lumen endotracheal tube? Are there any alternatives? What are the possible complications during coarctation repair? What methods are you aware of for spinal cord protection? Which are proven effective? How do you manage hypertension during aortic cross clamping? How will you con-trol systemic hypertension during emergence from anesthesia?

10. Shone's complex, strictly defined, is the combination of supravalvular mitral ring and parachute mitral valve (mitral stenosis), subaortic stenosis, and coarctation of the aorta. Pulmonary hypertension is the direct result of left atrial (LA) hypertension that in turn is the consequence of obstruction to both LV inflow (mitral stenosis and LVH) and outflow. The CXR will show pulmonary edema if LA pressure is high. If the LA is very large there may be upward deviation of the left main stem bronchus. In the presence of pulmonary hypertension hypotension and tachycardiac must be avoided as RV ischemia will result; thus an inhalation induction is not recommended. These patients are very difficult to resuscitate. Without an atrial or ventricular level communication (ASD or VSD) elevations in PVR will reduce delivery of blood to the systemic ventricle and severe reductions in cardiac output will result. Dexmedetomidine in combination with a low concentration of an inhalation agent would be a suitable approach to functional bronchoscopy.

11. In patients presenting beyond infancy, upper extremity hypertension or a murmur is the most common presentation for coarctation of the aorta. The systolic murmur of a narrowed descending thoracic aorta may be best heard along the left paravertebral area between the spine and scapula. Continuous murmurs may be heard along the chest wall due to collateral vessels supplying tissues beyond the coarctation. These collaterals may originate from the internal thoracic, intercostals, subclavian, and/or scapular arteries. Other murmurs can be due to coexistent aortic valve stenosis and/or VSDs. In the setting of extensive collateral development it is not uncommon for even a severe coarctation to be completely asymptomatic. Symptoms when present include exercise intolerance, headache, chest pain, nosebleeds, and lower extremity claudication. There is an increased incidence (as high as 10%) of cerebral artery aneurysms. Similar abnormalities may occur in the spinal arteries. Intracranial hemorrhage or subarachnoid bleeds are a risk for these patients.

The smallest double lumen tube (DLT) is a 26 French with an external diameter similar to a 6.0 mm cuffed ETT. This DLT is appropriate for use in child 8–10 years old. Alternatives would be a bronchial blocker or a 3.5 or 4.5 Univent tube. There are no proven methods of spinal cord protection although mannitol administration and mild systemic hypothermia (34–35°C) are popular.

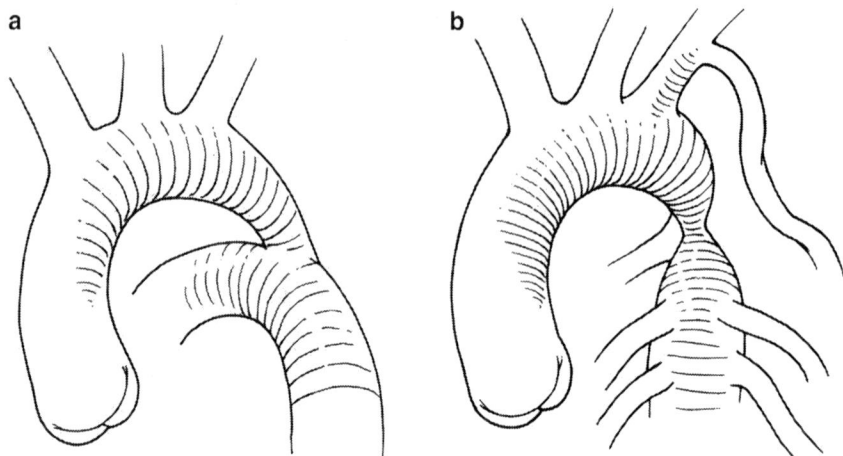

Typical appearances of coarctation of the aorta. (**a**) Coarctation associated with hypoplasia of the aortic isthmus and ductal-dependent perfusion of the descending aorta present at birth. Closure of the ductus arteriosus will likely result in LV afterload mismatch, compromise of somatic perfusion and oxygen delivery, and presentation in infancy. (**b**) Coarctation of the aorta in a patient who has tolerated ductal closure and developed extensive collateralization. Extensive fibrosis in the juxta-ductal region in association with growth of the native aorta has produced a discrete hourglass constriction. Presentation will be as a child or young adult.

General References

1. DiNardo JA (2008) Anesthesia for congenital heart disease. In: DiNardo JA, Zvara DA (eds) Anesthesia for cardiac surgery, 3rd edn. Blackwell Publishing, Oxford, pp 167–251
2. Kussman BD, DiNardo JA (2008) The cardiovascular system. In: Holzman RS, Mancuso TJ, Polander DM (eds) A practical approach to pediatric anesthesia. Lippincott Williams and Wilkins, Philadelphia, pp 306–374

Chapter 11
Gastrointestinal Disease

A 6-year-old, 14-kg girl, status/post repair of a tracheoesophageal fistula in infancy, is scheduled for a colon esophagus. In addition to her TE fistula, she had an imperforate anus and a tetralogy of Fallot, all repaired in infancy. She has intermittent wheezing and currently refluxes at night. She takes Protonix® daily and uses her Albuterol inhaler on a weekly basis. Vital signs are BP = 100/70 mmHg, P = 95 bpm, R = 16/min, T = 37°C. Her hemoglobin is 10.5 g/dL.

R.S. Holzman et al., *Pediatric Anesthesiology Review: Clinical Cases for Self-Assessment*,
DOI 10.1007/978-1-4419-1617-4_11, © Springer Science+Business Media, LLC 2010

Preoperative Evaluation

1. Of what significance is reflux in this patient? What additional information is important about the reflux? Is any additional chemoprophylaxis of her reflux necessary?

2. Of what importance is the history of tetralogy of Fallot? What additional information would you like? Is a preoperative ECG indicated? Any other tests indicated? Would an echocardiogram help?

Preoperative Evaluation

1. The diagnosis of gastroesophageal reflux (GER) is important in any patient coming to the OR. These patients may be a significant risk for aspiration of gastric contents or they may be at only slightly greater risk than children without the diagnosis. A detailed history will help clarify the severity of the GER. Once the clinical situation is known, a plan for induction of anesthesia can be developed [1]. Pantoprazole (Protonix®) suppresses secretion of gastric acid by inhibiting the gastric parietal cell hydrogen/potassium pump. It is used to treat erosive esophagitis associated with GER. Metoclopramide, which promotes gastric motility and accelerates gastric emptying, can be given IV prior to induction of anesthesia and may decrease the volume of the gastric contents. The onset of action of IV metoclopramide is 1–3 min. Drowsiness sometimes follows rapid IV administration and extrapyramidal symptoms are likely with larger doses. The usual antiemetic, antireflux dose is 0.1 mg/kg for children <6 years of age and 2.5–5 mg for 6–14 years of age.

2. The components of tetralogy of Fallot are right ventricular outflow obstruction (pulmonary stenosis), ventricular septal defect, overriding of the aorta onto the ventricular septum, and right ventricular hypertrophy [2]. The parents may not appreciate the important distinctions between palliation in the neonatal period followed by eventual repair of tetralogy of Fallot vs. complete repair in the newborn period. Palliation is intended to improve pulmonary blood flow. Generally, an aortic to pulmonary shunt is performed. The most common type of systemic to pulmonary connection done for these children is a Blalock–Taussig shunt. In this procedure, a 3–5 mm diameter Gore-Tex graft is used to create a side-to-side connection between a subclavian artery and the ipsilateral pulmonary artery. Later a complete repair is undertaken, with patch closure of the VSD, realignment of the aorta, and removal of the obstruction to pulmonary blood flow. The complete repair often involves a ventriculotomy but a transatrial–transpulmonary approach that avoids a ventricular incision is also done. Conduction disturbances are common postoperatively. The VSD is close to the AV node and bundle of His. Permanent complete heart block is unusual but other, less serious, conduction abnormalities can persist beyond the postop period. It is unlikely that cardiovascular function will be normal in children who have had congenital heart disease repaired in infancy and extremely unlikely if the CHD was palliated. An echocardiogram will give a good assessment of contractility as well as an indication of the degree of valvular insufficiency. The repair of the pulmonary outflow tract obstruction often leaves the pulmonary valve incompetent to varying degrees.

Intraoperative Course

1. What monitors will you choose? Where would you place the pulse oximeter probe? Why? What are the risks of central line placement in this patient? Would you place an arterial line?

2. The parents insist on having the patient fall asleep in their presence. Do you agree? How will you counsel them? Why? The surgeon wants to know what you think about a "single breath" sevoflurane induction. Do you agree? Why/why not?

3. What will be your primary anesthetic technique? Is nitrous oxide contraindicated? What is your choice of muscle relaxant?

Intraoperative Course

1. In addition to the usual ASA monitors, a foley catheter, an arterial, and a central line should be used. If the child had a previous Blalock–Taussig (BT) shunt, it is possible that the collateral flow around the shoulder to that arm could be insufficient to allow good oximeter function. In this case, another extremity should be chosen for the oximeter probe. With the surgical procedure planned, a colon-esophagus, there will be a large thoraco-abdominal incision generally on the left. Depending upon the level of the prior anastamosis, the surgeon may also have to enter the neck. Prior to insertion of a CVL in the neck, the surgical plan needs to be discussed with the surgeon. An internal jugular or subclavian line may be in the area prepped by the surgeons or possibly become kinked when the patient is positioned. A femoral venous line will be away from the surgery but will of necessity be quite long to have the tip of the catheter at the IVC right atrial junction. Care should be taken in assessing the adequacy of arterial circulation prior to cannulating a peripheral artery. The child will have had several arterial lines as part of her anesthetic and postoperative care for prior surgeries. Nevertheless, arterial access is important for this case, both for hemodynamic measurements and blood gas, electrolyte and hemoglobin measurement.

2. This child has gastroesophageal reflux (GER) at night. Although not an absolute contraindication to an inhalation induction, it certainly is a relative contraindication to one. It does not make medical sense to pull an anxious child from her parents and drag her into the OR. If the child is anxious, as expected, a premedication with an oral anxiolytic such as midazolam will help calm her. With forethought, EMLA could have been applied over a vein and a peripheral IV started in the preop holding area. Intravenous sedation/anxiolysis will very likely safely satisfy the parents' request that she fall asleep in their presence. If, after consideration of the risks and benefits, an inhalation induction were chosen, a single breath induction with sevoflurane would not be a good choice. Although much better tolerated than halothane, this vapor drug is still irritating to the airway and starting the induction by exposing the larynx to 8% could precipitate laryngospasm. A slow inhalation induction with sevoflurane using precautions against reflux could be done. The child could be kept seated upright, when unconscious mask ventilation, if needed, should be particularly gentle and done while using cricoid pressure.

3. Anesthesia can be maintained with inhaled or intravenous drugs or both. During the procedure, the right lung will be retracted away, necessitating the use of a high FiO_2. In addition, there will be manipulation of the bowel in this lengthy procedure, another relative contraindication to the use of nitrous oxide. The child likely has normal renal and hepatic function, making the choice of muscle relaxant easier. Histamine release should be avoided. The tachycardia that results from pancuronium, while not harmful per se, is not helpful. The procedure is rather lengthy so the use of an intermediate-acting nondepolarizing relaxant offers no advantages and a possible disadvantage since frequent dosing will be needed. Vecuronium has a good combination of characteristics for this patient for this case.

4. During surgery, the pulse oximeter reading drops from 99 to 82% and the inspiratory pressure increases from 25 to 45 cm H_2O. What might be going on?

5. The previous maneuvers are ineffective and the patient progresses to worsening saturations accompanied by bradycardia and widening of the QRS complex. What is your differential diagnosis? How would you confirm your leading diagnosis? What interventions would you make at this time?

Postoperative Course

1. Would you extubate deep to avoid emergence bronchospasm and/or laryngospasm? At the end of the surgery, during planned "awake" extubation, the bronchospasm recurs. Your management of the bronchospasm?

2. You are called to the PACU half an hour later to evaluate this patient's stridor. She is breathing 40 times per minute and retracting. How else will you evaluate the patient? What might be causing the stridor? How will you treat it? How would you decide to re-intubate this patient?

4. Increased inspiratory pressure accompanied by hypoxemia can have several causes in this case. The child could be wheezing, she could be resisting ventilation due to inadequate anesthesia, and could have inadequate neuromuscular blockade; there could be problems with the endotracheal tube and/or ventilator circuit. The FiO$_2$ should be increased to 1.0 and ventilation by hand begun while the surgical field is quickly scanned. The tracing on the capnograph can give useful information about the quality of ventilation. If Albuterol is administered, several puffs should be given since much of the drug will adhere to the inner walls of the endotracheal tube and not reach the lungs. It may be necessary for the surgeon to release the retracted lung to decrease the shunt and improve oxygenation.

5. The rhythm disturbance is due to the continued hypoxemia.

Postoperative Course

1. It is entirely possible that the best course for this case would be ventilation for the first postoperative night. Extubation could be considered after careful review of the intraoperative course of events, fluid and blood product administration, the length of the procedure, the extent of the surgical incision, and the plan for analgesia. If extubation is planned, an awake extubation offers a greater degree of safety. It is quite possible that the patient will have PONV and after a deep extubation, airway protection is absent until the child fully emerges from anesthesia. The time from the deep extubation to return of airway protection could be 10–15 min. Management of bronchospasm at this point is difficult. Albuterol should be administered through the endotracheal tube. IV lidocaine could be given. It is possible that the best course of action would be extubation. The wheezing is in response to the tracheal foreign body and once the OETT is removed, the child may no longer wheeze.

2. Stridor can occur during inspiration, exhalation, or both. The obstruction can be fixed, meaning the caliber of the airway does not change with breathing, or variable. Inspiratory stridor is due to extra-thoracic airway obstruction such as subglottic airway narrowing (croup) while expiratory stridor is due to an intrathoracic obstruction. In this case, the causes most likely are subglottic edema following intubation or vocal cord paresis as a result of surgical trauma. Although risk factors for the development of postintubation stridor (croup) have been identified, some patients with no obvious risk factor swill nevertheless exhibit this problem in the PACU [3].

Additional Topics

1. How do you preoperatively assess free water and electrolyte deficits in babies with gastrointestinal obstruction? How is a hypochloremic hypokalemic metabolic alkalosis generated? How do you calculate your therapy? How do you judge the efficacy of therapy? In what setting would hypertonic and hypernatremic dehydration present? What are the risks of treatment of this condition?

2. What is the pathognomonic radiographic finding in duodenal atresia? Are there any known syndrome associations? When do you expect this lesion to present? How do you expect it to present? Will there be bile-staining of the vomitus?

Additional Topics

1. Dehydration in children is generally divided into mild, moderate, and severe [4]. In mild dehydration, the child has lost approximately 5% of body weight and has a fluid deficit of 50 mL/kg and generally appears alert and thirsty, perhaps restless. Vital signs are normal, urine output is 1–2 mL/kg/h and specific gravity of the urine is approximately 1.020. In cases of moderate dehydration, the child has lost 10% of body weight and has a fluid deficit of 100 mL/kg. The heart rate is increased, pulse is weak, and the BP is low. An infant will be lethargic but arouseable and an older child will be thirsty and exhibit postural hypotension. Urine output will be <1 mL/kg/h with a specific gravity of 1.025–1.030. With severe dehydration, the child has lost 15% body weight and has a fluid deficit of 150 mL/kg. The child has the clinical appearance of shock. The heart rate is very high, and the pulse is very weak with accompanying tachypnea. The child is very lethargic or comatose and has cold clammy skin with very decreased turgor. Urine output is scanty with a specific gravity >1.030.

   With GI obstruction, the child vomits fluid, hydrogen and chloride, which leads to a hypochloremic metabolic acidosis. Although serum potassium levels may be normal, there is often total body potassium depletion. The alkalosis is worsened by the production of a paradoxical aciduria. This occurs for two reasons. Depletion of potassium results, in the distal tubule of the kidney, in the exchange of potassium for hydrogen. In the proximal tubule, when sodium is retained to maintain intravascular volume, the only anion present to accompany sodium is bicarbonate due to the severe chloride depletion.

   Hypertonic, hypernatremic dehydration can occur in Diabetes Insipidus, or severe diarrhea. In newborns and infants, excessive evaporative water losses can lead to hypernatremia. The hypertonic state itself can lead to CNS damage in the form of cerebral hemorrhages and subdural effusions. Correction of hypernatremic dehydration is quite difficult [5]. While the patient is hypertonic, the intracellular sodium content of the cells in the brain increases and intracellular idiogenic osmoles (taurine) raise the intracellular osmolality. If the extra cellular fluid osmolality decreases too rapidly, water accumulates in the cerebral cells resulting in cerebral edema. Seizures often occur either while the patient is hypernatremic or during treatment of hypernatremic dehydration.

2. Duodenal obstruction is most often due to atresia. Other causes of duodenal obstruction include stenosis, compression by an annular pancreas, or a web. The pathognomonic radiographic finding in duodenal atresia is the "double bubble" that is caused by the gas filled stomach and proximal duodenum. When the obstruction is complete, there is no gas distal to the double bubble. An important aspect of the clinical presentation of duodenal atresia is bilious vomiting on the first day of life. Associated problems seen in these patients are Down's syndrome with associated cardiac defects and low birth weight. Jejunoileal atresia is another cause of bilious vomiting in the newborn, often due to an in-utero mesenteric vascular accident. Affected newborns have abdominal distention and radiographs show distended loops of bowel.

3. What is the basic defect in prune belly syndrome? Why should this produce abnormalities of the abdominal wall? What are the respiratory implications of prune belly syndrome? If the patient's history was accompanied by polydipsia and polyuria, what would you consider in your review of systems? Why does congenital pulmonary hypoplasia occur with this syndrome? Are there any facial anomalies that you must consider for airway management?

3. The basic defect in Prune Belly syndrome (Eagle–Barrett syndrome) is likely severe urethral obstruction during fetal development. As a result of these problems, affected children come to the operating room for many procedures throughout their lives [6, 7]. The massive dilatation of the bladder leads to deficiency of the abdominal muscles and cryptorchidism. Oligohydramnios leads to pulmonary hypoplasia. If the patient reported polyuria and polydypsia it is possible that he had developed nephrogenic DI as a result of the in-utero urinary obstruction. Oligohydramnios can be associated with Potter syndrome: flat nose, epicanthal folds, low set ears, limb abnormalities and importantly for an anesthesiologist, a recessed chin [8]. Another source of respiratory difficulty these patients have is the inability to produce an effective cough as a result of absence of abdominal wall muscles.

Annotated References

1. Greenbaum, LA (2006) Fluids and electrolytes. In: Kliegman R, Marcdante K, Jenson H, Behrman RE (eds) Nelson essentials of pedaitrics. Elsevier Saunders, Philadelphia Section VII

    This section reviews, in addition to the referenced chapters on dehydration and disorders of sodium, maintenance fluid therapy, disorders of potassium, acid base disorders, and also parenteral nutrition. Tables summarize important concepts such as etiologies of the electrolyte and acid–base abnormalities mentioned above.

2. Greenbaum, L (2007) Pathophysiolgy of body fluids and fluid therapy. In: Kliegman RM, Jenson HB, Stanton BF, Behrman RE (eds) Nelson textbook of pediatrics, 18th edn. Elsevier Saunders, Philadelphia Sect. VI, pp 267–319

    The author here reviews in appropriate detail, the composition of body fluids in children, regulation of intravascular volume and osmolality, disorders of sodium, potassium, and acid base aberations.

3. Orenstein S, Peters J, Kahn S, Youssef N, Hussain S (2007) Gastroesophageal reflux disease (GERD). In: Kliegman RM, Jenson HB, Stanton BF, Behrman RE (eds) Nelson textbook of pediatrics, 18th edn. Chapter 320, pp 1547–1550

    This chapter reviews the epidemiology, pathophysiology, and clinical manifestations of GERD. Various diagnostic tests are discussed as well as general aspects of medical and surgical management. The chapter concludes with a discussion of the complications of GERD and mention of atypical clinical presentations of the condition.

References

1. Ng A, Smith G (2001) Gastroesophageal reflux and aspiration of gastric contents in anesthetic practice. Anesth Analg 93(2):494–513
2. Shinebourne EA, Babu-Narayan SV, Carvalho JS (2006) Tetralogy of Fallot: from fetus to adult. Heart 92(9):1353–1359
3. Koka BV, Jeon IS, Andre JM, MacKay I, Smith RM (1977) Postintubation croup in children. Anesth Analg 56(4):501–505
4. Greenbaum L (2006) Fluids and electrolytes. In: MK KRM, Jenson HB, Behrman RE (eds) Nelson essentials of pediatrics, 5th edn. Elsevier/Saunders, Philadelphia, pp 160–165
5. Greenbaum L (2006) Disorders of sodium. In: MK KRM, Jenson HB, Behrman RE (eds) Nelson essentials of pediatrics, 5th edn. Elsevier Saunders, Philadelphia
6. Denes FT, Arap MA, Giron AM, Silva FA, Arap S (2004) Comprehensive surgical treatment of prune belly syndrome: 17 years' experience with 32 patients. Urology 64(4):789–793, discussion 793–4
7. Fusaro F, Zanon GF, Ferreli AM et al (2004) Renal transplantation in prune-belly syndrome. Transpl Int 17(9):549–552
8. Baris S, Karakaya D, Ustun E, Tur A, Rizalar R (2001) Complicated airway management in a child with prune-belly syndrome. Paediatr Anaesth 11(4):501–504

Chapter 12
Renal

A 3-month-old male, 4.2 kg with chronic obstructive nephropathy as a result of bilateral megaureter presents for megaureter repair and bilateral ureteral reimplant. His hematocrit is 29%, with electrolytes $Na^+ = 132$ meq/dL, $K^+ = 4.0$ meq/dL, $Cl^- = 103$ meq/dL, $HCO3^- = 19$ meq/dL, BUN = 8 mg%, and Cr = 1.7 mg%. He is on sulfamethoxazole/trimethoprim once a day. Heart rate is 110 bpm, BP 110/70 mmHg, and RR 20/min.

R.S. Holzman et al., *Pediatric Anesthesiology Review: Clinical Cases for Self-Assessment,*   301
DOI 10.1007/978-1-4419-1617-4_12, © Springer Science+Business Media, LLC 2010

Preoperative Evaluation

1. Why is this patient hyponatremic? Why? What does this have to do with the obstructive uropathy? Why is the HCO_3 low? Will this patient's urine be concentrated, dilute, or isosthenuric? Is a hematocrit of 29% normal? What is the GFR of a 3-month old with a creatinine of 1.7? Is renal function normal at 3 months of age?

2. Cardiovascular findings in renal failure. Is this patient hypertensive? Why? How is this mediated in this patient? How will you assess this patient's volume status?

3. Antibiotic prophylaxis. Why is this patient on antibiotics? Is prophylaxis effective? Would infection make this problem worse? How so? Any particular implications for your anesthetic management?

Preoperative Evaluation

1. This child has chronic obstructive nephropathy, which is associated with renal salt wasting. Obstructive uropathy causes distension, ischemia, and necrosis of the renal tubules and glomeruli. Obstructive uropathy also produces hydronephrosis, urine stasis, and recurrent urinary tract infection, which in turns causes necrosis and scaring of the renal tubules and eventually the glomeruli. The plasma bicarbonate is low due to acidemia. In chronic renal failure the total renal tubular mass is reduced and the kidney is unable to excrete adequate hydrogen ions in the distal tubule. This patient's urine will be dilute because of failure of the tubules to concentrate the urine leading to both salt and water wasting. The hematocrit is low for age probably due to reduction in erythropoietin production by the kidneys. The GFR at 3 months is much lower than normal for age if the plasma creatinine is 1.7 mg/dL. After the first month of life the plasma creatinine is expected to be approximately 0.6 mg/dL or lower when GFR function is normal at 3 months of age. A rough estimation of GFR can be calculated as follows: GFR (mL/min/1.73 $M^2 = 0.55 \times$ length(cm)/plasma creatinine). Renal function, as measured by GFR, approaches adult renal function by the end of the first month of life.

2. This patient is hypertensive. The expected blood pressure at this age is 80/45. The increased level of angiotensin II is a potent systemic vasoconstrictor. It is mediated through primary activation of renin–angiotensin–aldosterone system and/or depletion of the extracellular fluid due to salt and water wasting. The best way to assess hydration status in patients with renal failure is by examination for clinical signs of dehydration such as weight loss greater than 3% of body weight, increased thirst, a dry mouth and tongue, increased heart rate, fast breathing and cool extremities, sluggish capillary refill longer than 2 s, impaired skin turgor, and sunken eyes and/or fontanel.

3. This patient is on antibiotics because patients with obstructive uropathy have urinary stasis and are at risk for urinary tract infection. The use of prophylactic antibiotics is effective for the prevention of recurrent UTI prior to definitive surgical treatment. Chronic kidney infection can worsen obstructive uropathy, hydronephrosis and cause kidney damage because of the chronic inflammation of the glomeruli and tubules resulting in scarring. If the infection is not controlled preoperatively it may spread in to the bloodstream causing bacteremia and septic shock under general anesthesia or in the immediate postoperative period.

Intraoperative

1. Does this patient need an arterial line? Is the intravascular volume normal? Would a central venous line be helpful?

2. How will you induce this patient? Why? What metabolic and electrolyte effects will this patient experience if there is laryngospasm on induction, and the patient desaturates, and in the meantime, the end-tidal CO_2 increases to 65 mmHg? Are these of significance to your anesthetic management?

3. Which muscle relaxant will you choose? Why? What if there is laryngospasm prior to starting the IV? Is there a problem using succinylcholine? What if the K^+ was 5.0, 5.5 or 6.0 meq/L? Is muscle relaxant use influenced by the presence of renal failure? How so?

4. Is a regional anesthetic indicated for perioperative pain management? Specifically how and where would you place the catheter? Is coagulopathy a significant concern? Which drugs would you dose the epidural with? Why? Are your considerations any different with regard to the patient's underlying problems?

Intraoperative

1. This patient does need an arterial line but not a central line for reasons discussed below. His intravascular volume might be normal.

2. I will induce general anesthesia with intravenous anesthetics because of the elevated serum potassium and metabolic acidosis that can be aggravated by hypoventilation and respiratory acidosis or laryngospasm. Laryngospasm in this patient can produce severe metabolic and respiratory acidosis, acute hyperkalemia, cardiac arrhythmias, and even cardiac arrest. The outcome of cardiac arrest in the presence of severe acidosis is poor and resuscitation drugs such as epinephrine and other catecholamines may not be as effective.

3. I will use cisatracurium because its elimination is not dependent on renal clearance. If laryngospasm occurs I will use intramuscular succinylcholine to treat the laryngospasm. There is a risk of using succinylcholine because it can increase the serum potassium by 0.5–1 meq/mL acutely in the presence of a normal serum potassium. A higher baseline serum potassium will predispose to the hyperkalemia that may ensue after the administration of succinylcholine. A high serum potassium in chronic renal failure reflects severe renal failure, more severe metabolic acidosis and a greater potential for exaggerated hyperkalemia.

4. The use of combined epidural and general anesthesia may improve intraoperative pain control, reduce the need for intravenous opioids and inhaled anesthetic agents and facilitate immediate postoperative tracheal extubation. I will place the epidural catheter after the induction of general anesthesia at an upper lumbar or lower thoracic spinal interspace and advance the catheter tip to approximately T10. The presence of coagulopathy, particularly platelet dysfunction related to renal failure, and the use of heparin postoperatively are major concerns for the use of regional anesthesia in chronic renal failure patients. I will use a combination of bupivacaine and fentanyl or morphine infusion because fentanyl is primarily metabolized in the liver. Bupivacaine and morphine are metabolized in the liver; however, the amount of morphine used for epidural analgesia is smaller and the resulting active metabolites are lower than for parenteral morphine use. The low quantities of metabolites of both morphine and bupivacaine are of little concern in patients with CRF with mild-to-moderate, stable, reduced renal function. If the CRF is moderate-severe with abnormalities of coagulation I will avoid epidural analgesia.

Emergence

1. The anesthetic vapor has been off for 30 min, the ET agent concentration is 0, and the patient is completely unarouseable. You have just looked at the pupils following waiting in the OR for half an hour after the case is over, and the pupils are fixed and dilated. What is your differential? Approach? Concerns?

Additional Questions

1. What is the role of the kidney in vitamin D metabolism? Calcitonin metabolism? Parathormone metabolism? Why is this more of a problem in children than adults?

2. Nephrotic syndrome. A 2-year old with nephrotic syndrome is scheduled for ultrasound-guided kidney biopsy. What is the basic ultrastructural lesion? How does this account for the manifestations of the disease? What are the anesthetic implications? Is albumin administration of any help?

Emergence

1. My differential diagnoses are total spinal anesthesia, cerebral edema, intracranial hypertension from a space-occupying lesion such as a subdural or intracranial bleed, cerebral stroke, brain stem ischemia/anoxia, or drug-induced effects, e.g., anticholinergics and sympathomimetics. If the condition does not resolve within the expected duration of total spinal anesthesia and drug-induced pupillary dilation is ruled out, neurology consultation is obtained and brain MRI and/or EEG is considered. The major concern is brain edema, brain stem ischemia/anoxia, or an intracranial space-occupying lesion that may need immediate neurosurgical intervention.

Additional Questions

1. The kidney synthesizes calcitriol, the most active metabolite of Vitamin D, which is the rate-limiting factor in promoting intestinal absorption of calcium. Impaired calcium absorption from the gut will result in bone demineralization. Calcitonin hormone antagonizes the effect of parathormone by reducing the tubular reabsorption of calcium and phosphate and inhibition of osteoclast activity. In CRF as the GFR deteriorates, phosphate excretion is reduced and hyperphosphatemia stimulates the release of parathormone, which in turn will mobilize the calcium and phosphate from the bone to maintain normal serum calcium at the expense of bone demineralization. Renal osteodystrophy during skeletal growth in childhood can result in significant skeletal growth failure, fractures, and deformities as opposed to skeletal demineralization of the fully matured skeletal system in adulthood.

2. The basic ultrastructural lesion on biopsy is absence of glomerular inflammation and the active sediments. On electron micrographs the glomerular basement membrane appears normal, there are no immune deposits and characteristic widespread fusion of the epithelial cell foot processes. Focal glomerulosclerosis is seen in some patients. There is abnormally increased permeability of the glomerular basement membrane filtration of large particles including serum albumin which results in proteinuria of greater than 50 mg/kg/day (hypoalbuminemia with serum albumin less than 3 g/dL) and water and salt retention. Clinically, patients present with fluid and salt retention manifested as generalized edema, pleural effusion, irritability, fatigue, and hypertension. The anesthetic implications in these patients are increased total body fluid by 3–5% or higher, pleural effusion, pericardial effusion, hypertension, reduced cardiac output due to fluid overload and hypertension, impaired renal function, potential for cerebral edema due to reduced or absent cerebral autoregulation with volatile anesthetics. Nitrous oxide could cause hypertension by activation of the podocyte receptors. The administration of albumin may not be of help in these patients because it will be filtered out in urine by the impaired glomeruli but it can be harmful if an acute rise in oncotic pressure expands the intravascular volume potentially leading to acute heart failure and cerebral or pulmonary edema.

3. What is the difference between distal and proximal renal tubular acidosis?

4. How are the lungs compromised in the prune belly syndrome? Why is this so?

3. The difference between the two types of renal tubular acidosis is that in proximal tubular acidosis the tubules fail to reabsorb bicarbonate resulting in bicarbonate wasting. In distal tubular acidosis, the renal tubules fail to filter or excrete hydrogen ion and acids in urine resulting in systemic acid load accumulation.

4. In patients with prune belly syndrome, the lungs are hypoplastic and fail to expand and development because of oligohydramnios during early fetal development. Oligohydramnios results from inadequate urine production by the hypoplastic kidneys. In addition, oligohydramnios causes mechanical compression of the chest wall causing deformities and a restrictive chest wall disorder.

General References

1. Roth KS, Koo HP, Spottswood SE, Chan JC (2002) Obstructive uropathy: an important cause of chronic renal failure in children. Clin Pediatr (Phila) 41:309–314
2. Laing CM, Toye AM, Capasso G, Unwin RJ (2005) Renal tubular acidosis: developments in our understanding of the molecular basis. Int J Biochem Cell Biol 37:1151–1161
3. Salusky IB, Kuizon BG, Juppner H (2004) Special aspects of renal osteodystrophy in children. Semin Nephrol 24:69–77
4. D'Addessi A, Bongiovanni L, Racioppi M, Sacco E, Bassi P (2008) Is extracorporeal shock wave lithotripsy in pediatrics a safe procedure? J Pediatr Surg 43:591–596
5. Sanchez CP (2008) Mineral metabolism and bone abnormalities in children with chronic renal failure. Rev Endocr Metab Disord 9:131–137
6. Holder JP (1989) Pathophysiologic and anesthetic correlations of the prune-belly syndrome. AANA J 57:137–141
7. Donckerwolcke R, Yang WN, Chan JC (1989) Growth failure in children with renal tubular acidosis. Semin Nephrol 9:72–74
8. Martinez JR, Grantham JJ (1995) Polycystic kidney disease: etiology, pathogenesis, and treatment. Dis Mon 41:693–765
9. Kemper MJ, Harps E, Muller-Wiefel DE (1996) Hyperkalemia: therapeutic options in acute and chronic renal failure. Clin Nephrol 46:67–69

Chapter 13
Genitourinary System

A baby in the first day of life presents for closure of an exstrophy of the bladder. The product of a 36-week gestation, he is 2.3 kg, preop hematocrit 56%, BP 65/35 mmHg, HR 130 bpm, and RR 24/min.

R.S. Holzman et al., *Pediatric Anesthesiology Review: Clinical Cases for Self-Assessment*, DOI 10.1007/978-1-4419-1617-4_13, © Springer Science+Business Media, LLC 2010

Preoperative Evaluation

1. Is this baby premature?

    (a) How can you differentiate premature from small for gestational age (SGA) babies?

    (b) What difference would it make in your anesthetic technique?

    (c) What problems would you expect related to prematurity?

Preoperative Evaluation

1. Yes, this baby is premature because he was born before 37 weeks gestational age. Infants born between 36 and 37 gestational age are categorized as borderline premature. Those born between 31 and 36 weeks GA are considered moderately premature and those born between 24 and 30 weeks gestation are considered severely premature.

    (a) Small gestational age (SGA) babies have a body weight less than 2.5 kg whereas the babies with normal gestational age have body weight of 2.5 kg or greater at birth.

    (b) The more premature infants are the greater the risk for perioperative complications.

    (c) Premature babies are born with underdeveloped vital organs, structurally and functionally, therefore, are at increased risk for morbidity and mortality for the following reasons:

        1. These neonates are unable to maintain body temperature due to labile thermoregulation. Hypothermia increases the metabolic rate linearly between 28 and 36°C and increases oxygen consumption leading to hypoxemia, acidosis, apnea, and respiratory depression and an increased mortality rate. Exposure to cold may aggravate the physiological rise in the metabolic rate that normally occurs during the first 2 weeks of life; a minimum metabolic rate of 4 mL/kg/min on the first day of life to 8 mL/kg/min on the 14th postnatal day. Unlike older infants, premature infants tend to lose body heat at a faster rate because of higher body surface/volume ratio and lack of insulating fat. Heat stress is equally detrimental because premature infants are unable to sweat (dissipate heat by evaporative heat loss) and body heating causes dilation of peripheral vessels, passive evaporative water loss which is inversely related to body size and dehydration. Therefore, during anesthesia, an infant's body and head should be covered with plastic or cotton wrap to avoid heat and water loss. Inspired anesthetic vapors and gases should be warm (34–37°C) and humidified (preferably 100%).

        2. Infants are unable to sustain ventilation due to poorly developed ventilatory centers in the brainstem and inefficient respiratory mechanics.

        3. Infants are at risk for respiratory distress syndrome, due to impaired availability or lack of surfactant.

        4. Infants may develop intraventricular hemorrhage from high blood pressure or cerebral ischemia from hypoperfusion due to impaired cerebral autoregulation.

        5. Infants are at risk for left to right shunting via the patent ductus arteriosus soon after birth (within 3–5 days after birth) due to less musculature in the pulmonary arteries and low pulmonary compliance leading to pulmonary hyperperfusion and congestive heart failure.

2. Should a regional anesthetic be utilized?

3. Would you use narcotics? Why/why not?

4. Would you hope to extubate this baby at the end of surgery?

5. Is it common for bladder exstrophy to occur in males?

    (a) What do we call bladder exstrophy in a female?
    (b) Why does this happen?

    (c) Are there any future problems the patient can expect?
    (d) Is early closure better than later closure? Why/why not?

    (e) Is it likely that there is more surgery in the future for this baby? What type? Why?

6. Premature infants born before 34 weeks gestational age have a decreased glomerular filtration rate (GFR). Even term neonates have only 40% of the adult GFR, resulting in decreased tubular reabsorption capacity, an inability to absorb water, salts, glucose, protein, phosphate, and bicarbonate. Glucosuria can act as an osmotic diuretic and cause sodium and water loss.

7. Hepatic catalyzing enzymes are less active in premature infants. Oxidizing, reducing, and hydrolyzing enzymes are relatively inactive. Conjugation enzymes (conjugation with acetate, gylcine, sulfate, and glucuronic acid) are also less active except for sulfonation. Therefore, the metabolism of various drugs, particularly opioids, can be impaired. These enzymes mature to adult capacity within 6–12 months.

2. Yes, whenever feasible to minimize the need for opioid analgesia.

3. Narcotics could be used with caution, in reduced doses, and the infant's respiration monitored closely in a high dependency (neonatal intensive care unit) environment.

4. Yes, if successful epidural analgesia is attained and minimal or no narcotics are administered intraoperatively.

5. Yes, male:female ratio is 2:1.
   (a) Cloaca.
   (b) At 5–6 weeks of gestation, the cloacal membrane prevents normal migration of mesoderm (germ layer of anterior abdominal muscles and pelvic bones) of the infraumbilical area resulting in failure of fusion of recti muscles and the pubic symphysis. As a result the urethra fails to close dorsally (epispadias) and bladder's anterior wall may remain open. Urinary tract is everted exteriorly.
   (c) Yes, bladder exstrophy can cause incontinence and sexual dysfunction.
   (d) Early closure (within 24–48 h of life) of the bladder and abdomen is better to achieve an optimal anatomical and functional outcome.
   (e) Yes, this child will require further reconstructive surgeries to correct epispadius at age 2–3 years and urinary continence (bladder neck) by age 4–5 years. Other possible procedures include bladder augmentation if the bladder is of small capacity, ureteral reimplantation for ureteral reflux, and creation of a Mitrofanoff stoma.

Intraoperative Course

1. Monitoring:

   (a) Does this baby need an arterial line? Why/why not?
   (b) Should a central line be placed?
   (c) Where would you place the IVs? Why?
   (d) You can only get an IV in the foot – what next?

   (e) If the case will take 8 h, do you need to obtain surveillance blood gases? Why/why not?

   (f) Would you treat if the pH was 7.34? 7.22? 7.14? Why?

2. Intraoperative management:

   (a) Can you do this case with an epidural or caudal catheter and sedation? Would you choose to do so? Why/why not?

   (b) A general anesthetic with an endotracheal tube is chosen. Would you place an oral or a nasal tube? Why?
   (c) Should narcotics be avoided? Which would you choose? Why/why not?

   (d) What about muscle relaxants? (Surgeon wants you to avoid them; why do you think?)
   (e) Is nitrous oxide contraindicated? Relatively contraindicated?
   (f) What problems might you expect?
   (g) When would you expect them?

3. Intraoperative positioning:

   (a) The surgeon has turned the baby *prone* to do bilateral iliac osteotomies. The saturation drops to 94% and the end-tidal CO_2 has disappeared from the screen.
   (b) What do you think is going on?
   (c) The Dinamap is not reading, but recycling. The ECG heart rate is 110 bpm then it becomes 80 bpm. What is Durant's maneuver?
   (d) Should the baby be placed in the left or right lateral decubitus position?

Intraoperative Course

1. (a) The arterial line is necessary if the surgery is expected to be prolonged and involves blood loss and extensive third space losses.

   (b) A central line for this procedure is not necessary.

   (c & d) I will place intravenous canulae in the upper extremities if possible. The lower extremities are usually unavailable for IV access and prepared and draped within the surgical field. A disadvantage of placing the IV in the lower extremity is the potential for loss of infusate from iliac veins within the surgical field. Other options include venous cutdown of the upper extremities or a central line.

   (e) Yes, ABG surveillance could be helpful for long surgical procedures to accurately monitor blood pressure, blood loss and large fluid shifts and their biochemical effects as well as the adequacy of ventilation and oxygenation.

   (f) I would treat a pH less than 7.22 because it is below two standard deviations (7.37 ± 0.03) for age and is associated with deleterious acidosis.

2. Intraoperative management:

   (a) No, because the use of surgical concentrations of local anesthetics in premature infants could result in systemic toxicity. The hepatic enzymes that metabolize amide and ester local anesthetics are immature and elimination of these local anesthetics is prolonged, exposing the newborn infants to potential CNS and cardiovascular toxicity. The use of sedatives is not advisable because they can depress the immature brainstem in these infants leading to hypoventilation, periodic breathing, and even apnea.

   (b) I will use a nasal tube because it is secured better than an oral tube and is more comfortable for the infant who requires postoperative ventilation support.

   (c) No, narcotics should not be avoided. I would choose fentanyl because it is metabolized effectively by mixed enzyme oxidase enzymes which are active in early infancy.

   (d) The surgeon might request avoiding muscle relaxants if he/she is contemplating stimulation of the perianal sphincter or identification of major nerves.

   (e) Not absolutely contraindicated; probably relatively contraindicated.

   (f) Nitrous oxide is not contraindicated; however, its use during long surgical procedures may result in accumulation in the bowel causing distension and can be problematic if an ostomy is planned.

3. Intraoperative positioning:

   (a & b) Most likely cause could be air entrainment and air embolism but also could be due to endotracheal tube occlusion, dislodgement, or severe hypotension.

   (c & d) I suspect significant air embolism and hypoperfusion of the lungs. Positioning the patient in steep head down and left lateral decubitus (Durant's maneuver) will allow buoyant foam to remain in the right ventricle and prevent it from occluding the pulmonary arteries.

Postoperative Course

1. Tracheal extubation:

    (a) Should this patient be extubated? What criteria would you use?

    (b) The patient is vigorous, and you extubate, but the saturation is 92% on supplemental O_2 by face shield? Your next move?
    (c) Facemask fails to improve saturation; would you be happy with 93%?

    (d) What if it was 91%? Should patient be reintubated?
    (e) For a respiratory rate of 24/min? 34/min? 54/min? What could be going on to account for the findings?
    (f) How would you manage V/Q mismatch at this time?

2. Postoperative pain management:

    (a) How would you manage a continuous morphine infusion for pain relief?

    (b) How would you constitute the epidural solution? With fentanyl or Dilaudid? Why?

    (c) A colleague stops by as you are putting in the epidural needle, and says that he always gets a spine film in babies with bladder exstrophy because he is worried about what? Is he right?
    (d) What difference would it make in your anesthetic management?
    (e) Could you place a continuous caudal catheter instead? Or would you just stay away from the back?

Additional Questions

1. How does the presence of chronic renal failure influence your choice and use of volatile anesthetic agents?

Postoperative Course

1. (a) Yes, this patient should be extubated if awake, exhibiting adequate strength (lifting heels for 5 s, tight fists, strong bite, furrowing the forehead/supraorbital muscles), the muscle relaxant is reversed (return of train-of-four and no fade at 50 Hz for 5-s tetanus), breathing regularly, and has an empty stomach.
   (b) Provide 100% oxygen with a facemask and monitor for periodic breathing and apnea.
   (c) If the infant maintains adequate, regular breathing with a saturation of 93%, then that would be acceptable.
   (d) If the saturation was 91% then I will consider intubating the trachea.
   (e) A low respiratory rate of 24 bpm may indicate impending respiratory depression due to hypoxemia and hypercarbia.
   (f) The V/Q mismatch can be corrected by controlled ventilation after re-intubation of the trachea.

2. Postoperative pain management:
   (a) I will start the morphine infusion at 10 mcg/kg/h after intubation or 5–8 mcg/kg/h in a nonintubated, spontaneously breathing infant.
   (b) I would avoid the use of opioids in epidural solutions for newborn infants. If the infant is intubated, I will use a solution of bupivacaine 0.1% with fentanyl 1 mcg/mL, or chloroprocaine 1.5% if the infant is extubated and spontaneously breathing. If the infant is extubated it is prudent to avoid neuraxial opioids in order to avoid the potential for inducing periodic breathing and central apnea. I will avoid the use of hydromorphone because of the very high risk of apnea in newborn infants and the absence of data on its use.
   (c) He might be worried about possible associated vertebral anomalies because of the high incidence of spinal vertebral anomalies and possible tethering of the spinal cord that may increase the risk of spinal cord injury.
   (d & e) I will review the neuroimaging of the spine and if there are no vertebral or spinal cord anomalies I will place a caudal catheter.

Additional Questions

1. My first choice is desflurane because it is the least fluorinated volatile agent and extremely resistant to defluorination. Ingoranic fluoride accumulation from metabolism of fluorinated volatile agents can cause direct nephrotoxicity. My second choice is isoflurane because its metabolism is not associated with clinically significant release of inorganic fluoride even when used for MAC sedation in the pediatric ICU for few days.

2. Patient with neuroblastoma:

   (a) What is the difference between neuroblastoma and nephroblastoma (Wilms tumor)?

   (b) Any other syndromes associated with neuroblastoma?

   (c) Can both be endocrinologically active?

   (d) What is the difference between a ganglioneuroma and a neuroblastoma?

   (e) What makes a neonatal Wilms tumor (congenital mesoblastic nephroma) different from a regular Wilms tumor?

3. "Infantile" polycystic kidney disease:

   (a) What is the natural history of "infantile" polycystic kidney disease?

   (b) How does it affect anesthetic management?

   (c) What are the nonrenal considerations for perinatal form?

4. A 4-year old post repair of exstrophy of the bladder in infancy and a subsequent ureteral reimplant has a ureteral stone at the ureteropelvic junction of the implanted ureter. The surgeons and radiologists would like to use the extracorporeal lithotripter, but need your help for the patient to be motionless.

   (a) What are the issues?

   (b) What kinds of lithotripter devices are currently used?

   (c) What problems can you expect postoperatively relative to the use of a lithotripter?

   (d) The PACU nurses call you for blood in the urine; your response?

2. (a) Neuroblastoma is a malignancy that arises from primitive blast cells of the postganglionic sympathetic chain and suprarenal adrenal glands, whereas nephroblastoma (Wilms Tumor) is a malignancy that arises from anomalous metanephric differentiation of renal blastema (undifferentiated renal cells).

   (b) Neuroblastoma can be associated with pheochromocytoma and von Recklinghausen disease which is a neurofibromatosis disease. About 75% of neuroblastomas secrete catecholamines. Wilms tumors can also secrete catecholamines as well as renin.

   (c) Ganglioneuroma is a benign tumor arising from well-differentiated and mature sympathetic ganglia.

   (d) Neonatal Wilms tumor is a benign nephroma arising from metanephric blastema or secondary mesenchyme whereas regular Wilms tumor (nephroblastoma) is a malignant tumor of the undifferentiated metanephric blastema.

3. (a) Infantile polycystic kidney disease varies in severity. When oligohydramnios presents early in pregnancy the outlook is extremely poor due to associated pulmonary hypoplasia in addition to renal insufficiency. The condition sometimes presents later in infancy with reduced renal function. It may not become manifest until adolescence, when it represents a milder expression of disease.

   (b) The extent of pulmonary hypoplasia determines the difficulty of ventilation. The degree of renal impairment determines the clearance of anesthetic agents' metabolites.

   (c) Obstetricians may consider cesarean section, particularly in bilateral disease, because of a large body size and the risk of renal rupture during vaginal delivery. The newborn may require control of ventilation and treatment of high blood pressure.

4. (a) The primary issue is the positioning of the patient and the requirement for motionlessness, as well as the pain involved in the procedure.

   (b) There are several shock wave generator devices that include piezoelectric, electromagnetic, electrohydraulic and microexplosive sources.

   (c) The use of the lithotripter results in less postoperative pain than an open
   &   surgical procedure. The piezoelectric source is commonly used because it
   (d) delivers low energy and focused shock waves and does not require a water bath. The patient can be placed on a multifunction table to allow performance of other procedures such as cystoscopy, placement of stents etc.

(e) The PACU nurses call you half an hour later because the patient says his chest hurts when he breathes; your response?

(f) The nurses call from the floor at 1:00 AM because the patient complains of intense belly pain that is like a spear going through her; they would like your narcotic order. Your response?

(g) What if it hurt her belly every time she breathed? What if her serum amylase was 1,200? 3,000?

5.Chronic renal failure:

What is likely to be occurring at the membrane level in this patient with chronic renal failure?

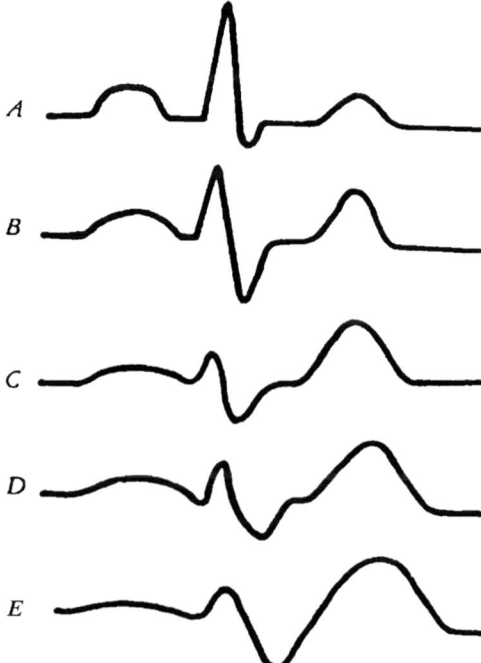

The passage of shock wave energy through body tissues produces little damage and depends on the amount of energy to which the tissues are exposed. Hematuria is expected in most patients even to the point of acute anemia. Other potential adverse effects are abdominal pain and distention, nausea and vomiting due to punctate hemorrhage of the stomach and gastrointestinal tract. Hemoptysis and respiratory distress may also occur due to rupture of alveoli as a result of shock wave energy dissipation at the air-water interface within alveoli. Cardiac arrhythmias occur in a small percentage of patients either due to lack of synchronization of the shock energy with the refractory period of the cardiac cycle. The mechanism of arrhythmias is presumably due to mechanical stress of the shock energy on the conduction system.

(e) Lithotripter shock waves may damage cortico-medullary tissue and cause flank pain. If the pain primarily involves the chest, I would administer oxygen via mask, auscultate breath sounds for rales, crepitation and a focal decrease in breath sounds, If these findings are present I will obtain a chest X-ray to exclude large areas of alveolar hemorrhage.

(f & g) Prior to the administration of narcotics I will examine the patient's abdomen for distention and auscultate for bowel sounds; lithotripter shock wave energy can, although rarely, cause hemorrhage and perforation of the stomach and intestine. The potential for retroperitoneal organ damage such as pancreas is also possible.

5. (a) Normal appearing depolarization, repolarization and conduction tracing on ECG.
   (b) Tall peaked T-wave "tenting," depressed ST-segment and widening of the QRS wave as a result of hyperkalemia progression.
   (c) Further widening of QRS wave and loss of depolarization potentials. Usually occurs with serum potassium of 8 mEq/L or greater.
   (d) Hyperpolarization, further widening of QRS wave and pending ventricular standstill.
   (e) Loss of depolarization and merging of QST and T-waves to form the so called "sine wave" and impending ventricular fibrillation or standstill.

6. You wish to perform a peripheral nerve block for hypospadias repair. Which nerves do you wish to block, and what anatomic structures will your needle pass through on the way to those nerves?

6. Penile tissues are innervated by the dorsal penile nerve (S 2,3,4) and perineal cutaneous nerve at the root of the penis. The dorsal penile nerve is best reached at the base of penis shaft from the dorsal surface. The needle has to traverse the skin, subcutaneous tissue, and Buck's fascia.

General References

1. Messeri A, Romiti M, Andreuccetti T, Busoni P (1995) Continuous epidural block for pain control in bladder exstrophy: report of a case and description of technique. Paediatr Anaesth 5:229–232
2. Kain ZN, Shamberger RS, Holzman RS (1993) Anesthetic management of children with neuroblastoma. J Clin Anesth 5:486–491
3. Eisenhofer G, Rivers G, Rosas AL, Quezado Z, Manger WM, Pacak K (2007) Adverse drug reactions in patients with phaeochromocytoma: incidence, prevention and management. Drug Saf 30:1031–1062

Chapter 14
Bone and Connective Tissue

An 11-year-old boy with achondroplasia presents for an Ilizarov leg lengthening procedure. His admission vital signs are: HR = 92 bpm, BP = 110/80 mmHg, RR = 16/min, Hct = 34%. There is no prior history of surgery.

R.S. Holzman et al., *Pediatric Anesthesiology Review: Clinical Cases for Self-Assessment*,
DOI 10.1007/978-1-4419-1617-4_14, © Springer Science+Business Media, LLC 2010

Preoperative Evaluation

1. The patient has a large head:

    (a) Is this normal? Why/why not?

    (b) How could you evaluate the presence or absence of hydrocephalus?

    (c) Is this important? Why/why not?

    (d) How would it alter your anesthetic management if he had normal pressure hydrocephalus?

    (e) What if this patient had progressive difficulty walking; what would this suggest?
    (f) How would you evaluate it?
    (g) How could this be distinguished from his short-limb difficulties?

2. Bony abnormalities:

    (a) What are the anesthetic implications of his bony abnormalities?

    (b) Is the spinal defect only a mesodermal defect, or does it involve neuroecto-derm as well?

    (c) The parents want to find out about a spinal anesthetic; what would you tell them?
    (d) Is it likely to be easy to perform a spinal in this patient (aside from psychological issues)?
    (e) What level would you choose to perform the block?

Preoperative Evaluation

1. (a) Yes, large head is normal in achondroplasia dwarfism. It is typical of the syndrome but could also be from hydrocephalus which occurs with a higher incidence in these patients due to foramen magnum stenosis.
   (b) The presence of hydrocephalus can be detected by head radioimaging studies such as MRI to examine the possible presence of dilated ventricles.
   (c) It is important to investigate the presence of hydrocephalus because it reflects foramen magnum stenosis, which predisposes to brainstem compression and respiratory arrest.
   (d) The presence of normal pressure hydrocephalus does not rule out the presence of foramen magnum stenosis and the risk of brainstem compression from manipulation of the neck during tracheal intubation and intraoperative positioning.
   (e, The evaluation of spinal cord/brainstem compression and spinal stenosis
   f, could be determined by obtaining radioimaging studies such as CT and MRI scans.
   & If the patient is having difficulty walking due to spinal cord compression from
   g) thoraco-lumbar stenosis, the patient will have sensory and/or motor dysfunction on clinical neurological examination. Lumbar spine stenosis will also cause bladder and rectal sphincter dysfunction. If the difficulty walking is due to short limbs, the neurological examination will be normal.

2. (a) Failure of bone growth in this syndrome may result in stenosis of the foramen magnum and spinal canal and vertebral malalignments that may predispose the brainstem, spinal cord, and peripheral nerves to compression during larygeal intubation maneuvers and intraoperative positioning, particularly if neuromuscular blocking agents are used.
   (b) The primary defect is of the mesoderm, i.e., the failure of the cartilage to form bone.
   (c) Lumbar spinal anesthesia has been performed safely in patients with spinal stenosis and vertebral malalignment but is associated with a potentially high incidence of direct neural injury by the block needle or neural tissue compression by anesthetic volume or accidental epidural hematoma mass effect. Therefore, it is advisable to perform spinal anesthesia only if it offers distinct advantages over general anesthesia in a particular patient. In this particular patient, there is no obvious benefit of spinal anesthesia over general anesthesia.
   (d) Performance of spinal anesthesia is likely to be difficult in this patient due to the typical lordotic deformity and vertebral malalignment.
   (e) I will choose a site that is not involved with lordosis, kyphosis, stenosis, or vertebral malalignment after reviewing the neuroimages and documenting any preprocedural neurological deficit. Spinal interspace L5-S1 may be safe because the deformities are usually located above this level. Nevertheless, the risk of cord compression is possible with the use of a large volume of local anesthetic and in the event accidental epidural venous bleeding or hematoma should occur.

3. Short neck:

   (a) Should he have a neck radiograph? Why/why not?

   (b) Does this patient need an airway MRI?

   (c) Does this patient need cervical spine films to evaluate the abnormal airways? Why/why not? How will it affect your anesthetic management?

Intraoperative Course

1. Intraoperative monitoring:

   (a) What kind of monitoring would you choose for this case? Why/why not?

   (b) Does this patient need an arterial line? Why/why not?

   (c) A CVP?

   (d) A precordial doppler? Why/why not?

2. Anesthesia induction:

   (a) Your colleague walks by the room, takes a look in as you are placing monitors, and suggests that you consider a rapid sequence induction because the patient is a preteen, and "they all have full stomachs." What do you think?

   (b) How would you decide which approach to use?

   (c) Would you use succinylcholine for a rapid sequence induction? Why/why not?

3. (a) No, it is not necessary for this patient to have a cervical radiograph if he has no neurological disease and the fact that patients with achondroplasia are expected to have underdevelopment of bone and deformities including the potential for cervical spine stenosis.

   (b) No, this patient does not need an airway MRI because midface hypoplasia is expected with this disorder. MRI of the airways can be helpful to determine the extent of airways involvement.

   (c) No this patient does not need cervical spine films if he is neurologically asymptomatic. Achondroplasia is a disease of underdevelopment and malalignment of bones and can be associated with dysgenesis of the odontoid process that produces atlanto-axial instability. Atlanto-axial instability requires protection of the spinal cord from compression by stabilization of the spine in extension during tracheal intubation maneuvers and throughout the perioperative period. Difficult tracheal intubation should be anticipated due to midface hypoplasia, micrognathia, or macrognathia. If available, fiberoptic intubation should be considered.

Intraoperative Course

1. (a) I will choose standard ASA monitors: ECG, end-tidal carbon dioxide ($ETCO_2$), inspired oxygen (F_iO_2), end-tidal anesthetic vapor concentration, and temperature.

   (b) No, this patient does not need invasive arterial blood pressure or CVP monitoring because this procedure is not associated with extensive blood loss, extracellular third space fluid loss and the patient does not have known cardiovascular disease.

   (c) Yes, I will use a precordial Doppler to monitor for venous air entrainment via deformed bones during surgery.

2. (a) I disagree with my colleague's assessment. Achondroplasia is associated with difficult tracheal intubation due to midface hypoplasia and micrognathia. Minimal manipulation of the cervical spine is advisable because of the potential of atlanto-axial joint instability. Fiberoptic laryngoscopy may be necessary to secure tracheal intubation with minimal cervical spine manipulation.

   (b) A careful evaluation of the airway during the preoperative visit by clinical examination and review of radioimages to assess the ease or difficulty with which tracheal intubation could be performed is warranted. In the operating room, airway access could be further assessed after providing sedation or an inhaled anesthetic in a spontaneously breathing patient.

   (c) No, I will not use succinylcholine in this patient because the fasciculation may produce atlanto-axial instability and spinal cord compression. Achondroplasia is also associated with hypotonia and the use of succinylcholine potentially may produce clinically significant hyperkalemia.

(d) Any association with malignant hyperthermia?

(e) The patient can extend his neck through an arc of 15–20°. Does this influence your choice of anesthetic induction techniques?

(f) How will you do an awake intubation?

(g) Would a light wand be just as good as a fiberoptic bronchoscope? Would an anterior commissure scope work just as well for this problem?

(h) What are the advantages and disadvantages. of each in patients with odontoid hypoplasia and decreased neck extension?

(d) There is no known association of this syndrome with malignant hyperthermia syndrome.

(e) The limited cervical extension may make direct laryngoscopy and tracheal intubation difficult; therefore, I will consider an inhalation induction and fiberoptic intubation.

(f) I will administer intravenous sedation, with incremental doses of midazolam 25 mcg/kg followed by a short-acting opioid such as fentanyl 0.5 mcg/kg IV at 5 min intervals, to effect. Alternatively, supplementation with IV droperidol 75–100 mcg/kg in divided doses instead of or in addition to midazolam to achieve a state of anxiolysis, antegrade amnesia, and adequate sedation while maintaining patient's ability to maintain a patent airway and respond to verbal command. In addition, I will anesthetize the airway mucosa of the nares, oropharynx, and supraglottic area with topical local anesthetic and/or superior laryngeal nerve block if anatomically permissible to markedly reduce the discomfort associated with instrumentation and reduce the requirement for intravenous sedation. Lidocaine 1% or cocaine 4% spray is an effective topical anesthetic of the mucosa. Cocaine 4% is also applied to the nasal mucosa with cotton tipped applicators and the advantage of cocaine over lidocaine is that it produces vasoconstriction and minimizes the bleeding from instrumentation of the nasal turbinates. The oropharynx is anesthetized by intraoral glossopharyngeal nerve blocks with submucosal infiltration, 3–5 mL of 1% lidocaine into each palatoglossal fold. The supraglottic mucosa, including the epiglottis, is anesthetized by bilateral superior laryngeal nerve blocks. This is accomplished by percutaneous injection of 2–3 mL of 1% lidocaine at the junction of the greater cornu of the thyroid cartilage and the lateral aspect of the hyoid bone, percutaneously through the thyrohyoid membrane. Alternatively, a supraglottic transmucosal approach is achieved by placing a lidocaine-soaked gauze pad into the pyriform fossae bilaterally.

(g) The light wand can be used for blind oral intubation while the neck is stabilized and the glottis is not too anteriorly placed. An anterior commissure scope may not be useful because of restricted neck mobility during stabilization; often excessive neck extension is required to visualize the glottis with an anterior commissure scope.

(h) The advantage of the light wand is that it allows blind oral intubation without the need for excessive neck extension and flexion. The disadvantage is that advancing of the endotracheal tube beyond the glottis may require flexion of the neck, which may result in spinal cord compression in the presence of atlanto-axial instability. The advantage of the anterior commissure scope is that it facilitates visualization of an anteriorly placed larynx. The disadvantage is that it requires hyperextension of the neck.

3. Intraoperative events:

(a) After the first 3 h of the case, six transfemoral Ilizarov struts have been placed; the pulse oximeter reads 94% on 50% nitrous and oxygen. What do you make of this?

(b) There are at least three more hours of distraction to go. What will you do?

(c) Is positive end-expiratory pressure (PEEP) effective for fat embolism syndrome?

(d) How would you choose the most effective PEEP level?

(e) What are the problems with PEEP?

(f) Any particular problems with this patient? What are they? Is this different than any other patient?

(g) After the first 4 h of the case, you note that the nasopharyngeal temperature is 39.7°; the heart rate, which started at 100 bpm, is now 140 bpm. What do you think is going on? What else could it be?

(h) How will you evaluate?

(i) Is there any way to test?

(j) Would you place an arterial line at this point?

(k) Give dantrolene prophylactically?

(l) What if the end-tidal CO_2 was 43 mmHg? 57 mmHg?

(m) What if you increased the minute ventilation by 100% and the end-tidal CO_2 decreased from 53 to 50 mmHg? What could this be? Why?

3. (a) Acute oxygen desaturation could be due to venous air or fat embolism.

   (b) Optimize ventilation. Increase the inspired oxygen to maintain transcutaneous oxyhemoglobin saturation above 95%. Acutely, notify the surgeon, cover the surgical wound with saline and lower the surgical wound below the heart level. Place an arterial cannula to monitor arterial blood gasses.

   (c) PEEP can be effective for ventilation/perfusion mismatch, particularly for venous air embolism. Serial blood gasses would help to determine an optimal PEEP value for oxygenation should fat embolism be suspected.

   (d) I will increase the PEEP gradually to optimal arterial saturation without compromising hemodynamics.

   (e) High PEEP may compromise right ventricular function by increasing intrapulmonary (and pulmonary artery) pressure and left ventricular function by interventricular septal shift causing reduced LVEDV and cardiac output.

   (f) The hemodynamic effect of PEEP could be exaggerated in this patient due to scoliosis, a restrictive chest wall and limited intrathoracic capacity.

   (g) Malignant hyperthermia should be suspected on the top of the differential diagnosis list. However, most likely it is due to passive body heating and heat retention because the torso, upper limbs, and head are covered with insulating surgical drapes. Other less likely causes are a blood transfusion reaction, drug induced pyrexia, and intracranial bleed from fat embolism.

   (h & i) Monitor for progressive rise of $ETCO_2$, obtain a venous or arterial blood gas analysis to rule out malignant hyperthermia, hypercarbia, and initiate active cooling of the patient. Hypercarbia grossly out of proportion to the minute ventilation and tachycardia, muscular rigidity, profound metabolic and respiratory acidosis contribute to the clinical diagnosis of malignant hyperthermia.

   (j) Yes, I will place an arterial line at this point.

   (k) I will administer dantrolene if the arterial blood gas analysis confirms uncompensated metabolic and respiratory acidosis and a wide A-a oxygen gradient despite increased minute ventilation and 100% inspired oxygen, i.e., hypermetabolic state.

   (l) These values of $ETCO_2$ are not suggestive of MHS. These low values could be due to hypoventilation or increased dead space and do not reflect a hypermetabolic state.

   (m) An inability to reduce $ETCO_2$ despite doubling the minute volume is suggestive of inability to compensate for excessive production of carbon dioxide and a hypermetabolic state. This could very well suggest MHS; a state of progressive hypermetabolic process and excessive CO_2 production unresponsive to compensatory increased ventilation.

Perioperative Care

1. Tracheal extubation:

   (a) Should this patient be extubated (assume odontoid hypoplasia and decreased neck range of motion). Why/why not?
   (b) Is it safer if he pulls his tube out in the middle of the night in the ICU?
   (c) What criteria will you use for extubation? Why?

   (d) Do you think this patient would meet spirometric or inspiratory force criteria for extubation? Why/why not?

   (e) Is there any reason for him to have weak muscles?
   (f) Should he be extubated in the operating room?

2. Postoperative pain management:

   (a) Is this patient at any higher risk with PCA methods of pain management?

   (b) Would a preoperative blood gas have been likely to reveal this problem?

   (c) How would you write the orders for his PCA?

Additional Questions

1. A 1½-year old with osteogenesis imperfecta is on the add-on list for open reduction internal fixation of a femur fracture. His temperature preop is 39.4°C.

   (a) How will you evaluate this?
   (b) What if he has no signs of a cold? Urinary tract infection? Is this temperature normal? Why?

   (c) What else will you evaluate preoperatively?

Perioperative Care

1. (a) No. If the patient's airways are compromised postoperatively and he requires emergency re-establishment of the airway, uncontrolled extension of the neck may cause spinal cord compression.

   (b) No.

   (c) I will ensure that the patient is alert, comfortable, and responds appropriately to commands. There should be a leak around the endotracheal tube, and he should not have any residual effect of neuromuscular blockade (sustained tetanus at 50 Hz for 5 s or sustained double burst stimulation prior to administration of cholinesterase antagonists). The patient should be capable of maintaining a patent airway and spontaneous ventilation.

   (d) This patient may not fulfill the spirometric or inspiratory force criteria due to restrictive chest wall disease secondary to scoliosis, and hypotonia. Many patients with achondroplasia are cognitively impaired and may not cooperate with spirometric assessment.

   (e) Yes, patients with achondroplasia have poor muscle tone.

   (f) Yes, this patient had a peripheral orthopedic procedure not associated with significant blood loss or airway compromise.

2. (a) No, this patient is not at higher risk for PCA methods of pain management provided that the dose and frequency are adjusted to lower values than a standard regimen.

   (b) Preoperative blood gas analysis may uncover carbon dioxide retention in this patient if severe scoliosis, chest wall restrictive disease, hypotonia, and obesity are present.

   (c) I would use a conservative dosing regimen and may prescribe Nurse Controlled Analgesia (NCA) if there is concern about developmental delay/impairment.

Additional Questions

1. (a) Preoperative evaluation should rule out pulmonary and other sources of infection.

   (b) Hyperthermia occurs in OI patients due to a baseline hypermetabolic state from chronically elevated rates of bone degeneration and reformation. Hyperthermia probably occurs due to thermoregulation instability that does not progress to MHS. In this particular patient, I would consider the possibility of fat embolism.

   (c) I will evaluate the airway status, severity of scoliosis, chest wall restriction, coagulation abnormalities (easy bruisability), cardiac disease, and the presence of multiple fractures.

(d) What if his platelet count is normal, but he has a history of easy bruising (as well as easy breaking)?

(e) How can platelet aggregation abnormalities be evaluated?

(f) How will platelet abnormalities affect your anesthetic management? Hematologic support?

(g) Does he need platelets?

(h) What if he is 6 kg; how will you manage his fluid therapy?

(i) Would you use succinylcholine to gain rapid control of the airway?

(j) What are the drawbacks?

(k) Does this patient need an arterial line instead of a blood pressure cuff?

2. Radial dysplasia and associated syndromes: Identify and briefly describe with regard to anesthetic implications.

   (a) Radial aplasia and Hallerman–Strieff Syndrome

   (b) Radial aplasia and Cornelia de Lange syndrome

   (c) Radial aplasia and Holt–Oram syndrome

(d) Easy bruising could be due to a defect in platelet adhesion so the platelet count could be normal.

(e) Bleeding time is a good clinical indicator of impaired platelet aggregation.

(f) Defective platelet aggregation can cause excessive bleeding during surgery. Transfusion of platelets will improve coagulation function and minimize surgical bleeding.

(g) Platelet transfusion is indicated if there is unexpected excessive intraoperative bleeding.

(h) Fluid replacement requires careful management because some patients with OI may experience hyperhydrosis and may need addition fluid replacement for insensible loss.

(i) If this patient was 6 kg, the fluid management requires closer monitoring because of the higher extracellular fluid content relative to the total body weight compared with older children.

(j) I will not administer succinylcholine in this patient because it can induce muscular fasciculation and contractures that increases the risk of fracture of the brittle bones.

(k) An arterial line is a safe alternative to the use of an oscillometric blood pressure cuff if the OI is severe in order to avoid fractures of the brittle bones. Alternatively, the use of an ultrasonic Doppler or aneroid strain gauge blood pressure device allows the use of the lowest inflation pressures.

2. Radial dysplasia and associated syndromes: identify and briefly describe with regard to anesthetic implications.

(a) Hallerman–Strieff syndrome is characterized by narrow upper airways, obstructed nares, micrognathia, tracheomalacia, OSA and cor pulmonale, and structural heart disease.

(b) Cornelia de Lange syndrome is associated with a short neck (66%) and heart defects; difficult airway access should be anticipated.

(c) Holt–Oram syndrome is an autosomal dominant heart disease associated with skeletal malformations including hypoplastic thumb and a short forearm. Patients may have radio-ulnar synostosis, accessory carpal bones, and carpal or tarsal coalition. Additional anomalies seen in some patients include hyperphalangism and preaxial polydactyly. It also shares some features with Fanconi's anemia.

(d) Radial aplasia and Fanconi syndrome

(e) TAR (Thrombocytopenia-Absent Radius) syndrome

(f) VATER syndrome

3. A 6-month old comes in for a hernia repair; he has rickets.

   (a) What are the anesthetic implications?

   (b) Any lab tests needed for this particular patient? Which ones?

   (c) Is there any particular anesthetic technique that would be safer than any other? Why/why not?

   (d) Risk of postoperative mechanical ventilation?

(d) It is caused by a proximal tubular defect that results in an excess loss in the urine of amino acids, glucose, phosphate, magnesium, potassium, bicarbonate, and sodium. Growth failure and the development of rickets in childhood and osteomalacia in adults occur. Dehydration occurs due to excess urination. Individuals with FA may feel extremely tired or have frequent infections due to immune system compromise. They may bruise easily and experience nosebleeds. Blood tests may reveal low red, white, or platelet cell counts. Approximately 75% of affected subjects have one or more of the following physical characteristics: café au lait spots (light brown birth marks), short stature, thumb and arm abnormalities (missing, misshapen, or extra thumbs or an incompletely developed/missing forearm bone), low birth weight, short stature, small head or eyes, abnormalities of the kidneys, genitals, gastrointestinal tract, heart, and central nervous system. Sometimes leukemia or myelodysplasia is the first sign of FA. Individuals with FA may only have a few of the clinical features described above or none at all.

(e) TAR (Thrombocytopenia-Absent Radius) syndrome is a rare congenital disorder with a complex inheritance characterized by low levels of platelets and aplasia of the radii. Additional skeletal defects include absence or underdevelopment of the ulnae, congenital heart defects, and renal dysplasia. It is believed to be inherited as a complex autosomal recessive trait.

(f) VATER syndrome or VACTERL associate a cluster of congenital (not genetic) defects that are linked to other syndromes such as Klippel Feil, Trisomy 18, and Goldenhar Syndromes. The acronym CARROT captures the various defects: Cardiac (TOF, VSD, ASD, AVC, HPLHS); Anal: imperforate anus; Radial dysplasia with missing or duplicate fingers, Renal dysplasia (polycystic kidney, bladder exstrophy, cloaca, hypospadius); Oesophageal defect: usually atresia and tracheal defect (most commonly Tracheo-esophageal fistula). The estimated incidence is approximately 16 cases per 100,000 live births and it occurs more frequently in infants born to diabetic mothers.

3. (a) Patients with rickets usually have hypocalcemia that may cause arrhythmias and potentiate nondepolarizing muscle relaxants. Patients with untreated rickets may have soft bones, which are predisposed to fracture with mild pressure or awkward positioning. Poor muscle tone is associated with kyphosis and ventilatory compromise.

(b) Yes, serum ionized calcium, phosphorus and alkaline phosphate concentrations, and parathyroid hormone.

(c) Avoidance of muscle relaxants may reduce the risk of enhancing the muscle weakness. Both hypocalcemia and hypophosphatemia potentiate nondepolarizing muscle relaxant effect.

(d) The potential for postoperative ventilatory support is high in this patient due to baseline poor muscle tone, restrictive chest wall disease from a pectus, scoliosis, and weak muscle tone that could be affected by any residual inhalation anesthetic effect, and postoperative opioid-induced suppression of central respiratory drive.

(e) Why is the serum calcium level typically normal?

(f) Then how is the metabolic component of the diagnosis made?

4. A patient with spine scoliosis.

   (a) With what degree of curvature in scoliosis would you counsel a family for postoperative mechanical ventilation? Why?

   (b) How will this influence your choice of monitors?

   (c) At what degree of curvature would you expect to have to use a pulmonary artery catheter?

   (d) Would a TEE do just as well to follow the patient intraoperatively?

   (e) Would you use TEE postoperatively? Why?

5. A 16-year old is scheduled for a saggital split osteotomy and mandibular advancement; she has severe juvenile rheumatoid arthritis.

   (a) What are your airway considerations?

   (b) Why do these patients have airway problems?

   (c) Are these mainly at the level of the mandible, the temperomandibular joint, or the larynx?
   (d) Is there any cervical spine problem?

(e) The serum calcium could be normal because of a compensatory increase of parathormone secretion in response to the initial low serum calcium. Increased parathormone secretion mobilizes the calcium and phosphorus from the bone (producing osteomalacia), normalizes serum calcium, raises the serum alkaline phosphatase, and lowers serum phosphorus due to inhibition of re-absorption of phosphorus from the renal tubules.

(f) The metabolic component of rickets is completed by analysis of plasma calcium, phosphorus, alkaline phosphatase, and vitamin D hepatic and renal components (Vitamin D3, D2, 25(OH)D3, 1,25(OH)2D3, 24,25(OH)2D3).

4. (a) The patient and family should be counseled with a curve of 65° or greater because a significant decline in ventilation–perfusion distribution occurs when the deformity progresses beyond than 65°. Postoperative mechanical ventilation may be required because of the increased dead space to tidal volume ratio ($V_d/V_t > 0.6$) and widening of the alveolar to arterial oxygen tension ratio (>350 mmHg).

(b) If the scoliosis curvature progresses beyond 65°, the adequacy of ventilation should be monitored with serial arterial blood gas analyses because the $ETCO_2$ will be falsely low due to increased alveolar dead space.

(c) I will use pulmonary artery catheter in the presence of a curve of 90° and greater, evidence of right ventricular compromise, or the presence of pre-operative hypoxemia and carbon dioxide retention.

(d) TEE is not a substitute for a pulmonary artery catheter; it may provide information about ventricular function and to a lesser extent about volume status. It is employed when pulmonary artery catheter placement is contraindicated or cannot be accomplished. Doppler monitoring provides beat-to-beat blood flow waveform of blood flow in the descending aorta that is proportional to left ventricular stroke volume.

(e) Yes, TEE in the postoperative period can be very useful to monitor right ventricular function during positive pressure ventilation and to guide fluid and inotropic therapy.

5. (a) In advanced or severe rheumatoid arthritis the airway can be compromised. The earliest manifestation is micrognathia due to ankylosis of temporomandibular joints. Other manifestations are ankylosis of the cricoarytenoid joint and a small glottic aperture, cervical spine ankylosis, flexion deformity, and subluxation of atlanto-axial joint.

(b) These patients can have airway problems due to a small mouth opening, limited range of motion of the neck, severely restricted neck extension, and a small glottis due to restricted movement of cricoarytenoid joint.

(c) The airway problems occur at all levels of the upper airway passages.

(d) Yes, there are problems of the cervical spine due to flexion deformity and subluxation of the vertebral bodies and atlanto-axial joint.

General References

1. Horton WA, Hall JG, Hecht JT (2007) Achondroplasia. Lancet 370:162–172
2. Sisk EA, Heatley DG, Borowski BJ, Leverson GE, Pauli RM (1999) Obstructive sleep apnea in children with achondroplasia: surgical and anesthetic considerations. Otolaryngol Head Neck Surg 120:248–254
3. Monedero P, Garcia-Pedrajas F, Coca I, Fernandez-Liesa JI, Panadero A, de los Rios J (1997) Is management of anesthesia in achondroplastic dwarfs really a challenge? J Clin Anesth 9:208–212
4. Krishnan BS, Eipe N, Korula G (2003) Anaesthetic management of a patient with achondroplasia. Paediatr Anaesth 13:547–549
5. Barros F (1995) Caudal block in a child with osteogenesis imperfecta, type II. Paediatr Anaesth 5:202–203
6. Mather JS (1966) Impossible direct laryngoscopy in achondroplasia. A case report. Anaesthesia 21:244–248
7. Goldfarb CA, Wall L, Manske PR (2006) Radial longitudinal deficiency: the incidence of associated medical and musculoskeletal conditions. J Hand Surg [Am] 31:1176–1182

Chapter 15
Orthopedics: Scoliosis

Introduction

A 13-year-old female with idiopathic scoliosis is scheduled for instrumentation and posterior fusion. She has a history of asthma and a remote history of strabismus repair. Weight 40 kg, $P = 92$ bpm, BP = 108/62 mmHg, RR = 20/min, and $T = 36.7°C$.

Preoperative Evaluation

1. Evaluation of scoliosis deformity:

   (a) Her curve is 60°. Is this cause for concern?
   (b) Do you need pulmonary function tests?

   (c) Do you need more information on her cardiac status?
   (d) With two muscle abnormalities, is she at risk for malignant hyperthermia?

2. Evaluation of the respiratory status:

   (a) Her asthma is worsened by exercise, allergies, and colds. Her normal medications are an albuterol (Ventolin®) inhaler TID and beclomethasone (Vanceril®) inhaler BID. What are these medications?
   (b) Do inhaled steroids require perioperative coverage?

   (c) She has received three pulses of oral steroids over the last year. Will she need perioperative steroids?
   (d) How will you prepare her for the operating room?

3. Preoperative blood donation:

   (a) Should she predonate blood? Is she too small?

   (b) How often can she donate?

   (c) How long will it last?

Preoperative Evaluation

1. (a) Yes, curves of 65° or greater can cause significant restriction of ventilation.

   (b) Yes. Although the curvature is below 65°, the associated pulmonary hypoplasia may cause marked ventilation–perfusion uneven distribution.
   (c) No, not if the patient has good tolerance to physical activity.
   (d) Yes, based on statistical probability, patients with congenital strabismus are at slightly higher risk for malignant hyperthermia. The causes of congenital strabismus and idiopathic scoliosis are unknown. Idiopathic scoliosis is a genetically determined musculoskeletal disorder and congenital strabismus is presumably due to either a neurogenic or muscle disorder. The presence of two possible myopathic conditions in this patient raises the likelihood of generalized subclinical myopathy. Malignant hyperthermia is a subclinical generalized myopathy that is triggered by pharmacologic agents including anesthetics.

2. (a) Albuterol is a selective beta-2 agonist, is a bronchodilator, and is useful for prevention and treatment of reversible bronchospasm. Beclomethasone is a synthetic corticosteroid used for treatment of asthma and allergic rhinitis.

   (b) There is no need for perioperative coverage or additional steroid in this patient, because a very small amount of the inhaled corticosteroid is absorbed systemically. Compared with systemic corticosteroids, inhaled corticosteroids administered in the recommended doses cause less adrenal suppression, although beclomethasone 300–800 mcg/day is reported to cause adrenal suppression in children.
   (c) If the last oral pulse steroid dose she received was a year ago she does not need perioperative steroid coverage.
   (d) A major anesthetic consideration is optimization of asthma control. I will obtain a pulmonary medicine consult to evaluate pulmonary function tests before and after bronchodilator treatment and also obtain a baseline chest radiograph.

3. (a) Her body weight is too small and she should not predonate blood. Current predonation requirements are a body weight of 50 kg and greater, a minimum Hct of 33% to qualify for an average donated volume of 250 mL. A lower body weight between 40 and 50 kg body weight may be acceptable provided that the amount of predonated blood volume is proportionately smaller.
   (b) She may donate every 4 days provided that she does not experience vasovagal instability symptoms due to hypovolemia.
   (c) Whole blood can be stored for 35 days when collected in CPDA-1 anticoagulant. Red blood cells can be stored for 42 days if preserved in Adsol or Nutricel.

(d) What other methods are available to avoid blood transfusion?

(e) Are DDAVP or erythropoietin cost effective?

(f) Should you take off a unit of blood at the start of the case?

4. Induction of anesthesia:

   (a) She is incredibly scared; she is crying and keeps pulling her hand away as you try to look for an IV. How do you premedicate?

   (b) Would you use nitrous oxide to help start the IV?

Intraoperative Course

1. Intraoperative monitoring:

   (a) What monitors do you need?

   (b) Is CVP monitoring important?

   (c) What are the disadvantages?

   (d) What are somatosensory evoked potentials (SSEPs)?

   (e) What do they measure?

(d) Other methods to avoid blood transfusion in addition to preoperative blood donation with or without the use of erythropoietin are intraoperative acute normovolumic hemodilution, intraoperative blood salvage procedures including the use of a Cell-Saver®, and the use of antifibrinolytic agents.

(e) DDAVP is cost effective but its effectiveness is questionable for idiopathic scoliosis spinal fusion. Erythropoietin is an effective bone marrow inducer of red blood cell production and when combined with preoperative blood donation could be effective in avoiding allogenic blood transfusion but the cost is prohibitive.

(f) Intraoperative blood salvage and acute hemodilution is an option if the hemoglobin is greater than 11 mg/dL.

4. (a) I will offer oral midazolam as a premedication, 0.5–1 mg/kg, and use a topical anesthetic prior to insertion of an intravenous needle.

(b) Yes, if the patient prefers inhalation induction with a mask, the use of 70% nitrous oxide in oxygen is an alternative method to alleviate anxiety and pain associated with intravenous catheterization.

Intraoperative Course

1. (a) In addition to the standard ASA monitors of ECG, blood pressure, $ETCO_2$, and pulse oximetry, I will use intra-arterial blood pressure monitoring and urine output.

(b) The use of a CVP is of little value if the patient has normal cardiac function.

(c) CVP will not offer additional information beyond the monitors mentioned above and is not without the potential risks of air embolism, hemo-pericardium, pneumothorax, and arrhythmias.

(d) SSEP measures electrical activity in ascending sensory pathways. Intraoperative SSEP monitors the integrity of the sensory neural pathways from site of sensory neuron stimulation (caudal to the surgical site) to a site cephalad to the surgical site such as the brainstem or the prefrontal sensory cortex. The principal goal of intraoperative monitoring is to promptly identify acute spinal cord function impairment at the operative site so that the surgeon can take quick corrective action and prevent permanent deficits.

(e) SSEP measures evoked electrical wave configuration, peak-to-peak intervals, absolute and interpeak latencies, and comparative latency delays between the ipsilateral and contralateral pathways. They measure the proximal neural electrical responses (brachial plexus, spinal cord, brainstem, or cerebral cortex) to peripherally applied standard sensory stimuli (such median or posterior tibial nerves), thereby testing the integrity of sensory neural pathways.

  (f) Does this assure normal neurological function postoperatively?

  (g) Does a wake-up test?
  (h) Are there alternatives to the wake-up test?
  (i) How do you perform motor evoked potentials?

  (j) Are they likely to be more specific and/or sensitive than somatosensory evoked potentials?

  (k) A wake-up test?

2. Anesthetic management:

  (a) What agents will you use? Why?

  (b) Are any induction agents less of a problem for SSEP monitoring?

  (c) Does it matter?

  (d) What muscle relaxant will you choose?
  (e) How will you place and secure the ETT?

  (f) What will you choose for maintaining the anesthetic?

(f) The use of SSEP does not ensure normal neurological function postoperatively because of the potential for false positive and false negative results.

(g) The wake-up test evaluates gross motor function but does not assess sensory deficit.

(h) The alternative to a wake-up test is the motor evoked potential (MEPs).

(i) MEPs are performed by electrical stimulation of the motor neurons in the dorsal spinal columns directly in the epidural space within the surgical wound or indirectly by transosseous stimulation.

(j) MEPs are a more specific test of descending motor pathways but by themselves are not more specific or sensitive than SSEPs in detecting spinal cord injury during surgery. The use of both MEPs and SSEPs during spinal surgery provides optimal sensitivity and specificity in detecting neurological impairment of spinal cord during surgery.

(k) The wake-up test is a specific test for gross motor function of the spinal cord to assess patient volitional motor function integrity across the spinal surgical site but it has its own limitations. The wake-up test is warranted and a reliable test if MEPs are absent or SSEPs are abnormal. If simultaneous recordings of MEPs and SSEPs are normal during spine surgery, these are of sufficient sensitivity and specificity to negate the need for wake-up test.

2. Anesthetic management:

(a) I will use an opioid-based balanced anesthetic, with an inhalation agent at less than 0.25–0.5 MAC in N_2O 50%, combined with a continuous infusion of propofol and infusion of a short acting opioid such as fentanyl and/or remifentanil. I will use a short-acting muscle relaxant if MEPs are not used. The above combination of agents has minimal effect on suppressing the motor and sensory evoked potentials.

(b) The combination of propofol and short acting opioids such as fentanyl and a short or intermediate acting muscle relaxant has the least suppressive effect on SSEP.

(c) Yes, agents that considerably suppress the SSEP are sodium thiopental, which selectively suppresses the evoked potentials to a greater extent than propofol and etomidate. Inhalation agents cause dose-dependent suppression of SSEP. It is critically important to obtain a reliable baseline recording after the induction of anesthesia and prior to surgical manipulation to establish a steady-state maintenance anesthetic that does not interfere with monitoring neurological testing.

(d) I will use cisatracurium or vecuronium.

(e) I will place the endotracheal tube via the nasal route which is more firmly secured against accidental dislodgement than via the oral route in patient positioned prone during surgery.

(f) I will use isoflurane between 0.25 and 0.5 MAC in N_2O 50%, a continuous infusion of fentanyl (15 mcg/kg initial loading dose followed by infusion of 2–3 mcg/kg/h), propofol (infusion 25–50 mcg/kg/h), and intermittent doses of vecuronium while maintaining one to two twitches by train-of-four monitor.

(g) Will this choice affect the SSEP monitoring?

(h) How will you assure amnesia?

3. Intraoperative blood pressure control:

(a) The surgeon asks for the blood pressure to be decreased.

(b) How can you do this?

(c) How low can you safely go?

(d) Would this change if you had acutely hemodiluted her to a hematocrit of 29% while taking off a unit of blood?

(e) Which are more effective in controlling blood loss: nitroprusside and other vasodilators or beta blockers that decrease cardiac output?

(f) What about using the volatile anesthetics to lower the blood pressure?

(g) You give labetalol and within minutes notice that the peak inspiratory pressure, which had been 24 cm H_2O, has risen to 52 cm H_2O. Tidal volume (exhaled) is decreased to 200 mL. Oxygen saturation falls to 92%. What is the differential diagnosis?

(h) How do you determine and correct the problem?

(g This combination has the least effect on the SSEP and will ensure adequate
& amnesia. If the use of inhaled agents interferes with SSEP and is not used
h) then I will administer small doses of IV midazolam 0.25 mg/kg every 2–3 h
to ensure amnesia. Alternatively, a BIS monitor can be used to maintain an
adequate hypnotic level.

3. (a) Controlled blood pressure reduction can be accomplished with titration of
small doses of labetalol (2.5–5 mg).
(b I would slowly induce hypotension over 15–20 min prior to surgical incision. The
& optimal level of hypotension depends on many factors for this particular patient.
c) The systolic blood pressure may be allowed to decrease lower than 80 mmHg,
which is close to two standard deviations for her age. Alternatively, a mean blood
pressure between 55 and 66 mmHg would be safe.
(d) If hemodilution is performed, I will maintain blood pressure near normal
systolic blood pressure for her age (100 mmHg) to ensure adequate tissue
oxygen delivery.
(e) The use of short-acting vasodilators is probably safer than beta blockers
because their effect can be rapidly reversed in the event of sudden blood
loss. The disadvantage of beta blockers is myocardial depression and
decreased compensatory autonomic responses to acute hypovolumia. There
are no controlled trials in children to address this controversy and its possible effectiveness in different ages. In this particular patient, beta blockers
should be avoided given the history of asthma. I will choose an arteriolar
vasodilator such as sodium nitroprusside.
(f) I will not use the volatile agents to control blood pressure because of the
dose-dependent myocardial depression and peripheral vasodilation effects
of high concentrations of these agents. This will expose the child to an
increased risk of hemodynamic instability during the rapid blood loss phase
and also will interfere with MEP and SSEP monitoring.
(g) The beta blocker component effect of labetalol may have caused
brochospasm.

(h) To confirm that the airway pressure rise and desaturation are due to bronchospasm rather than other causes I will assess the patient for the following
conditions:

1. Pnuemothorax (asymmetry of breath sounds and shift of precordial api-
cal pulse).
2. Blood transfusion reaction (hives, rashes, fever, darkening of urine, and
direct and indirect Coomb's test).
3. Endobronchial intubtation (asymmetric breath sounds); this is remedied by
withdrawal of the endotracheal tube until breath sound are symmetrical.
4. Obstruction of the endotracheal tube due to secretions (insertion of suction catheter into the endotracheal tube).

4. Intraoperative blood loss:

   (a) The surgeon notes that his field is "rather wet." You send a hematocrit sample which comes back 28%. Do you transfuse? For a hematocrit of 25%; 23%; 20%; 17%?

   (b) You are using a cell saver. What efficiency of blood salvage can you expect to obtain with this device?

   (c) What are you giving back to the patient when you transfuse "cell saver blood?"

   (d) What is the hematocrit on "cell saver blood?"

   (e) Should you use DDAVP? What is DDAVP?

5. Intraoperative "wake-up test":

   (a) The surgeon asks for a wakeup test. Should you reverse the muscle relaxant before the test?

   (b) How do you perform a wakeup test?

   (c) What are the risks?

5. Kinking of the endotracheal tube is confirmed by failure to advance a suction catheter through the length of the endotracheal tube. If the head position correction fails to rectify the kinking, the endotracheal tube must be replaced.

4. (a) I will transfuse when the Hct is 25% or lower.
   (b & c) The amount of blood that can be salvaged with the use of Cell Saver device ranges from 50 to 70% of the shed blood primarily in the form of salvaged intact red blood cells.

   (d) The hematocrit of the re-transfused salvaged RBC is high, in the range of 50–70%.
   (e) DDAVP is desmopressin, a synthetic analog of natural arginine-vasopressin, with the de-amination of homocysteine in position 1 and substitution of D-arginine for L-arginine at position 8. This difference in chemical structure enhances the pressor to antidiuretic potency (2,000–4,000:1), and prolongs the duration of action of the compound due to its resistance to enzymatic cleavage. As with arginine–vasopressin, desmopressin stimulates the endothelial cells to release factor VIII, prostaglandin I2, and tissue plasminogen activator but is more potent than arginine–vasopressin. It may also increase platelet adhesiveness.

5. (a) No, I will not reverse the muscle relaxant unless the muscle twitch response to nerve stimulation is completely suppressed.

   (b) I will lighten the anesthetic depth to the extent that the patient responds appropriately to verbal command. This is accomplished by discontinuing the inhaled agent, nitrous oxide, and propofol and fentanyl infusions while maintaining muscular twitch response at two twitches in train-of-four nerve stimulation. When the patient starts to awaken as indicated by an increase in heart rate, blood pressure and spontaneous breathing, or limb movement, she/he is asked to squeeze the anesthesiologist's fingers to ensure that the patient understands and follows commands appropriately, and then instructed to move the toes or the feet.
   (c) The risks of a wakeup test are usually associated with abrupt and too light a depth of anesthesia. Vigorous and deep spontaneous breathing may entrain venous air or fat from the surgical field and produce systemic embolism. Muscle strength reversal to three and four twitches in the train-of-four may enable the patient move vigorously and fall off the surgical frame or cause undue spine extension that may break or dislodge the metal rods and injure the spinal cord. If the arms are not restrained the patient may pull out the endotracheal tube and/or the vascular lines.

Postoperative Course

Tracheal extubation:

(a) Would you extubate the patient at the end of the procedure? On what would you
     base your decision?

(b) Does the patient need to be in an ICU postoperatively? Why?

(c) What are you particularly concerned about?

Additional Topics

1. A patient with Gaucher's Disease needs an anterior/posterior (AP) spinal fusion.
    What is Gaucher's Disease and how will it affect your anesthetic plans?

Postoperative Course

(a) Yes, I will plan to extubate the trachea if the patient is awake, breathing spontaneously, comfortable, and follows commands appropriately. Reversibility of
neuromuscular blockade can be assessed by full recovery of the muscle twitch
response to nerve stimulation in the train-of-four and sustained tetanus at 50 Hz
for 5 s or sustained double burst stimulation prior to administration of cholinesterase antagonists. $ETCO2 < 50$ mmHg, head lift for >5 s and an ability to
generate maximum inspiratory pressure of greater than -25 mmHg are the
desirable respiratory endpoints.
(b) No, this patient does not need the ICU if she maintains adequate spontaneous
gas exchange, has stable hemodynamics, and is producing an adequate urine
output.
(c) Major concerns about the postoperative care of this patient are the moderate
restrictive chest wall disorder due to a $60°$ curvature, respiratory depression
from a large amount of postoperative opioid requirement, the potential for a
flare-up of her asthma, and a low postoperative Hct; all these factors can
compromise tissue oxygenation.

Additional Topics

1. Patients with Gaucher disease exhibit a deficiency of an enzyme called glucocere-
brosidase that catalyzes the first step in the biodegradation of glucocerebroside.
Except for the brain, glucocerebroside arises mainly from the biodegradation of old
red and white blood cells. In the brain, glucocerebroside arises from the turnover of
complex lipids during brain development and the formation of the myelin sheath of
nerves. Absence of this enzyme leads to deposition of glucocerebroside in the histio-
cytes of spleen, liver, bone marrow, and other tissues causing impairment of coagulation function, anemia, low platelet count, enlarged liver and spleen, weakening of the
skeleton, and sometimes impairment of liver and kidney function. In severe types,
the brain is involved resulting in developmental delay and seizures.

2. A patient with Duchenne Muscular Dystrophy needs an anterior/posterior (AP) spinal fusion.

   (a) What is Duchenne Muscular Dystrophy and how will it affect your anesthetic plans?

   (b) Is this patient at risk for Malignant Hyperthermia?

2. (a) Duchenne muscular dystrophy is a hereditary muscle disease associated with skeletal muscle weakness and abnormal function of smooth muscles including cardiac muscles. It is due to defects in the dystrophin gene, on the X chromosome. The dystrophin defect is inherited as an X-linked recessive; therefore, only males are affected and female relatives of affected males may be carriers. The defective skeletal muscles are at risk for breakdown (rhabdomyolysis) from succinylcholine and inhalation agents. The defective heart muscles result in dilated and occasionally restrictive cardiomyopathy. Some patients may have a right bundle branch block and other rhythm defects. In adolescence, degeneration of the tongue musculature and replacement with fatty infiltrate may make direct laryngoscopy and visualization of the glottis extremely difficult. When muscle weakness is moderate to severe patients usually require postoperative mechanical ventilation. Because of the extensiveness of posterior spinal fusion surgery these patients tend to lose substantial amount of blood, ranging from 50 to 200% of the circulating blood volume.

   (b) A small percentage of patients with DMD probably are at risk for MHS based on clinical case reports and demonstration of a higher incidence of positive halothane–caffeine contracture test but there is no genetic testing performed in these patients to identify the defective MHS gene.

General References

1. Gibson PR (2004) Anaesthesia for correction of scoliosis in children. Anaesth Intensive Care 32:548–559
2. Tucker SK, Noordeen MH, Pitt MC (2001) Spinal cord monitoring in neuromuscular scoliosis. J Pediatr Orthop B 10:1–5
3. Noonan KJ, Walker T, Feinberg JR, Nagel M, Didelot W, Lindseth R (2002) Factors related to false- versus true-positive neuromonitoring changes in adolescent idiopathic scoliosis surgery. Spine 27:825–830
4. Anand N, Idio FG Jr, Remer S, Hoppenfeld S (1998) The effects of perioperative blood salvage and autologous blood donation on transfusion requirements in scoliosis surgery. J Spinal Disord 11:532–534
5. Doherty GM, Chisakuta A, Crean P, Shields MD (2005) Anesthesia and the child with asthma. Paediatr Anaesth 15:446–454
6. Lieberman JA, Lyon R, Feiner J, Diab M, Gregory GA (2006) The effect of age on motor evoked potentials in children under propofol/isoflurane anesthesia. Anesth Analg 103:316–321, table of contents
7. Hayes J, Veyckemans F, Bissonnette B (2008) Duchenne muscular dystrophy: an old anesthesia problem revisited. Paediatr Anaesth 18:100–106
8. Sethna NF, Rockoff MA (1986) Cardiac arrest following inhalation induction of anaesthesia in a child with Duchenne's muscular dystrophy. Can Anaesth Soc J 33:799–802
9. Sethna NF, Rockoff MA, Worthen HM, Rosnow JM (1988) Anesthesia-related complications in children with Duchenne muscular dystrophy. Anesthesiology 68:462–465
10. Shapiro F, Sethna N, Colan S, Wohl ME, Specht L (1992) Spinal fusion in Duchenne muscular dystrophy: a multidisciplinary approach. Muscle Nerve 15:604–614

Chapter 16
Skin/Connective Tissue/Metabolic Disease

A 15-year-old female, 38 kg, is scheduled for a total shoulder replacement. She has a history of juvenile rheumatoid arthritis, status post bilateral total hip replacements and bilateral total knee replacements. She also had a tracheostomy for one of her hip replacements following intubation attempts that lasted 3 h. Vital signs are BP 90/60 mmHg, P 92 bpm, and T 37°C. Her hemoglobin is 11.5 g/dL. She has been on gold therapy, but currently is only on methotrexate and prednisone 20 mg, qod.

Preoperative Evaluation

1. How will you evaluate this patient's airway? What else are you concerned about in this particular patient with regard to airway management? Why? Should the tracheostomy be reopened? What is the risk of lung disease? Why? How will you evaluate? Are PFTs helpful? If so which ones? Is this obstructive or restrictive lung disease?

2. What are the implications of joint disease for this patient and your anesthetic management? Is there a greater risk of peripheral neuropathy? Why? What can you do about it? Would a regional anesthetic help?

Preoperative Evaluation

1. The airway should be evaluated for abnormalities of temperomandibular ankylosis and inability to open the mouth, mandibular hypoplasia, and cricoarytenoid joint arthritis. Symptoms include a feeling of fullness or tightness in the throat or a foreign body sensation, hoarseness, stridor, dysphagia, and pain on swallowing. Neck mobility and atlantoaxial or low cervical subluxation is evaluated by imaging studies. My concerns are restricted neck mobility and an inability to open the mouth wide enough to allow adequate visualization and instrumentation of the glottis. Tracheostomy reopening may be necessary because of difficult or impossible fiberoptic-guided intubation or if the patient refuses fiberoptic intubation with sedation.

   The disease affects the pulmonary system. The inflammatory process involves the sternocostal and costovertebral joints leading to a stiff rib cage and restricted chest wall motion. In advanced disease, inflammation of the lung parenchyma results in interstitial fibrosis with a reduction in lung volumes and compromised gas exchange. Pulmonary function tests may initially show restrictive lung disease. With progression of the disease, PFTs may show both restrictive and obstructive patterns. The vital capacity is usually preserved or minimally affected early in the course of the disease if the diaphragm activity is unimpeded. In addition to FVC, FEV_1, FEV_1/FVC, PEF, FEF_{25-75}, and flow-volume loops are of value in defining the site of airway obstruction.

2. Excessive motion of stiff and inflamed joints may result in joint dislocation or muscle and tendon stretch injury. Excessive motion of the cervical spine may compress the spinal cord or roots leading to neurological complications. Difficulty positioning the limbs due to stiff joints may cause excessive stretch of ligaments, muscles, nerves and postoperative discomfort, and paresthesias. With direct and prolonged pressure over bony prominences, soft tissue may suffer from ischemia and necrosis. Malpositioning of the limbs and prolonged compression of superficial nerves against bony prominences can cause neuropraxia and variable degrees of peripheral neuropathy. Compression of veins and/or arteries may cause a compartment syndrome, pain, compression neuropathy, muscle breakdown, myoglobinemia, myoglobinuria, and increased CPK. I would pay careful attention to proper positioning, soft padding of the pressure points, and periodically changing the position of pressure points to relieve pressure. Regional anesthesia may reduce the potential of pressure-related adverse effects of body regions not anesthetized by regional blockade and avoid airway manipulation. Upper extremity nerve blockade and neuraxial anesthesia are desirable for surgery involving the lower extremity and lower abdomen, but may not be feasible to perform due to loss of mobility of the spine and fusion of the vertebrae

364 Skin/Connective Tissue/Metabolic Disease

3. What are the anesthetic implications of prior treatment with gold? Current treatment with methotrexate? What about steroids? What problems may be a consequence of steroid use in this disease? If this patient was on aspirin, how could you evaluate for salicylism? Is acetaminophen indicated for long-term treatment of juvenile rheumatoid arthritis in children? Why/why not?

4. Should this patient be premedicated? With what? Why?

Intraoperative Course

1. Would an arterial line be a good idea? Why/Why not? Would you place it preinduction? Why? Any other special monitors you would choose?

3. The most common adverse effects of gold salts are dermatitis, stomatitis, and pruritic rash. Membranous glomerulonephritis is another serious side effect, with its earliest manifestation being proteinuria and hematuria. Bone marrow toxicity may present with aplastic anemia, agranulocytosis, and thrombocytopenia with severe marrow depression. Methotrexate is a cytotoxic drug and can cause bone marrow depression with severe leukopenia, infection, and hepatotoxicity. Long-term steroid therapy may cause a host of side effects including Cushing syndrome, osteopenia, platelet dysfunction, hyperglycemia, gastritis, hypertension, myopathy, and adrenal suppression. Salicylism manifests with sweating, vomiting, epigastric pain, tinnitus, and blurring of vision and later metabolic acidosis in moderate salicylism syndrome. In a severe overdose, the acidosis reduces the ionization of salicylic acid enhancing tissue penetration particularly in the CNS, which can manifest as agitation, tremor, and convulsions and eventually lead to coma and respiratory depression. Acetaminophen is an antipyretic and analgesic drug; its mode of action is not known. It is commonly used in JRA because it has no known drug interaction with anti-inflammatory agents and other agents used for treatment of JRA. The drawback of using acetaminophen in standard doses for an extended period of time is hepatotoxicity. Therefore, it is used on an as needed basis and not on an "around the clock" schedule.

4. Premedication should be used judiciously because of the potential for respiratory depression in the presence of severe restrictive respiratory disease and airway compromise. For anxiolysis, midazolam can be used and titrated to effect. Flumazenil should be readily available to reverse any excessive effect of midazolam.

Intraoperative Course

1. An arterial line is a good idea for monitoring the adequacy of controlled ventilation in this patient with chronic restrictive/obstructive respiratory disease. While it is preferable to place the arterial line prior to induction for monitoring purposes, it may not be practical if the patient is anxious and uncooperative. The shoulder procedure is usually performed in a semi-sitting position and there is an increased risk of air embolism; therefore, a precordial Doppler would be helpful for early detection.

2. Should you give an anticholinergic prior to induction? Why/why not? Should intravenous induction agents be avoided? Why/why not? What about a rapid-sequence intravenous induction? Is propofol better than thiopental for induction? The parents insist on a mask induction because of the patient's fear of needles and her multiple experiences with surgery. Your response? What about a regional anesthetic without general anesthesia? What would you choose? How can you provide surgical anesthesia for shoulder joint surgery?

3. What is your choice for anesthetic maintenance? Why? How would the use of halothane compare to isoflurane? Would desflurane be a good choice after induction and during maintenance? Is MAC different in this age group? In what way? Is ketamine a choice? Why/why not? Would a nitrous–narcotic technique be better? Why/why not?

4. What muscle relaxant would you choose? Should you use succinylcholine? Why/why not? Does this patient have a significant risk for reflux?

2. Anticholinergic agents should be avoided in patients with JRA who have keratoconjunctivitis sicca (Sjogren's syndrome) and associated fibrosis of the tear glands. These agents could further aggravate the dry eyes. Intravenous drugs should be avoided because they may cause respiratory depression, apnea and in the presence of compromised airways, manual controlled ventilation could be difficult if not impossible. Propofol is preferable to thiopental because of its rapid onset and offset. A mask induction without intravenous access is not advisable because of apnea or larygospasm. In addition, patients with JRA have a high incidence of gastroesophageal reflux, which may predispose them to aspiration of gastric contents. The use of regional anesthesia without general anesthesia is possible if the patient is cooperative and motivated. Nevertheless, performance of regional anesthetic techniques such as interscalene block could be associated with the potential for accidental intravascular injection of the local anesthetic, which may result in seizures, apnea, and cardiotoxicity. I would perform an awake-sedated fiberoptic tracheal intubation and general anesthetic supplemented with an interscalene block for perioperative pain relief.

3. My choice is either sevoflurane or isoflurane to minimize cardiovascular depression. Halothane can depress the myocardium more than sevoflurane or isoflurane and may aggravate preexisting hepatic dysfunction or cause hepatitis. Desflurane is a good choice for maintenance of anesthesia because of its low blood-gas solubility and rapid offset. It is not a good agent for induction of anesthesia because it has a pungent odor, irritates the airways, and is associated with a high incidence of laryngospasm and bronchospasm. Ketamine is not a good choice because it causes tachycardia and hypertension. There is high incidence of cardiac involvement in JRA (left ventricular enlargement, congestive heart failure, coronary artery disease due to vasculitis) particularly when complicated with Sjogren Syndrome. A nitrous oxide–narcotic-based technique is safer in the presence of cardiac involvement but may delay emergence from anesthesia and may necessitate postoperative ventilatory support.

4. I would use cisatracurium. I would not use succinylcholine because fasciculations caused by succinylcholine may lead to subluxation of joints and possibly neurological complications in the presence of cervical spine subluxation. Yes, this and other patients with JRA are at increased risk for gastroesophageal reflux due to fibrosis of the esophagus and incompetence of gastroesophageal sphincter. In addition, these patients have increased gastric acid production secondary to chronic intake of NSAIDs and steroids.

5. What are the advantages of allowing this patient to breath spontaneously throughout the entire case? Would you do it? Why/Why not? What breathing system would you choose? Why? Does it matter which breathing system you use if the patient is breathing spontaneously as opposed to through a circle absorption system? How do you ventilate someone with restrictive lung disease? Why? What will you set your I:E ratio at? Why? Is it better to ventilate with frequent short breaths or a slower respiratory rate with long breaths? Why?

Postoperative Course

1. When would you extubate? Why/why not? You extubate, and the patient is stridorous in the OR...what will you do? How do you evaluate? What are you concerned about?

2. You are called to the PACU to evaluate this patient for aphonia without stridor 1 h later. What is your differential? What will you do? Should this patient go back to the operating room?

5. The advantage of preserving spontaneous ventilation is that it avoids any potential trauma associated with instrumentation of the airway and potential barotrauma to the lungs. However, I would not advocate spontaneous breathing because of the presence of restrictive lung and chest wall disease and the high likelihood of hypoventilation during inhaled anesthesia. The drawback of spontaneous ventilation is the potential for aspiration pneumonitis due to GE reflux and the inability to secure the airway if gastric aspiration occurs. I would choose a nonrebreathing system such as Mapelson D to enhance efficient CO_2 elimination. The choice of a nonrebreathing vs. rebreathing system matters because certain systems such as the Mapelson D system are efficient in eliminating CO_2 and decrease the work of breathing because of being a valveless system. The valved circle system presents at least a theoretical concern of increased work of breathing because of the valves. I would set a longer inspiratory time with an I:E ratio of 1:1.5 to allow a sustained inspiratory flow to aerate the stiff alveolar tissue at a relatively slow ventilatory frequency. This strategy should generate adequate intra-alveolar distending pressures and gas mixing.

Postoperative Course

1. I would extubate the trachea when the patient is fully awake and the residual effect of the neuromuscular blocking agent has dissipated or has been fully reversed. Patients must be able to generate an inspiratory force greater than 20 cm of water and a vital capacity of 10 mL/kg or greater, and require a FiO_2 less than 0.5. For stridor, I would consult an otolaryngologist to perform direct/flexible laryngoscopy to assess the possible causes, such as subluxation of the arytenoid cartilages, swelling of the vocal cords or the subglottic region and examine the vallecula, epiglottis, pyriform sinuses, false vocal cords, true vocal cords, and the subglottic area.

2. Acute aphonia postextubation could be due to either bilateral subluxation of the arytenoid joints with the vocal cords immobile in abducted position or edema from traumatic laryngeal instrumentation that may worsen the chronically inflamed stiff arytenoid joints leading to immobility and full abduction of the true vocal cords. This patient should go back to the operating room and be thoroughly evaluated under direct laryngoscopy by an otolaryngologist and intubated to protect against aspiration.

Additional Topics

1. What are the anesthetic induction considerations in the patient with *epidermolysis bullosa*? Of what specific airway implications are the two broadly recognized forms of EB? Would you recommend a regional anesthetic for an otherwise healthy 5-year old having heel cord lengthening? How would you secure an epidural catheter? Prone position?

2. A 5-year old with *Hurler Syndrome* needs a recurrent umbilical hernia repaired. What are the anesthetic considerations? During mask anesthesia, the patient develops crowing, then laryngospasm…your next move? Would an LMA help? Would a blind nasal intubation help?

3. A 12-year-old boy with neurofibromatosis is scheduled for scoliosis surgery, posterior instrumentation, and spinal fusion. The surgeons keep asking you to lower the blood pressure so that they can get on with the surgery, but you have tried labetalol, esmolol, hydralazine, and some nitroprusside, all without significant effect. What could be going on? Which is the most likely cause?

Additional Topics

1. The major anesthetic induction consideration with epidermolysis bullosa is the risk of seriously traumatizing the facial skin and oropharyngeal and laryngeal mucosa with the use of a facemask and airway manipulation that can lead to severe airway compromise and pulmonary infection secondary to cross contamination. Airway manipulation should be avoided whenever possible. The facemask should be used with care and contact sites should be padded with cotton or foam. Tracheal intubation, when necessary, should be performed with extreme gentleness, using an endotracheal tube that is smaller in size than predicted by age. Any pressure or friction caused by monitors and airway management may cause blisters. Pressure causes less significant blisters than friction; application of a pulse oximeter clip probe is less hazardous than an adhesive probe. Barbiturates should not be used because of the increased risk of porphyria. There are two types of EB, the polyplastic form and the lethalis variant that invariably involves the mucosa of the gastrointestinal and respiratory systems. Regional anesthesia offers the benefit of not manipulating the airway and is feasible with effective premedication and a low dose infusion of propfol during the surgery. I would secure the epidural catheter by applying cotton or foam padding at the site of the catheter insertion and support it with a cotton (Webril) bandage wrapped around the trunk. I would take extra caution in positioning the patient, supporting pressure points and contact points with cotton or foam padding.

2. Anesthetic considerations for Hurler's syndrome are (1) lack of cooperation because of developmental delay, (2) difficulty maintaining the airway and during intubation due to macroglossia and stiff joints, (3) risk for bronchospasm due to reactive airway because of chronic respiratory infections, (4) difficulty with ventilation due to kyphosis, hepatosplenomegaly, and chronic obstructive lung disease, tracheo-bronchomalacia from mucopolysacharide deposits, and (5) potential for congestive and ischemic heart failure due to biventricular dilation, valvular incompetency, and coronary artery occlusion from infiltration of the mucopolysacharide deposits. If the patient develops laryngospasm I would administer rocuronium, 1.2 mg/kg to facilitate rapid airway patency. If it were difficult to ventilate the patient by facemask I would place an LMA to secure ventilation. It is not advisable to perform blind nasal intubation because it could cause trauma and bleeding of the swollen turbinates, adenoids, and naso-oral mucosa from chronic infection and muscopolysaccharide deposits.

3. Failure of various antihypertensive drugs may raise the possibility of pheochromocytoma or severe renal artery stenosis.

4. An otherwise healthy 5-year-old boy with vesicoureteral reflux was started on Bactrim 2 days earlier for uroprophylaxis. He was admitted to the intensive care unit with malaise, fever, headache, sore throat, vomiting, diarrhea, and extremely painful erosive bullae surrounding the mouth, lips, nares, and conjunctivae. He is not intubated. He needs a central line for better vascular access, and has a 24-gauge IV. How will you evaluate and manage his airway? What fluid/electrolyte problems can you anticipate? Nutritional problems? How long will this problem take to resolve? Can it recur?

5. A 14-month old has a mixed *cavernous and capillary hemangioma* involving the right side of the face, distributed in the forehead, orbit, cheek, lip, and mandibular area. He looks like the picture below, and is scheduled for a vascular study with possible embolization vs. sclerosant injection in the interventional angiography suite. Is this an unusual problem? What are your considerations? What does your laboratory work-up include? What if his platelet count was 75,000; what would you make of that? Should he receive a platelet transfusion? What is the Kasabach–Merritt syndrome? Would you expect that this patient would have been receiving any medications chronically? Is this likely to be a problem? Does he require steroid coverage?

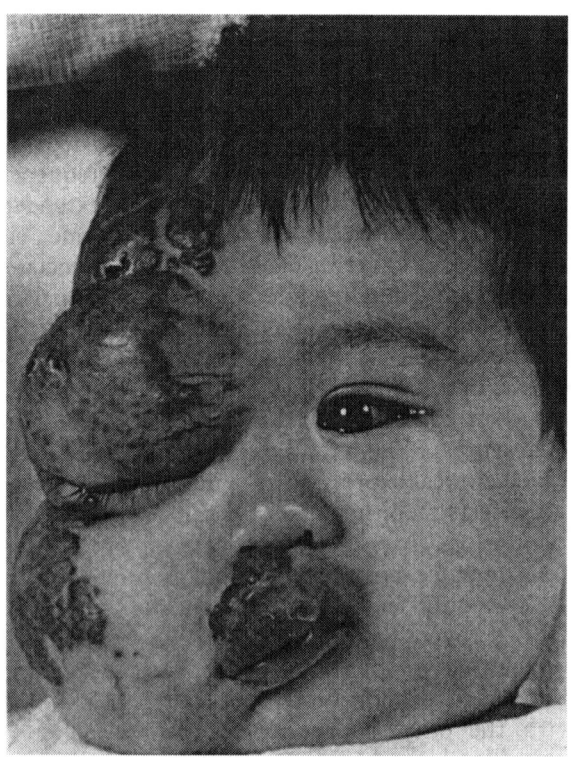

4. Tracheal intubation should be avoided in erythema multiforme major (Stevens–Johnson syndrome) if possible because this syndrome is characterized by blistering necrolytic bullous eruption of the skin and mucus membranes. Airways can be evaluated by otolaryngology using a flexible laryngoscope under intravenous ketamine sedation. If pharyngeal and subglottic respiratory mucus membranes are moderate to severely involved in the disease process, ventilation could be managed by facemask. Excessive loss of mucus, interstitial fluid, and electrolytes through necrolytic blisters of the skin and mucus membranes are expected in this syndrome. Intravenous nutrition is necessary because of failure to absorb nutrients via the alimentary tract. Spontaneous healing usually occurs in the mild form. In severe cases, it may take 6–8 weeks for the condition to resolve. Recurrence is reported with reactivation of herpes simplex virus infection.

5. Cavernous–capillary hemangioma is a rare condition and commonly affects the head and neck area early in infancy. This type of vascular anomaly may cause platelet destruction leading to thrombocytopenia and microangiopathic hemolytic anemia. Patients should be examined for ecchymoses, petechiae, and rapid enlargement of the hemangioma that may indicate local hemorrhage and consumption coagulopathy. Laboratory workup should include CBC, platelet count, and fibrinogen concentration. This platelet count is not terribly low but indicates intravascular trapping and destruction of platelets. Kasabach–Merritt syndrome is a type of cavernous hemangioma that rapidly enlarges and causes thrombocytopenia, microangiopathic hemolytic anemia, and acute or consumption coagulopathy. It manifests early in infancy, usually involves the head and neck and may compromise the upper airways but can involve viscera and other tissues and may grow rapidly causing local tissue destruction, disfigurement, and life-threatening coagulopathy. These patients chronically receive blood product transfusions of FFP, platelets, and packed red blood cells. Digitalization may be necessary if arteriovenous shunts are large enough to cause high-output heart failure. Other medications include recombinant interferon-alpha that may inhibit proliferation of vascular endothelial and smooth muscle cells, steroids, and antifibrinolytic agents. Steroid coverage is necessary if the patient is receiving steroids chronically.

6. What is the most important consideration for a patient coming from the ICU to the OR for a central line if he has *toxic epidermal necrolysis*?

7. A 14-year-old patient with *Ehlers–Danlos Syndrome* is coming to the OR for posterior spinal fusion. Preop considerations? Special anesthetic requirements? Laboratory evaluation? How much blood would you set up for him? You find a 3/6 holosystolic murmur at the cardiac apex – any special thoughts? Are there any consequences to invasive cardiovascular monitoring in this patient? How would you judge the risk/benefit ratio of invasive monitoring when you explain it to the patient and parents? What contribution can an anesthesiologist make to the special perioperative considerations for wound healing in these patients?

8. You are called to the radiology suite for a patient with a history of panic attacks. He has a history of congenital *C1-esterase inhibitor deficiency*. You arrive in a darkened room. He just received a contrast injection, and is complaining of a fullness in his throat. You turn on the light, and find facial, lip, and eyelid swelling. He is complaining of abdominal pain. Your assessment? Treatment? Airway management? Plans following intubation? How long will he likely have to stay in the ICU? Medical therapy? Would antifibrinolytics like Amicar or tranexamic acid be of any help? Why/why not? Should he receive FFP to increase his level of C1 esterase inhibitor?

6. The most important consideration for this patient is airway management and intubation of the trachea.

7. Preoperative considerations for the patient with Ehlers–Danlos syndrome include a comprehensive history and physical evaluation of (1) excessive joint laxity particularly in the neck and temporomandibular joint, (2) the presence of fragile blood vessels may indicate difficult vascular access, (3) the potential for arterial aneurysms, (4) cardiac valve prolapse and dilated ventricles, (5) the potential for involvement of the lungs (blebs), and (6) glaucoma. Laboratory evaluation should include platelet function and bleeding time. Since EDS is a connective tissue disease, a subtype of this syndrome can affect platelet function and predispose to excessive surgical bleeding. The holosystolic murmur at the apex most likely is due to mitral valve regurgitation. I would set up at least 6 units of blood in anticipation of excessive blood loss due to platelet dysfunction and microvascular bleeding from impaired vascular contractility as a result of the thin vascular wall and weakened smooth muscle. All monitors should be applied with caution particularly invasive cardiovascular monitors because the vessel walls are thin and fragile due to collagen deficiency and are prone to injury with mild trauma. Patients and parents should be made aware of the risk of rupturing major vessels during placement of vascular needles and indwelling catheters and the potential for creating aneurysms. The selection of a particular invasive monitoring strategy should be guided by whether it provides clear information that would assist interventions that could reduce the risk of cardiovascular complications in the perioperative care. Wound healing is a major issue due to impaired collagen function; therefore, considerable care is needed in positioning the patient prone and in protecting all the pressure points and skin contact areas with cotton and foam pads to avoid skin ischemia, breakdown, and infection. Meticulous care and patience should be observed during airway management (TMJ dislocation, airway soft tissue injury), vascular access, and application of other monitoring devices such as blood pressure, temperature probe, and bladder catheter. The positive pressure ventilation parameter should also be modified to avoid delivery of high intrathoracic pressures to minimize the potential for barotrauma and pneumothorax.

8. Most likely, this patient is developing an acute episode of hereditary angioedema that involves the skin and mucosa of the respiratory and gastrointestinal systems. The treatment in acute angioedema is to secure the airway by placement of an endotracheal tube. After intubation, supportive therapy is instituted until C1 inhibitor esterase concentrate or FFP is available. The patient will have to stay in the ICU until laryngeal edema as well as other inflammatory manifestations of this disease resolve with treatment. Medical therapy during an acute attack consists of administration (1) of C1-inhibitor concentrate infusion during the acute episode and (2) aerolized heparin to bind to activated complement within the lung parenchyma. For long-term therapy, parenteral androgens are useful to boost the production of C1-inhibitor or antifibrinolytic agents. Prophylaxis treatment with two units of FFP is advised immediately prior to surgery or manipulation of the airways. FFP may decrease autoantibody production and increase solubilization and removal of

immune complexes. Antifibrinolytic agents like aminocaproic acid or tranexamic acid are useful for treatment of the acute attack or as prophylaxis. They act by inhibiting plasmin action and thereby blocking the activation of the fibrinolytic system by C1-inhibitor. No, this patient should not receive FFP during an active episode because it may worsen the condition by providing complement components that may accelerate the angioedema process.

General References

1. Miller M, Cassidy J (2004) Juvenile rheumatoid arthritis. In: Behreman R, Kliegman R, Jenson H (eds) Nelson textbook of pediatrics, 17th edn. WB Saunders, Philadelphia, pp 809–813
2. Ciarallo C, Galinkin J (2008) Metabolic diseases and inborn errors of metabolism. In: Holzman R, Mancuso T, Polaner D (eds) A practical approach to pediatric anesthesia. Lippincott Williams and Wilkins, Philadelphia, p 560
3. Holzman R, Worthen H, Johnson K (1987) Anaesthesia for children with junctional epidermolysis bullosa (letalis). Can J Anaesth 34:395–399
4. Lane G, Polaner D (2008) Integumentary system. In: Holzman R, Mancuso T, Polaner D (eds) A practical approach to pediatric anesthesia. Philadelphia, Lippincott Williams and Wilkins, pp 511–514
5. Walport M (2001) Complement: first of two parts. N Engl J Med 344:1058–1066

Chapter 17
Inborn Errors of Metabolism

A 5-year old with Hurler syndrome needs a recurrent umbilical hernia repaired. He cannot come in for evaluation prior to surgery, but will be coming in early on the day of surgery for his preop work-up. He is not yet in school, and is 24 kg.

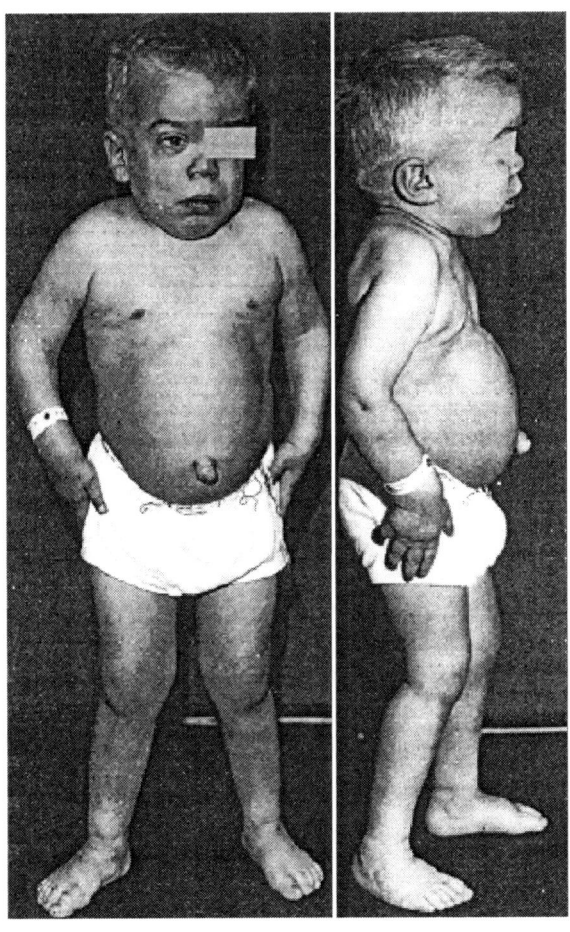

Preoperative Evaluation

1. What is Hurlers syndrome? What is/are the metabolic defects in this condition?

2. He has a large head. Is this of any concern to you? Why/why not? Why is the head large in this disorder? How would you evaluate his airway? What is the significance of the macroglossia? The nasal obstruction? Is there anything about the neck that concerns you? Would it be easy to do an emergency bronchoscopy or tracheostomy, if the need arose?

3. What is the significance of the protuberant abdomen and enlarged liver and spleen?

4. How might this disease affect the cardiovascular system? What evidence would you look for? How can you distinguish right from left ventricular dysfunction in this patient? Is it important to do so? How do you know that the patient does not have any significant coronary artery disease? Why might he?

5. Does this patient have restrictive or obstructive lung disease? How do you know? Can you quantify it? Should arterial blood gases be obtained preoperatively? If not, what would you study to quantify the extent of disease preoperatively?

Preoperative Evaluation

1. Mucopolysaccharidosis 1 H, called Hurlers disease, is one of a group of inherited disorders resulting from defects in degradation of complex mucopolysaccharides now called glycosaminoglycans. Affected patients lack the lysosomal hydrolases (specifically lysosomal alpha-L-iduronidase) responsible for degradation of these compounds. The lysosomes become engorged with mucopolysaccharides. The compounds dermatan and heparan, formed in excess as a result of defects in degradation of the glycosaminoglycan, accumulate in virtually all tissues of the body. Hurler's syndrome is inherited as an autosomal recessive.

2. The syndrome is characterized by growth retardation with enlargement of the skull. The head has frontal bossing and prominent metopic and sagittal sutures. Dermatan and heparan accumulate in virtually all tissues of the body. The children have nasal obstruction and an enlarged tongue due to accumulation of heparan and dermatan. Affected children are usually mouth breathers as a result of the nasal obstruction. The laryngeal inlet and trachea itself may be narrowed by accumulated glycosaminoglycans. The exaggerated kyphosis is typical of affected children. The cervical spine, as all joints, will have impaired mobility. The enlarged chest makes performing tracheostomy, particularly in an emergency, very difficult [1–3].

3. The liver and spleen are enlarged as a result of accumulation of incompletely degraded glycosaminoglycans, similar to the tongue and other connective tissues.

4. There is distortion of the valves and coronary arterial deformation, again caused by accumulation of incompletely degraded glycosaminoglycans. All valves are affected, but in postmortem examinations, the mitral valve is the most severely affected. In addition, the walls of the coronary arteries are thickened in these patients. Cardiac function is impaired as a result of coronary artery disease and deposition of glycosaminoglycans in the myocardium [4].

5. The ribs are flared and these patients have frequent respiratory infections. Accumulation of material in the chest wall may lead to a restrictive pattern of disease while airway narrowing due to accumulation of the same by-products may give an obstructive pattern. This child will not cooperate with measurement of pulmonary function. If the serum bicarbonate is elevated, measurement of blood gases will help quantify the degree of preoperative respiratory insufficiency.

Intraoperative Course

1. Other than standard noninvasive monitors, which additional monitors would you choose? Why? Does this patient need an arterial line for this umbilical hernia repair? Why/why not? Central line or PA line for monitoring cardiac function? What about a transesophageal echo? What would you look for? How would it show up on echo?

2. Mom asks if the patient can be premedicated in the holding area because she is the only one who can comfort him. Your response to her request? Is IM ketamine a reasonable alternative if he is so hard to manage? Why/why not? What would you be concerned about specifically? Would you "breathe him down" given the fact that he has a high likelihood of significant cardiac dysfunction? What agent would you choose in this setting? Why?

3. You begin your anesthetic induction, smell a pungent odor, and immediately notice that the desflurane vaporizer was left on; the patient has just gotten 6% desflurane at a 10 L fresh gas flow and now has solid, unremitting laryngospasm. How to manage? What are your considerations? Is succinylcholine indicated or contraindicated? What type of heart rate response would you expect? How and where to administer if there is no IV?

4. You have tried to do a direct laryngoscopy, anterior commissure scope and fiberoptic scope transorally, all without success. What next? Is a laryngeal mask airway (LMA) a reasonable choice? Why/why not?

Intraoperative Course

1. This case could be done with standard monitors. If, after induction, it becomes apparent that his cardiac function is impaired to a greater degree than previously thought, or if postop ventilation is considered, additional monitors may be useful. An arterial line will be helpful as much in the postoperative period when evaluation of the effectiveness of his respiratory function on clinical grounds will be difficult. TEE intraoperatively will give information about cardiac function but placement could be problematic. This monitor may show poor contractility due to ischemia, it may show valvular dysfunction or impaired contractility due to infiltration of the myocardium by mucopolysaccharides. Pulmonary hypertension secondary to cor pulmonale and longstanding hypoxemia may also be diagnosed with an ECHO. Placement of these additional monitors will be difficult, owing to the deposition of the glycosaminoglycans in the pharynx and on the extremities over the peripheral arteries.

2. Excessive sedation from premedication of this child can lead to hypoventilation and worsening of his airway obstruction [5]. Care must be taken in choosing a medication and dose. Vigilant monitoring is essential after the dose is given. Oral midazolam with an antisialogue is a reasonable option. Midazolam alone is unlikely to cause significant hypoventilation and may calm the child somewhat. Glycopyrrolate is an important addition to the premedication since airway management will be difficult in any case and even more so if excessive secretions are present. IM ketamine can certainly sedate this child but there are side effects that may worsen the situation. The direct myocardial depressant effect is generally not clinically significant in well children but this patient may have cardiac impairment that will worsen with administration of ketamine. In addition, the increased production of secretions and increased airway reactivity also may complicate airway management. If an inhalation induction is chosen, sevoflurane would be a good choice since it is generally well tolerated and causes relatively little cardiac depression.

3. Laryngospasm, the complete closure of the true and false cords, is an airway emergency. The oxygen remaining in the child's FRC is all that is available to sustain aerobic metabolism. Treatment is administration of a rapidly acting muscle relaxant as soon as possible. If there is an IV in place, atropine and succinylcholine should be given intravenously. If there is no IV, the clinician must decide immediately whether or not IV access can be secured very quickly. If not, the atropine and succinylcholine must be given intramuscularly.

4. An inhalation induction has proceeded smoothly, an IV is in place, and easy mask ventilation assured. In this situation, intubation has failed even with the use of anterior commissure scope and transoral fiberoptic scope. Nasal obstruction with mucopolysaccharide nasal passage infiltration often renders transnasal fiberoptic intubation impossible. Placement of an LMA may be possible but the size chosen should be smaller than usual, expecting the oropharynx to be smaller as a result of deposition of dermatan and heparan. However, if there is a satisfactory mask airway a reasonable choice may be to quickly finish the hernia repair with mask inhalational general anesthesia [6].

Postoperative Management

1. What are your recommendations for pain management?

2. What if the procedure was an exploratory laparotomy for incarcerated hernia?

What about parent-controlled PCA? Is an epidural a good idea? If an epidural is placed how will proper positioning be assured?

Additional Topics

1. A 3-year old presents for open liver biopsy with a suspected diagnosis of Glycogen storage disease type I (von Gierke). What problems might you expect with this disorder of carbohydrate metabolism? What physical characteristics might be of most significance in planning the anesthetic? Any particular considerations for intravenous fluid management? Does the hepatomegaly occur together with splenomegaly?

Postoperative Management

1. Children who undergo routine hernia repair generally require NSAIDs for analgesia once the immediate postoperative period is over. Perioperative analgesia can be accomplished by a variety of techniques. Another option is for the surgeon to perform the nerve blocks during the procedure itself. Intravenous ketorolac given near the end of the repair should provide adequate postop analgesia for several hours.

2. If the procedure were an exploratory laparotomy, it would have been important to secure the airway. Postop analgesia would require more than NSAIDs or Tylenol. In that case lumbar epidural analgesia is a good choice for this child. Placement would be accomplished after successful induction of general anesthesia and securing the airway and would be a technical challenge. Epidural placement in these patients can be as difficult as securing the airway [7]. Confirmation of proper placement with radiographs (epidurogram) or via nerve stimulation would be important. Even if the solution used is local anesthetic plus opioid, the opioid dose administered will be lower than if opioid were given IV. Local anesthetic alone might be sufficient if IV ketorolac were administered for 1–2 days postop in addition. IV nurse controlled analgesia (NCA) with opioid could be used to provide analgesia to this child following a laparotomy. Parent-controlled analgesia has been used, but in a patient with these risk factors for respiratory compromise, analgesic administration should only be performed by the RN.

Additional Topics

1. In glycogen storage disease type I (von Gierke's disease), deficiency of glucose-6-phosphatase and glycogen accumulates in the liver, kidneys, and intestines. This is the most common of the glycogen storage diseases. The spleen is not enlarged. Excess glucose-6-phosphate enters the anaerobic glycolosis pathway leading to accumulation of lactic acid. In addition, these children may have elevated cholesterol and triglycerides. When feedings are spaced or interrupted, hypoglycemia results. Some of these patients may have severe hypoglycemia and not show clinical signs and symptoms, perhaps because the brain can utilize the lactate as an energy source when glucose availability is limited. Intraoperatively, glucose-containing solutions should be given and glucose checked frequently. Muscle does not normally contain the enzyme glucose-6-phosphatase so neither cardiac nor skeletal muscle is involved in this disease. These children also may have impaired function of platelets and neutrophils and so may be subject to bacterial infection or have a prolonged bleeding time.

2. Why are infants tested for phenylketonuria? What are the consequences of a deficiency of phenylalanine hydroxylase? Can this be managed adequately by reduction of phenylalanine intake? Let us say that you had to do a gastrostomy in patient with phenylketonuria (PKU) who was 5 years old with an IQ of 20. Any special anesthetic considerations?

3. An 8-year old with a history of familial hypercholesterolemia type II B is scheduled for a portacaval shunt as a last-ditch treatment to lower his cholesterol; he is treated with cholestyramine and clofibrate. Dietary treatment has been of no benefit. His preoperative ECG shows Q waves in leads II, III, avF and leads V_4–V_6. What are your thoughts about management? Do you think he is homozygous or heterozygous for this disorder? What difference does it make? What if his brother was heterozygous?

4. A 2-year old with Lesch–Nyhan syndrome (absence of hypoxanthine–guanine phosphoribosyl transferase, with resultant uric acid accumulation) is scheduled for complete dental extractions. Why? What are your anesthetic considerations? How can you put this patient to sleep? How should you wake this patient up?

2. PKU is caused by absence of the enzyme phenylalanine hydroxylase, which degrades the essential amino acid phenylalanine via the tyrosine pathway. In PKU, the excess phenylalanine not used in protein synthesis is transaminated to phenylpyruvic acid or decarboxylated to phenylethylamine. These and other metabolites as well as phenylalanine itself disrupt normal metabolism and cause CNS damage. Affected newborns are normal at birth but if left untreated may lose as much as 50 IQ points in the first month of life [8]. Severe vomiting occurs early and the condition can be misdiagnosed as pyloric stenosis. Treatment is dietary, with rigid control of phenylalanine intake for at least the first 6 years of life and some control for life. An older child with PKU should not be seen in countries with screening. A 5-year old with untreated PKU may have severe mental retardation, microcephaly, increased tone, growth failure, a prominent maxilla, and widely spaced teeth. The airway may be difficult [9]. These children generally have fair skin with seborrhea and blue eyes.

3. Familial hypercholesterolemia is inherited as a dominant disorder. Patients who are heterozygous often do not develop coronary atherosclerosis until the third or fourth decade of life. By age 60, 85% of these individuals have suffered an MI. The rare (1:1,000,000) patient who is homozygous for the abnormality in lipoprotein metabolism has a much more severe form of the illness. These patients have plasma cholesterol levels of >600 mg%. Dietary management is of little or no help in lowering the cholesterol. Cholesterol-lowering medications also offer little benefit. Coronary disease is evident by 10 years of age and most patients die by 30 years of age. Therapies such as plasmapheresis, ileal bypass surgery, and portacaval shunt placement have had some success. Liver transplantation has helped several patients. There is a possible genetic treatment involving transfecting the patient's own hepatocytes with a gene for the missing receptor [10–12].

4. Lesch–Nyhan syndrome is a defect in purine and pyridimine metabolism transmitted as an X-linked condition. Affected infants appear normal at birth but show delayed motor development within a few months. Later, choreoathetoid movements appear accompanied by spasticity of the lower extremities but the most characteristic abnormality is compulsive self-destructive behavior [13]. These children bite and chew their fingers, lips, and buccal mucosa. Without restraints these children continue this self-destructive behavior. This patient would be scheduled for dental extractions because he is constantly biting himself. Cardiorespiratory function is normal and gastroesophageal reflux is not a problem in these children, leaving open the possibility of many induction and maintenance techniques. Prior to emergence, the child should be put back into his usual restraints and the IV particularly well covered and protected. Antiemetics should be given as part of the anesthetic since most children who have extensive dental work in the operating room swallow some blood [14, 15].

Annotated References

Nargozian C (2004) The airway in patients with craniofacial abnormalities. Paediatr Anaesth 14:53–59

This very thorough review includes an assessment of airway abnormalities analyzing various parts of the airway including the oral cavity, anterior mandibular space, temporomandibular joint, and vertebral column. In addition to the mucopolysaccharidoses, specific conditions such as Trisomy 21, Treacher–Collins syndrome, Klippel–Feil syndrome, and Beckwith–Weideman syndrome are discussed.

Seashore M (2006) Amino acid disorders. In: Kliegman RM, Marcdante KJ, Jenson HB, Behrman RE (eds) Nelson essentials of pediatrics, 5th edn. Elsevier Saunders, Philadelphia, pp 255–257

This chapter includes discussion of the treatment and outcome in children with these inborn errors of metabolism. Included are other conditions such as Maple Syrup Urine Disease and ornithine carbamoyl transferase (OTC) deficiency.

References

1. Nargozian C (2004) The airway in patients with craniofacial abnormalities. Paediatr Anaesth 14:53–59
2. Man TT, Tsai PS, Rau RH et al (1999) Children with mucopolysaccharidoses – three cases report. Acta Anaesthesiol Sin 37:93–96
3. Dearlove OR (1999) Anaesthesia for Hurler's syndrome. Hosp Med 60:71
4. Toda Y, Takeuchi M, Morita K et al (2001) Complete heart block during anesthetic management in a patient with mucopolysaccharidosis type VII. Anesthesiology 95:1035–1037
5. Gaitini L, Fradis M, Vaida S et al (1998) Failure to control the airway in a patient with Hunter's syndrome. J Laryngol Otol 112:380–382
6. Walker RW (2000) The laryngeal mask airway in the difficult paediatric airway: an assessment of positioning and use in fibreoptic intubation. Paediatr Anaesth 10:53–58
7. Vas L, Naregal F (2000) Failed epidural anaesthesia in a patient with Hurler's disease. Paediatr Anaesth 10:95–98
8. Williams RA, Mamotte CD, Burnett JR (2008) Phenylketonuria: an inborn error of phenylalanine metabolism. Clin Biochem Rev 29:31–41
9. Dal D, Celiker V (2004) Anesthetic management of a strabismus patient with phenylketonuria. Paediatr Anaesth 14:701–702
10. Huijgen R, Vissers MN, Defesche JC et al (2008) Familial hypercholesterolemia: current treatment and advances in management. Expert Rev Cardiovasc Ther 6:567–581
11. Marais AD (2004) Familial hypercholesterolaemia. Clin Biochem Rev 25:49–68
12. Kwiterovich PO (2008) Primary and secondary disorders of lipid metabolism in pediatrics. Pediatr Endocrinol Rev 5(Suppl 2):727–738
13. Chiong MA, Marinaki A, Duley J et al (2006) Lesch-Nyhan disease in a 20-year-old man incorrectly described as developing 'cerebral palsy' after general anaesthesia in infancy. J Inherit Metab Dis 29:594
14. Larson LO, Wilkins RG (1985) Anesthesia and the Lesch–Nyhan syndrome. Anesthesiology 63:197–199
15. Williams KS, Hankerson JG, Ernst M, Zametkin A (1997) Use of propofol anesthesia during outpatient radiographic imaging studies in patients with Lesch–Nyhan syndrome. J Clin Anesth 9:61–65

Chapter 18
Allergy/Immunology

An 8-year-old 25-kg boy is scheduled for functional endoscopic sinus surgery. He has a history of hypogammaglobulinemia diagnosed at 4 months of age with recurrent sinus and respiratory tract infections, and was seen in the emergency department 2 weeks ago requiring an epinephrine injection for moderate respiratory distress. He has a productive cough constantly, and bronchiectasis by X-ray. His medications include cromolyn, terbutaline, sulfamethoxazole/trimethoprim, and an inhaler. Vital signs are BP 90/60 mmHg, P 100 bpm, R 18/min, T 37°C and his Hb is 13 g/dL.

R.S. Holzman et al., *Pediatric Anesthesiology Review: Clinical Cases for Self-Assessment*,   387
DOI 10.1007/978-1-4419-1617-4_18, © Springer Science+Business Media, LLC 2010

Preoperative Evaluation

1. What is bronchiectasis? Of what importance is it to anesthetic management? Of what significance is the recent visit to ED? Do you desire additional information regarding his chronic lung disease? Specifically? Why? Is a chest X-ray necessary? Why/why not? Do you need to identify what inhaler he is using? Why? Relevance?

2. What effect does his lung disease have on his cardiovascular system? How will you evaluate this preoperatively? Why? What are the anesthetic implications? Are there tertiary effects of such cardiac disease on other organ systems?

3. The child is quite anxious and mother tells you anxiety can initiate asthma symptoms. Would you order premedication? If not, why not? If so, what? Rationale. Should this patient receive preoperative antibiotics? Why/why not?

Preoperative Evaluation

1. Bronchiectasis is characterized by weakness and loss of cartilaginous integrity of the bronchial wall as a result of chronic inflammation, infection, and abscess. It is usually the result of chronic focal or diffuse lung infections. Anesthetic management is influenced because of the chronic secretions, mucous plugging of the airways, impaired gas exchange, and air trapping affecting shunt as well as dead space. Patients often have chronic pulmonary disease such as cystic fibrosis or impaired immune defense mechanisms such as hypogammaglobulinemia. The recent visit to the ED suggests that the patient's compensation may be marginal. It would be helpful to know whether he is on bronchodilators and what those are, whether supplemental oxygen is required at home, whether he has been treated with steroids recently, and whether his respiratory difficulties are associated with any other medical abnormalities. A chest X-ray is helpful if the history points to an acute exacerbation above his usual baseline. It is important to identify the inhaler he uses because you might wish to employ additional inhalers or intravenous medications that may work additively or synergistically with his home medication.

2. Chronic pulmonary disease with resulting hypoxemia may result in gradual elevation of pulmonary artery pressure and pulmonary vascular resistance, with eventual right heart strain. Ultimately, right heart failure will affect not only pulmonary circuit volume but also systemic cardiac output and contribute to left ventricular failure and impaired perfusion. Because general anesthesia typically involves the use of positive pressure ventilation, which can adversely affect cardiac filling as well as cardiac performance and also involves the use of volatile anesthetics, myocardial performance can be severely affected. Tertiary effects of impaired cardiac disease include hypoperfusion to the splanchnic circulation and protein-losing enteropathies, hepatic and splenic congestion, and renal failure.

3. Mothers usually know their children best, and premedication may not be a bad idea for this patient. On the other hand, he is 8 years old and conversation may do well at this age; children younger than school age will need premedication more often. Oral midazolam would probably work well, but should be used in an effective dose; 15–20 mg seems reasonable to achieve a good anxiolytic effect. Other alternatives might include intramuscular ketamine, midazolam, and glycopyrrolate. Preoperative antibiotics, if given well in advance (e.g., 2–3 days), may aid in decreasing various sites of infection within ectatic segments of the patient's lungs. In addition, these patients may have other foci of infection, such as the sinuses, which may become important as a source of infection in the perioperative period.

Intraoperative Course

1. What monitors will you select? Why? How will your chosen monitors assist in evaluation of his pulmonary function? Will $P_{ET}CO_2$ accurately represent his $PaCO_2$? Explain. Would you consider an arterial catheter for ABG assessment? Why/why not? How will you place lines? What is the risk of infection? Is this patient colonized? Why?

2. This child is terrified at prospect of an IV and will not cooperate. How will you induce anesthesia? Rationale. Colleague suggests IM Ketamine. You respond? How will you prepare the skin? Why? Should antibiotics be administered before oral intubation? What is your choice? Why?

3. What agent(s) would you use to maintain anesthesia? Why? Would you avoid N_2O? Benefits? What is the role of nitrous oxide use with regard to immunosuppression? Methionine synthetase regulation? Would you favor spontaneous ventilation or would you control ventilation? Why? Would you use a muscle relaxant? Why/why not?

Intraoperative Course

1. At this point, standard noninvasive monitors should be sufficient for the planned procedure. SpO_2 should be sufficient to judge the efficiency of oxygenation and changes in shunting throughout the case and the $ETCO_2$ should be sufficient to judge the adequacy of ventilation and any changes in dead space. $PETCO_2$ should be a reasonable reflection of $PaCO_2$ because carbon dioxide is so much more diffusible than air; however, much depends on the extent of the bronchiectasis. While one lobe may not change the dead space to tidal volume ratio significantly, multilobe bronchiectasis could. If the bronchiectasis was extensive or perioperative ventilatory failure was anticipated, then an arterial line would be useful for following blood gases frequently. In this case, the line should be placed with good sterile technique because the risk of infection from opportunistic organisms as well as the patient's own colonized flora could be significant.

2. I do not think it would be bad to start off with a mask induction, but if he is terrified of the IV he may be terrified of the mask. Alternatives include an oral or intramuscular premed (but what about the needle stick with the IM shot?) or the use of eutectic mixture of local anesthetics (EMLA) cream applied about an hour in advance. Antibiotics may not be a bad idea, and a broad-spectrum antibiotic such as ampicillin, clindamycin, or Zosyn would probably be reasonable choices to cover a wide range of oral and respiratory flora.

3. Anesthetic maintenance should ideally be carried out with a balanced technique for a few different reasons. First of all, the volatile agent will act to attenuate bronchoreactivity and will also allow a higher F_iO_2 than would a high inspired concentration of nitrous oxide. The use of an opioid, on the other hand, would decrease the amount of postoperative coughing that would undoubtedly follow the anesthetic, and would also allow for more rapid emergence because of the decreased requirement for the volatile agent. If the patient remains well oxygenated then nitrous oxide need not be avoided, although nitrous oxide has been shown to worsen elevated pulmonary artery pressure in patients with known elevated pulmonary vascular resistance due to heart disease. Nitrous oxide has also been shown to interfere with methionine synthetase when used in inspired concentrations greater than 50%. There may be a role for spontaneous ventilation in decreasing turbulence in already turbulent airways and therefore enhancing gas exchange, but if the patient's airflow is that turbulent, one might be better off delaying the surgery anyway. The use of a muscle relaxant may allow a lighter plane of anesthesia and therefore faster emergence, but the lighter plane of anesthesia may worsen bronchoreactivity and bronchospasm. There is also a relationship between bronchospasm, airway reactivity, and laryngospasm, so it may nevertheless be worthwhile considering the use of muscle relaxants as an adjunct, but they are not intrinsically necessary to the procedure.

4. During surgery his breath sounds, which had been consistently coarse and rhonchorous, transform to a distinct expiratory wheeze. How would you proceed? Why? If you use an anticholinergic, is glycopyrolate as effective as atropine? Differences? Worried about drying and inspissation of secretions? What about aminophyllin? Efficacy of dosing regimen under general anesthesia? Would lidocaine be of any benefit? Your choice? Why?/Why not?

5. Toward the end of surgery the inspiratory pressure during controlled ventilation rises from a previous high of 24–60 cm H_2O, along with a drop in oxygen saturation to 85% and a drop in blood pressure to 72/40. Discuss your considerations? Diagnostic steps? Therapy? Defend.

4. The most likely consideration is bronchoreactivity and bronchospasm with an acute elevation in airway pressure and significant impairment of systemic cardiac output because of the mechanical effect of the increased intrathoracic pressure on left ventricular output (due to shifting of the interventriclar septum) and impaired venous return because of the increase in intrathoracic pressure. This picture would account for the acute elevation of airway pressure, the drop in oxygen saturation, and the drop in blood pressure. The differential would also include a pneumothorax and pneumo-hemothorax, an accidental mainstem intubation with resulting bronchospasm, and pulmonary edema, all of which should be carefully considered. A judgment should be made about any changes in the depth of the endotracheal tube, the chest auscultated, the length of the tube examined, and the beneficial effect of withdrawing the tube if deemed necessary. Pneumothorax should initially be evaluated by auscultation and a chest X-ray if needed; placement of a chest tube may be required and nitrous oxide should be discontinued. Pulmonary edema will likely be obvious because of the frothy material in the endotracheal tube and the copious secretions during suctioning.

5. The most likely consideration is bronchoreactivity and bronchospasm with an acute elevation in airway pressure and significant impairment of systemic cardiac output because of the mechanical effect of the increased intrathoracic pressure on left ventricular output (due to shifting of the interventriclar septum) and impaired venous return because of the increase in intrathoracic pressure. This picture would account for the acute elevation of airway pressure, the drop in oxygen saturation, and the drop in blood pressure. The differential would also include a pneumothorax and pneumo-hemothorax, an accidental mainstem intubation with resulting bronchospasm, and pulmonary edema, all of which should be carefully considered. A judgment should be made about any changes in the depth of the endotracheal tube, the chest auscultated, the length of the tube examined, and the beneficial effect of withdrawing the tube if deemed necessary. Pneumothorax should initially be evaluated by auscultation and a chest X-ray if needed; placement of a chest tube may be required and nitrous oxide should be discontinued. Pulmonary edema will likely be obvious because of the frothy material in the endotracheal tube and the copious secretions during suctioning.

Postoperative Course

1. Discuss your extubation sequence if compliance normal without wheezing. Awake vs. "deep"? Why?

2. In PACU, after extubation child becomes combative. How will you proceed? Why? What if you had given Ketamine? Why?

Additional Topics

1. What parts of the anesthesia machine can be stripped down and sterilized? Which parts cannot? Is everything proximal to the CO_2 absorption cannister safe for use in immunocompromised patients?

Postoperative Care

1. Here the data is controversial. Although many would prefer to extubate deep, I would tend to extubate awake, reasoning that if, at the end of surgery and with emergence, the patient was lightening and therefore bronchospasm worsened, I would remove the endotracheal tube with the expectation that the bronchospasm would resolve. The alternative would be to extubate and hope that the patient passes through the excitement stage uneventfully, which seems more hazardous, although both methods have been used successfully.

2. The combativeness can be difficult to deal with and dangerous for the patient because he can pull out IVs, etc. A rapid assessment must be made for hypoxia or any other cause of instability, pain, and/or delirium. If the patient is not conversing or answering questions, it is reasonable to try some pain medication first (morphine, fentanyl) before going on with the differential; however, if they seem delirious rather than in pain, a watch and wait attitude seems safest. Small doses (or continuous infusions) of propofol have been used to get through this stage of emergence, particularly following sevoflurane anesthesia, but in the end, the patient often ends up where he started off and one still needs mild (personal) restraint and careful protection of the patient to get through the emergence stage.

Additional Questions

1. Most parts of anesthesia ventilators can be steam autoclaved and most rubber bellows and tubing can be sterilized using ethylene oxide. Because microorganisms cannot typically survive the environment of the carbon dioxide absorbent, patients do not usually contaminate the absorber and disposable absorbers offer no greater protection than reusable absorbers for this reason. Unidirectional valves can be disassembled and cleaned with alcohol or a detergent; autoclavable cannisters are also available on newer anesthesia machines. The reservoir bag can be cleaned in an ethylene oxide sterilization machine. Breathing tubing, Y pieces and adapters as well as facemasks, if not disposable, can be cleansed by ethylene oxide. Autoclaving can be utilized for facemasks but it will shorten its life. Not everything proximal to the CO_2 absorption canister is necessarily safe for an immunocompromised patient, although the likelihood of significant bacterial contamination in the respiratory gas area of the ventilator bellows proximal to the CO_2 absorption canister is low.

2. What is the normal role of Helper T Cells in antibody formation? How is this different than B cells? Plasma cells? What is the consequence of a deficiency in Helper T Cells?

3. How should blood be prepared for a patient with severe combined immunodeficiency syndrome? Why? What if the blood was a month old? Other than the risks of infection, are there any other risks of transfusion in this patient?

4. The embryologic derivation of the thymus and the parathyroids has certain specific anesthetic implications besides an associated T cell dysfunction. Explain. What are the immunological implications? Why? What are the metabolic abnormalities you would anticipate? Why?

5. What is the basic defect in Kartagener's Syndrome? The most common presenting findings? Anything unique on their physical exam in addition to the pulmonary and upper respiratory findings? How about chest X-ray?

6. The mother of a 5-year-old spina bifida patient scheduled for tendon lengthening tells you that the child's lip swelled at the dentist recently. What else would you like to ask? How likely do you think it is that this patient is truly latex allergic? How would you test for this allergy? Is RAST testing as sensitive/specific as patch testing? What precautions will you take? If the patient develops wheezing and urticaria, how much epinephrine is effective?

2. Helper or inducer T cells serve to produce interleukins and lymphokines that are responsible for chemotaxis, activation, B cell growth and differentiation, and production of interferon. Short-lived B cells enter the circulation. They also have cell-surface antigens that, when cross-linked, promote B cell enlargement to a plasma cell capable of secreting IgE antibodies. A deficiency in helper T cells, while not completely preventing B cell activation or development of plasma cells will nevertheless significantly impair the efficacy of this process and for this reason will result in relative immunocompromise.

3. Severe combined immunodeficiency syndrome is a primary T cell abnormality that also results in failure of formation of the thymus. Patients are vulnerable to overwhelming viral infections and patients often die in the first few years of life. The risk of infection is constant, and because of chronic anemia, transfusions are often required. However, graft vs. host disease is a risk of transfusion. Lymphocytes in blood are viable for 3 weeks; therefore, blood must be irradiated prior to transfusion to kill lymphocytes. If the blood was a month old, then theoretically, lymphocyte viability should not be a significant clinical consideration, but other problems of using month-old blood should be considered.

4. The thymus and parathyroid are derived from the third and fourth pharyngeal pouches. Although anatomic abnormalities may result from congenital malformations, such as abnormalities of the tracheal or branchial cleft sinuses, these are rare in the third and fourth pouches. Concurrent abnormalities in other organ systems may include cardiac abnormalities, micrognathia, and low-set ears (from a concurrent failure of the second branchial pouch). However, failure of normal formation of the thymus and parathyroid results in the DiGeorge syndrome, with low parathormone levels, hypocalcemia, and immunological problems. If the thymic hypoplasia is minimal, T cell function may be almost normal; there may be variable degrees of severity. The decreased serum ionized calcium may result in tetany, myocardial depression, and seizures.

5. Kartagener's syndrome is characterized by immotile cilia, and as a result, patients have chronic otitis media, sinusitis, bronchitis, and bronchiectasis. Situs inversus is a consistent finding. Anesthetic management begins with good medical management of chronic respiratory tract infections and anesthetic plans directed to chronic respiratory disease with bronchospasm as a component. Placement of the ECG leads should take into account the situs inversus.

6. Children with spina bifida are at high risk for developing latex allergy. There is increasing evidence for a genetic predisposition, and in addition, patients who have catheterized for bladder emptying with natural rubber latex catheters have been chronically exposed to the latex antigen. Because dentists often use natural rubber latex dams, more than 50% of latex allergic patients will have their initial allergic presentation at the dentist's office. The suspicion for true latex allergy should be very high in spina bifida patients for the above reasons as well as for

their typical history of multiple surgical procedures. Testing for confirmation can consist of patch testing or epicutaneous (intradermal) testing, but probably the most common initial test is a latex RAST test, which is an in vitro test of the patient's IgE specific antibody for latex. It is almost as sensitive and specific as patch testing and is a good approximation for intradermal testing, which is more risky because of its in vivo nature. Epinephrine in doses of 0.1 mcg/kg intravenously can be used to treat anaphylactic reactions.

General References

1. Holzman R (1997) Clinical management of latex-allergic children. Anesthesia & Analgesia 85:529–533
2. Holzman R (2008) Anaphylactic reactions and anesthesia. In: Longnecker D, Brown D, Newman M, Zapol W (eds) Anesthesiology. New York, McGraw Hill, pp 1947–1963
3. Holzman RS (1993) Latex allergy: an emerging operating room problem. Anesthesia & Analgesia 76:635–641

Chapter 19
Infectious Diseases

A 6-month-old, 3.5-kg HIV positive boy is scheduled for bronchoscopy, washings and brushings, and possible open lung biopsy to confirm the diagnosis of *Pneumocystis carinii* infection. BP = 76/55 mmHg, $P = 150$ bpm, $R = 50$/min with retractions, and $T = 38.5°C$. Hematocrit is 25%, WBC count 3,500, and platelet count 35,000. He also has a pericardial effusion. Medications include zidovudine (AZT) and trimethoprim–sulfamethoxazole (Bactrim).

R.S. Holzman et al., *Pediatric Anesthesiology Review: Clinical Cases for Self-Assessment,*   399
DOI 10.1007/978-1-4419-1617-4_19, © Springer Science+Business Media, LLC 2010

Preoperative Evaluation

1. Is this patient in respiratory distress? Is this acute or chronic? Why? What difference does it make? How will you evaluate the patient's oxygenation and work of breathing? Would those assessments be of any importance to your anesthetic plan? Will a chest X-ray be of help?

2. Of what importance is the anemia? What additional information would you like to evaluate the anemia? Does this patient need a platelet transfusion? Are any other laboratory tests indicated? Which ones specifically?

3. How should his cardiac function be evaluated? Would an echocardiogram help?

Preoperative Evaluation

1. This child exhibits signs of respiratory distress such as tachypnea and retractions. Infection with HIV in this case was almost certainly through vertical transmission from mother to child, meaning that he has had HIV/AIDS for 6 months. Retractions are evidence of increased resistance to inspiratory flow and the tachypnea, in the presence of a smaller tidal volume, indicates decreased pulmonary compliance. An SpO_2 measurement on room air gives an indication of oxygenation but if the child is receiving supplemental oxygen, the oxygen saturation measurement can be normal in the face of significantly impaired pulmonary function. This child certainly has pulmonary disease. In addition to an infectious pneumonia, he also may have lipoid interstitial pneumonia (LIP), which can present with bilateral CXR infiltrates, wheezing, tachypnea, and cough [1–3]. The incidence of LIP in HIV-infected children is 20–30%. The most common opportunistic infection seen in children with AIDS is *Pneumocystis carinii* [4].

2. Children infected with HIV often have lowered counts of all the formed elements of the blood. As is the case with other chronic diseases, the anemia seen in these children is hypochromic and microcytic with low reticulocyte counts. The causes for the anemia are the disease itself, poor nutrition due to poor appetite and side effects of the medications used to treat AIDS. Based on the weight of 3.5 kg, it is likely that the infant is failing to thrive. A comparison with the birth weight will give information about the rate of postnatal growth. Thrombocytopenia is also seen commonly in these children. Both impaired production and increased destruction have been seen in HIV/AIDS patients. In addition, a lupus-like anticoagulant has been noted in up to 20% of HIV children undergoing coagulation testing. Blood products must be available for this child undergoing this procedure. Transfusion should be undertaken after discussion with the child's primary physician. Only CMV-negative, leukocyte-depleted RBCs should be given to AIDS patients. The need for additional platelets for this case depends upon the exact nature of the procedure. It may be prudent to have platelets available and to use them if the open lung biopsy is performed but withhold them if the bronchoscopy alone is done. Renal dysfunction is common in children with HIV/AIDS. A screening urinanalysis will detect proteinuria and hematuria. Given the child's poor nutritional status and failure to thrive, it is worthwhile to check the serum electrolytes and protein prior to inducing anesthesia. Abnormal sodium or potassium values would be a cause to delay proceeding and a knowledge of low serum protein would affect dosing of medication during the anesthetic.

3. Approximately 10–12% of children infected with HIV have significant cardiac involvement [5]. The infant's resting tachycardia may be due to HIV infection. The parent or caregiver should be asked about prior treatment for CHF and signs and symptoms of CHF should be sought when the history is taken. A cardiac ECHO will demonstrate LV hypertrophy and/or systolic dysfunction if present but diastolic dysfunction may not be apparent on a routine ECHO. An ECG will show a sinus arrhythmia, often seen in these children.

Intraoperative Course

1. What monitors will you choose? Is an arterial line indicated for this case? What are the risks of central line placement in this patient? Which lead would you choose to monitor on the ECG? Would a transesophageal echocardiogram be of any help? Why/why not?

2. The bronchoscopist requests "a little sedation only." Do you agree? Why? Why not? Your colleague stops by and suggests total intravenous anesthesia technique because the "lungs are so sick, and the heart is too." What do you think? You select an intravenous technique with small incremental doses of propofol; upon withdrawing the needle from the latex hub, you stick yourself and draw blood. What do you do next? Should you continue with the case? Ask someone to take over? Wash your hands in bleach, alcohol, betadine? Should you request to be started on AZT?

Intraoperative Course

1. Routine monitors are sufficient for the bronchoscopy, washings, and brushings. During these cases, drapes are ordinarily not used, the child is available to the anesthesiologist and the procedure can stop at any time. If the open lung biopsy is done, an arterial line is important in allowing assessment of blood gases. In this infant with pulmonary compromise, development of a pneumothorax during CVL placement would be very dangerous. If a CVL were planned, placement should certainly be done by the most experienced person and not until after induction of anesthesia. Lead II of the ECG should be monitored since that lead gives a good indication of the rhythm. TEE would not be particularly helpful in this case. If there is significant cardiac dysfunction and the open lung biopsy is undertaken, placement of a CVP and measurement of filling pressures will give adequate information about cardiac performance.

2. Sedation is not a good option for this child for several reasons. The infant has respiratory insufficiency, the bronchoscopist will obstruct part of the airway with the scope, and will then instill saline into the child's lungs after which s/he will suction out part of that saline, along with much of the FRC. With administration of general anesthesia through an LMA, a high concentration of oxygen and controlled ventilation can be delivered, if needed.

   Occupational exposure to the HIV virus is an important consideration in this case. Studies of hundreds of household contacts have confirmed that the risk of transmission from passive contact with an HIV-infected child is practically zero. Seroconversion is not a common occurrence following needle stick exposure. Hollow-bore needles used in drug administration give a much larger inoculum of blood than the solid needles used for suturing. After a parenteral exposure to a patient with HIV, the health care worker should undergo postexposure prophylaxis, postexposure treatment, and follow-up [6]. The wound should be immediately and thoroughly washed with saline. And the institutional "stick" team called. As prophylaxis is begun, the exposed person should be tested to document the HIV status. This testing should be repeated at 6 and 12 weeks after the exposure. Current recommendations are for exposed person to be treated with zidovudine with lamivudine or indinavir added. A CDC retrospective study of exposed health care workers had the following conclusions: a higher rate of conversion was associated with exposure to a greater quantity of blood, or exposure to a person in the terminal stages of AIDS and that there was a 76% decrease in seroconversion when zidovudine was begun after exposure.

3. What will be your primary technique be? Why? Will you use nitrous oxide? Why/why not? What is your choice of muscle relaxant? Why?

4. During surgery, the patient develops increasing difficulty, and the oximeter reading decreases from 93% to 87% with increasingly coarse breath sounds. What would you do? Why? Blood pressure is 60/40 mmHg with a heart rate of 160 bpm; how would you manage his depth of anesthesia? Why?

Postoperative Course

1. Would you extubate deep? Why/why not? What criteria will you use to decide about extubation? Why? At the end of the procedure, during planned extubation, the desaturation recurs while the patient is struggling, bearing down, and breath-holding. Your management?

3. There are several possibilities for maintenance for this case. The airway management is limited to the use of an endotracheal tube or an LMA. If an endotracheal tube is used, the size of the bronchoscope will be limited to a greater degree than if an LMA is used. The infant does not have a contraindication to an inhalation induction with oxygen and sevoflurane nor does he have a contraindication to an IV induction. Once anesthetized, an LMA can be placed. Once good air entry is assured, the adapter can be connected to the LMA and the procedure started. Anesthesia can be maintained with IV or inhalational agents. Since the procedure is of indeterminate length, an infusion or frequent small doses of a short-acting nondepolarizing relaxant would be a good choice. If an LMA is used, the anesthesiologist must be certain that adequate ventilation is possible with a peak inspiratory pressure <20 cm H_2O prior to the administration of a muscle relaxant in this patient.

4. The clinical deterioration could very well be a result of administration of excessive lavage fluid by the pulmonologist. Further attempts at suctioning the fluid from the lungs may not yield much and may worsen the hypoxia as gas is suctioned from the lung along with any residual lavage fluid. Hypotension in this case could be a result of impaired venous return as higher inflating pressures are used to combat the hypoxemia. If higher inflating pressures are needed to maintain gas exchange, increased preload with IV fluid administration may help increase the blood pressure. Another possibility is the development of a pneumothorax. Auscultation of the lungs and/or CXR will confirm or rule out this possibility. If a pneumothorax is the problem, it must be evacuated quickly. It may be necessary to administer vasoactive amines to support BP while the pneumothorax is being evacuated.

Postoperative Course

1. Prior to extubation, a suction catheter should be passed through the endotracheal tube to remove any lavage fluid. Once suctioning is complete, the infant should be kept on 100% oxygen for several minutes before extubation is considered. This infant should be extubated awake for several reasons. He should have a strong cough to clear residual saline lavage fluid, he should have as strong a respiratory drive as possible given the degree of preprocedure respiratory distress he exhibited, and he should be able to protect his airway. If the patient appears awake enough for extubation but is coughing and bearing down such that oxygen delivery is impaired, the best course of action may be to extubate and observe the child's degree of distress once the endotracheal tube is removed. Often, in such situations the child begins to breath more comfortably.

Additional Topics

1. What adjustments do you make in your anesthetic care plan for patients with increased body temperature? Does fever change MAC requirements? Should atropine be given prior to a rapid sequence induction in a febrile patient?

2. A 3-month old is admitted to the ICU in septic shock with meningococcal sepsis. There is considerable difficulty establishing an arterial line and the intensivist calls you for help; the parents want you to explain the risks and benefits of placing the line in their baby.

3. A baby with congenital rubella syndrome is scheduled for a percutaneous endoscopic gastrostomy. What problems can be anticipated?

Additional Topics

1. With temperature increases, oxygen consumption increases. The increase in metabolic rate is approximately 15%/°C. Thus a child with a temperature of 40°C will have an oxygen consumption of more than 150% of normal. In animal studies, hyperthermia has been found to increase MAC. Atropine has many pharmacologic effects mediated through blocking of the effect of acetylcholine; increased heart rate through its effect on the SA node, bronchodilation through its effect on muscarinic receptors in the bronchi, antagonism of gastric hydrogen ion secretion, and also inhibition of the activity of cutaneous sweat glands. This last effect can increase temperature although, in adults, hyperthermia is generally seen only with overdose of anticholinergic drugs. Increased body temperature and a cutaneous rash are sometimes seen in children who received only a therapeutic dose of atropine. Whether or not atropine should be given as part of a rapid sequence induction depends upon the clinical situation and the patient's body temperature should have very little, if anything, to do with that clinical choice.

2. Nearly all peripheral arteries have been used for direct monitoring of blood pressure in children. Common problems associated with arterial catheters include emboli, distal ischemia, thrombosis of the artery, and infection. In this setting, in which the child has sepsis, complications are more likely. The sepsis and vasculitis of meningococcemia will lower blood pressure generally and the inflamed intima of the cannulated artery will make the likelihood of thrombosis or embolism greater. On the other hand direct, instantaneous blood pressure monitoring is very important for these critically ill children. Considerations prior to placement include the patient's condition, whether or not the vessel has been damaged, and the amount of collateral flow. It is important to remember that the peripheral arteries of the lower extremity, the dorsalis pedis, and posterior tibial may exhibit pressure-wave amplification and may show a pressure higher than the aortic pressure.

3. The congenital rubella syndrome involves virtually all organ systems of the body. Intrauterine growth restriction (IUGR), often with associated microcephaly, is the most common finding. Manifestations of importance to anesthesiologists are myocarditis, patent ductus arteriosus, and pulmonary arterial stenosis. Assessment of cardiac function should be done prior to going to the operating room. Other findings are blueberry muffin skin rash, cataracts, sensori-neural hearing loss, and hepatosplenomegaly.

4. A child with a rash arrives in the Preop Clinic for evaluation. How will you differentiate between measles and chicken pox? What implications are there for this particular child with regard to an electively scheduled procedure? If you go ahead, are there risks to other patients in the operating room and the PACU?

5. You have difficulty waking up an otherwise healthy 8-year old after a 2½-h exploratory laparotomy for a ruptured appendix with significant peritonitis. Your anesthetic technique was impeccable, and could not possibly account for this situation. Triple antibiotics were used at the beginning of the case, which included ampicillin, gentamycin, and metronidazole (Flagyl®). What is your differential diagnosis? Would calcium be of any help? Another dose of neostigmine? Another anticholinesterase? What are the disadvantages of using additional doses of anticholinesterases? Does calcium have a direct effect on presynaptic portions of the neuromuscular junction? How long would you expect this problem to last?

6. Tuberculosis – what do you need to know as an anesthesiologist?

4. Chicken pox or varicella is a disease caused by human herpes virus. In the USA, most people acquire the disease during childhood. The AAP recommends vaccination for children >12 months who have not exhibited the clinical syndrome. There is a 10–21-day incubation period but most children develop a rash 2 weeks after exposure. The rash is often preceded for 1–2 days by fever, malaise, and headache. The typical rash of fluid-filled vesicles often begins on the trunk. The vesicles appear in crops and may be quite extensive or may be few in number. Varicella is contagious for 2 days prior to the appearance of the rash and until the lesions have crusted. Transmission is up to 90% in household contacts and 30% for classroom contacts. Measles, or rubeola, is another common infectious viral illness. It is also very contagious with 90% of household contacts becoming infected. The MMR (measles, mumps, rubella) vaccine is given at 12 months and again in early adolescence. The clinical course of the disease has three phases: a 10–12-day incubation period; a prodrome of 3–5 days characterized by Koplick spots on the buccal mucosa, moderate fever, cough, and conjunctivitis; and the final stage of 3–5 days with maculopapular rash on the neck, arms and legs, and high fever. This child does not have any particular increased risk if he were to undergo general anesthesia and a DSU procedure. However, varicella and rubeola are both quite contagious and infection can be quite serious in immunocompromised patients.

5. Antibiotics can enhance neuromuscular blockade. There has been evidence of both pre- and postjunctional effects attributed to antibiotics. It is likely that there is no common mechanism by which antibiotics cause neuromuscular blockade and thus there is no recommended standard therapy. If the recommended standard dose of neostigmine is not effective in reversing neuromuscular blockade, it is safer to provide mechanical ventilation until recovery has occurred. Administration of calcium is not recommended since the antagonism to neuromuscular blockade is temporary and calcium may inhibit the antibacterial activity of the antibiotics.

6. The incidence of tuberculosis is increasing worldwide. Recent immigrants to the USA, the homeless, and children with HIV/AIDS are specific groups of concern. Most children infected with *Mycobacterium tuberculosis* acquired the organism from close contact with an individual with active disease. Children with TB can have various presentations. Many are asymptomatic and are detected when a skin test is positive. Progressive pulmonary tuberculosis can occur with the development of lobar or bronchopneumonia. Children with pneumonia or pleural effusions may come to the operating room for placement of thoracostomy tubes, video-assisted thorascopic drainage of empyema (VATS) or bronchoscopy [7]. *M. tuberculosis* is a 1–5 µ-sized particle and disease transmission is by airborne spread. When children with the diagnosis of tuberculosis come to the operating room, prevention of infection of the caregivers and of contaminating the anesthetic equipment is of paramount importance. The CDC recommends protective masks be used that meet stringent filtering requirements. Filters are recommended for use in breathing circuits used on patients known to have TB [8].

Annotated References

van der Walt JH, Jacob R, Zoanetti DC (2004) Infectious diseases of childhood and their anesthetic implications. Paediatric Anaesthesia 14:810–819

The authors review the immunization schedule for children in Australia and the common infections affecting children. Incubation and infectious periods for measles, mumps, rubella, pertussis, varicella, and other common infections are listed. In addition, management issues of infected children in the perioperative period such as isolation and equipment disinfection are reviewed.

McGowan, CW Jr (2006) Congenital infections. Sect. XI, Chap. 66. In: Kliegman RM, Marcdante KJ, Jenson HB, Behrman RE (eds) Nelson's essential pediatrics, 5th edn. pp 329–335

The author, in 6 pages, reviews the clinical characteristics of congenital infections included in the TORCH designation and other perinatally acquired infections, *toxoplasmosis gondii*, cytomegalovirus (CMV), hepres simplex type 1 or 2, *treponema pallidum*, parvovirus, HIV, Hepatitis B, *Neisseria gonorrhea*, *Chlamydia trachomatis*, and *Mycobacterium tuberculosis.*

References

1. Larsen HH, von Linstow ML, Lundgren B et al (2007) Primary pneumocystis infection in infants hospitalized with acute respiratory tract infection. Emerg Infect Dis 13:66–72
2. Pitcher RD, Zar HJ (2008) Radiographic features of paediatric pneumocystis pneumonia – a historical perspective. Clin Radiol 63:666–672
3. Berman DM, Mafut D, Djokic B et al (2007) Risk factors for the development of bronchiectasis in HIV-infected children. Pediatr Pulmonol 42:871–875
4. Nesheim SR, Kapogiannis BG, Soe MM et al (2007) Trends in opportunistic infections in the pre- and post-highly active antiretroviral therapy eras among HIV-infected children in the Perinatal AIDS Collaborative Transmission Study, 1986–2004. Pediatrics 120:100–109
5. Leelanukrom R, Pancharoen C (2007) Anesthesia in HIV-infected children. Paediatr Anaesth 17:509–519
6. Diprose P, Deakin CD, Smedley J (2000) Ignorance of post-exposure prophylaxis guidelines following HIV needlestick injury may increase the risk of seroconversion. Br J Anaesth 84:767–770
7. Subramaniam R, Gupta S, Prasad CN (2005) Perinatal tuberculosis: implications of failure to isolate the lungs in an infant undergoing thoracotomy. Paediatr Anaesth 15:689–693
8. Tait AR (1997) Occupational transmission of tuberculosis: implications for anesthesiologists. Anesth Analg 85:444–451

Chapter 20
Neuromuscular Disease

A 14-year-old girl with juvenile myasthenia gravis has been treated with steroids and pyridostigmine for the past year; she now presents for thymus resection via median sternotomy. Her VS are BP 110/72 mmHg, HR 100 bpm, RR 28/min (at rest), and Hb 12.6 g.

R.S. Holzman et al., *Pediatric Anesthesiology Review: Clinical Cases for Self-Assessment*,   411
DOI 10.1007/978-1-4419-1617-4_20, © Springer Science+Business Media, LLC 2010

Preoperative Evaluation

1. Risks of intraoperative aspiration pneumonitis:

    (a) Is this patient at an increased risk of pulmonary aspiration of gastric contents?
    (b) How would you assess this preoperatively?
    (c) Should she receive pharmacologic prophylaxis? If so, which drugs?
    (d) Are there any interactive effects with her current medications? Why/why not?

2. Long-term steroid therapy:

    (a) Is it important to know which steroid she is on?
    (b) Should she be "covered" for surgery?
    (c) Is this clear-cut or controversial? Why/why not?
    (d) What would you do?
    (e) Should she receive her pyridostigmine preoperatively? Why/why not?
    (f) Would you base that on an assessment of her pulmonary function tests?

3. How would you go about assessing whether her PFTs were acceptable or unacceptable for surgery?

Preoperative Evaluation

1. (a) Yes, in general, patients with myasthenia gravis experience fluctuating weakness including weakness of the pharyngeal, laryngeal, and respiratory muscles. Swallowing and effective cough effort is impaired.

   (b) The patient's ability to protect and maintain a patent airway postoperatively should be assessed. General muscle strength is assessed by physical examination, evaluating the presence of ptosis, double vision, dysphagia, rapid fatigue with repetitive movement such as opening and closing of the hand. Pulmonary function testing showing a vital capacity less than 40 mL/kg, impaired expiratory effort (maximum static expiratory volume) and flow-volume loops in the supine and sitting position are a useful guide for evaluating the extent of the respiratory impairment.

   (c) Ranitidine and a nonparticulate antacid (Bicitra®) could be useful in diminishing the potential for aspiration pneumonitis.

   (d) Ranitidine is a weak and reversible inhibitor of cholinesterase and can augment the effect of pyridostigmine's anticholinesterase action.

2. (a) Yes, the hypothalamic–pituitary–adrenal axis could be suppressed by exogenous administration of glucocorticosteroid.

   (b) The perioperative stress steroid requirement depends on the maintenance dose. The patient will need a stress dose of steroid when the maintenance daily dose is greater than 10 mg of prednisone (or equivalent).

   (c) This guideline of steroid stress dose administration is controversial. There are arguments against the need for a stress dose of steroids if the patient has been on a daily maintenance dose of less than 10 mg of prednisone (or its equivalent) and for minor surgery.

   (d) If the patient has been on a daily maintenance dose of prednisone of 10 mg or greater I will administer a stress coverage dose of steroid. I will also administer steroid coverage for this particular patient because she is scheduled for a thoracotomy.

   (e) I will omit the morning dose of pyridostigmine because if the muscles are weak intraoperatively I do not have to administer nondepolarizing muscle relaxants (competitive inhibitor of cholinesterase). However, this may provoke the patient's anxiety due to subjective or actual weakness of her respiratory muscles.

   (f) I will not omit the morning dose of pyridostigmine if pulmonary function is impaired, despite optimal medical therapy.

3. The standard pulmonary function should be normal when the myasthenia is well controlled with medical therapy. If the myasthenia is not well controlled, the forced vital capacity and 1 s forced expiratory volume are decreased. If FVC is normal and the FEV_1 is decreased, it may indicate airway obstruction due to an enlarged thymus.

4. Preperative anxiety:

  (a) She is very anxious; how would you counsel her about preoperative sedation?
  (b) She wants a mask induction; is this okay?
  (c) What end-points will you look for?
  (d) What if she goes into laryngospasm during induction – how will you manage?

Intraoperative Course

1. Intraoperative monitoring:

  (a) What are your monitoring considerations?
  (b) Does this patient need an arterial line? Why/why not?
  (c) Should the patient have central access? Why/why not?
  (d) Are there circumstances for which a pulmonary artery catheter would help?

2. Induction of anesthesia:

  (a) Assume an intravenous induction; which agent will you choose? Any advantage for propofol, thiopental, or etomidate? Why/why not?
  (b) Should the patient undergo a mask induction with a volatile agent and breathe spontaneously?
  (c) Which inhalation agent would you choose? Why?

4. (a) Preoperative intravenous anxiolytics may be administered with caution and close monitoring.

   (b) Inhalation induction with a mask is safe provided the patient is appropriately NPO.

   (c) Lack of response to physical stimulation (such as intravenous cannula insertion and laryngoscopy) rather than loss of response to eyelash stimulation (which is muscle-dependent) is useful in this particular patient to determine the depth of anesthesia.

   (d) If the patient develops laryngospasm it may be amenable to positive pressure in the presence of weak pharyngeal muscles. Alternatively, a small dose of nondepolarizing muscle relaxant or a large dose of succinylcholine is administered to relax the glottic muscles.

Intraoperative Course

1. (a) I will use standard ASA recommended monitors: ECG, blood pressure, $ETCO_2$, and body temperature as well as a neuromuscular blockade monitor.

   (b) I will place an indwelling arterial catheter to monitor intraoperative blood pressure and perioperative blood gases to monitor ventilation.

   (c) Central venous access is not necessary for this particular procedure because it is not associated with significant blood loss or fluid shift.

   (d) Pulmonary artery monitor is indicated if cardiac dysfunction is of considerable concern.

2. Induction of anesthesia:

   (a) I will use propofol because of its advantages over etomidate and thiopental. Propofol is a shorter acting CNS and respiratory depressant than thiopental. The disadvantage of etomidate is that even a single induction dose can potentially suppress adrenal steroid synthesis and it may precipitate an adrenal crisis or unpredictably increase the requirement for a steroid stress dose.

   (b) Potent volatile agents in anesthetic doses can produce significant suppression of the weak muscles and cause apnea. Bearing this in mind, a mask induction is perfectly acceptable.

   (c) I will choose sevoflurane which has the least respiratory depressant effect, is less irritable to the airways, and has a faster onset and offset effect compared with other currently used volatile agents.

3. Anesthetic maintenance:

   (a) Assume that you have administered intravenous thiopental and turned on the isoflurane; the patient has not received a muscle relaxant. She is now in severe laryngospasm and her saturation is 85%. There is no $ETCO_2$ on the monitor. What would you do? Would succinylcholine be safe to give?
   (b) How do myasthenics respond to succinylcholine?
   (c) Should the patient be relaxed with a nondepolarizing agent? If so, how much?
   (d) Which one would you choose?

4. Intraoperative events:

   (a) The patient was intubated successfully and is oxygenating well. Your block-ade monitor indicates no twitches, yet the patient moves when the median sternotomy begins; the surgeon SCREAMS that you have to relax the patient and "the Hell with possibly needing to use a respirator at the end of the case." How much and which relaxant will you use?
   (b) How will you judge efficacy? (You call for another NMB monitor, but the tech says it will be 10 min before he can get to you).
   (c) How do you use a blockade monitor for a myasthenic patient?

5. During thymus dissection, the patient begins wheezing and you note a prolonged and slow upstroke to the exhalation CO_2 curve on the capnograph (assume no prior history of asthma).

   (a) Your considerations? How would you prove it?
   (b) You try some albuterol (Ventolin®) directly down the tube and it does not change a thing – the patient is still wheezing. The surgeons are having a difficult time with the dissection, and the wheezing is worse. On $F_iO_2 = 1.0$, the saturation is 92% and the expiratory CO_2 waveform is small and prolonged. Further considerations? It improves when the surgeons are not operating. Further considerations? Would endobronchial intubation help or hurt? Would a double-lumen tube help? What suggestions do you have for the surgeons?

3. (a) The administration of succinylcholine is safe to treat laryngospasm.
   (b) Patients with myasthenia are resistant to succinylcholine and may require a larger dose than nonmyasthenic patients and so they are at risk for phase II block with prolonged muscle relaxant effect.
   (c & d) The use of a nondepolarizing muscle relaxant in this patient is safe with the expectation that the onset of action could be delayed and the duration of relaxation could be very prolonged. It is reasonable to start with one half the ED_{95} for tracheal intubation, which is a much smaller dose than for a nonmyasthenic patient. I will choose cisatracurium because of its rapid elimination; furthermore, the patient may not require anticholinergic agents to reverse the cisatracurium effect.

4. (a) I will administer stepwise incremental doses of cisatracurium of 0.1 mg/kg to the desired clinical effect after ensuring adequate depth of general anesthesia.
   (b) Myasthenic patients have variable involvement of different body muscles and monitoring multiple sites such as facial muscles or posterior tibial nerve stimulation may be useful to evaluate a nondepolarizing agent's effect.
   (c) I will obtain a baseline T1/T4 ratio before administration of a nondepolarizing muscle relaxant and titrate the dose to maintain a visible T1 response. When T1 response strength is equal to T4 it will indicate no fade and adequate reversal of neuromuscular junction function should be expected.

5. (a) The wheezing could be due to airway obstruction by surgical manipulation and traction of the thymus and trachea. I will ask the surgeon to stop manipulation of the thymus and airways and remove any retractors. If the obstruction does not resolve it may indicate bronchospasm due to light general anesthesia.
   (b) I prefer placement of a double-lumen tube only if the surgery is performed via video-assisted thoracoscopy to facilitate the surgical procedure.

Perioperative Care

1. Reversal of neuromuscular blockade:

   (a) Should this patient have neuromuscular blockade reversed? Why/why not?
   (b) What are the hazards?
   (c) What is a cholinergic crisis?
   (d) What are the symptoms and signs?
   (e) How is it treated?

2. Are pulmonary function criteria helpful for deciding about extubation?

   (a) Which ones?
   (b) How would you judge?
   (c) What if PFTs are okay but there is a weak gag reflex while the patient is still intubated – should you extubate?

3. Should this patient's pain relief be managed with a thoracic epidural or a morphine PCA? Why/why not? What are the advantages and disadvantages of each?

Additional Questions

1. A farmer is brought into the ER from his field after the over flight of a crop duster 2 h earlier; he is weak, breathing quickly, delirious, and smells of stool.

   (a) What do you think is going on? What should you do?
   (b) Are there any specific pharmacologic agents you should use? Is there anything other than atropine?
   (c) How much atropine should you use?

Perioperative Care

1. (a & b) I will not reverse the neuromuscular blockade in this patient. It is not advisable to administer anticholinesterase drugs to reverse the neuromuscular blockade to avoid potential for cholinergic crisis. It is fatal if not treated in a timely manner.

   (c, d, & e) A cholinergic crisis is an excessive accumulation of acetylcholine at the nicotic and muscarinic cholinergic receptors in the CNS and in the periphery. It presents with salivation, lacrimation, nausea, vomiting, urinary incontinence, diaphoresis, rhinorrhea, bronchorrhea, muscle fasciculation, weakness and paralysis, laryngospasm, bronchospasm, respiratory failure, miosis, agitation, convulsions, and coma. It is best treated with support of the respiratory and cardiovascular systems and symptomatic treatment. Benzodiazepines can control seizures and atropine can reverse the bradycardia.

2. (a, b, & c) Pulmonary function parameters that are useful to guide tracheal extubation are a FVC volume greater than 10 mL/kg, maximum inspiratory pressure greater than -25 cm H_2O, a respiratory rate below 20 bpm, inspired oxygen requirement less than 50% and PEEP of 5 cm H_2O or less. In addition, the patient's bulbar muscle strength should be normal as reflected by the presence of gag and cough reflexes.

3. Pain control in this patient is best managed with thoracic epidural analgesia because it will minimize the need for systemic opioids that may suppress central respiratory drive. The disadvantage of epidural analgesia with local anesthetics is the potential for intercostal muscle weakness that can impair ventilation and may be confused with inadequate treatment of myasthenia or myasthenic crisis.

Additional Questions

1. (a) My preliminary diagnosis is pesticide toxicity. I will immediately deliver oxygen by mask, establish intravenous access, and assess hemodynamic status. If organophosphate toxicity is suspected, decontamination is initiated. The patient's clothing is removed and the intact skin cleansed gently with soap and water and ethyl alcohol; the eyes are irrigated, and clothing is disposed of as hazardous waste. Medical personnel decontaminating the patient should self-protect against accidental exposure to the pesticide dust by wearing protective gear (waterproof gowns, gloves such as neoprene, and eyewear protection).

   (b) I will also administer pralidoxime as a specific antidote to the organophosphate. It is effective when administered with 48 h of exposure. Diazepam is useful to control CNS excitation and seizures.

   (c) If a plan is made to administer pralidoxime the patient should be atropinized by repeated administration of 50 mcg/kg every 10–30 min to maintain a heart rate above 100 beats/min.

2. A 13-year-old boy with Duchenne Muscular Dystrophy (DMD) comes to the operating room emergently for an incarcerated umbilical hernia.

   (a) What are your airway considerations?
   (b) Are these patients "difficult airways?" Why/why not?
   (c) What are your considerations for doing an awake intubation in a DMD patient?
   (d) Is this "stressful?" So what?
   (e) Assuming that the patient cannot be intubated or can only be intubated with great difficulty and the surgeon cannot do the procedure with just local – would a mask anesthetic be a good idea? Any special considerations?
   (f) Any special precautions on your part?
   (g) For what specific problems?
   (h) Is a laryngeal mask airway with spontaneous breathing a reasonable alternative?
   (i) Using a potent inhalational agent technique? Why/why not?

3. A patient is scheduled for a muscle biopsy to confirm suspicion of "central core disease (CCD)."

   (a) What is that?
   (b) Any anesthetic concerns?
   (c) Is a spinal anesthetic likely to aggravate the condition? Why/why not?
   (d) Is this similar to multiple sclerosis?
   (e) Are these children developmentally delayed?

2. (a) A major concern in adolescents with DMD is difficulty swallowing which may predispose to aspiration during induction and a difficult tracheal intubation due to an enlarged and stiff tongue.

   (b) Some patients may develop an enlarged, stiff, and protruding tongue as a result of tongue muscle degeneration and replacement with fibro-fatty tissue.

   (c) An awake tracheal intubation is not a safe strategy if the patient has a cardiomyopathy or is intolerant to sedation due to restrictive chest wall disease.

   (d) Most children at this age are anxious and may not be cooperative. Stress-associated tachycardia and hypertension could be detrimental in DMD adolescents in the presence of cardiomyopathy.

   (e) If patient's trachea cannot be intubated, an LMA should be used to secure ventilation and tracheal intubation can be attempted via the LMA.

   (f & g) Patients with DMD are at risk for acute myocardial decompensation under stress and acute rhabdomyolysis in response to succinylcholine and possibly vapor inhalation anesthetics. An adequate depth of anesthesia should be maintained throughout the procedure to avoid myocardial decompensation and cardiac arrhythmias. Succinylcholine and all inhalation agents could cause acute rhabdomyolysis and death or acute myocardial failure in some patients with DMD.

   (h) The use of an LMA and spontaneous respiration is not a reasonable and safe strategy because of the risk of aspiration from a full stomach and the potential for larygospasm. In addition, the patient may not be able to maintain adequate tidal exchange during spontaneous breathing under general anesthesia due to severe restrictive chest wall disorder, particularly with the use of IV anesthetics.

   (i) Potent inhalation agents have been associated with acute rhabdomyolysis, myoglobinuria, renal failure, and death in some patients with DMD.

3. (a) Central core disease (CCD) is a congenital myopathy, and usually presents with hypotonia, hyporeflexia, generalized weakness that is more often proximal than distal and poor muscle bulk early in life and is relatively nonprogressive. It results from defects in the calcium channel that releases calcium to the myoplasm, causing muscle damage and weakness.

   (b) Approximately 25% of patients with CCD may also carry the defective gene associated with malignant hyperthermia syndrome (ryanodine allele on chromosome 19q13.1) on the same locus as the CCD gene. It is an autosomal dominant disease characterized by loss or dysfunction of genes that encode for muscle proteins. A severe variant of the disease could be inherited as autosomal recessive gene.

   (c) Spinal anesthesia may aggravate an existing muscle weakness and hip dislocation. CCD is a congenital muscle weakness that causes scoliosis and spontaneous hip dislocation.

   (d) The adult onset CCD may experience transient worsening with intense activity and present with clinical manifestations similar to multiple sclerosis.

   (e) In general, children with CCD have normal intelligence.

4. An infant with a family history of familial periodic paralysis is scheduled for a hernia repair.

   (a) Why is this family history important?
   (b) How should this patient be evaluated preoperatively?
   (c) Would an ECG help?
   (d) How about serum electrolytes?
   (e) What if the potassium was normal?
   (f) Should you include glucose in the IV?
   (g) What kind of IV fluid would you use?
   (h) What about muscle relaxants?
   (i) Does the muscle relaxant effect of volatile agents potentiate the weakness of familial periodic paralysis?

4. (a) Family history is important because familial periodic paralyses are inheritable neurological disorders caused by a mutation in genes that regulate sodium and calcium channels in the nerve cells. In early life, the most common types are the periodic paralyses due to hypokalemia and to a lesser extent hyperkalemia, an autosomal dominant disorder that occurs in approximately 1:100,000 people.

   (b) Preoperative evaluation includes the family history of the disorder and symptoms the infant may have that would indicate familial periodic hypokalemic paralysis. The periodic paralysis often presents with generalized weakness lasting minutes to hours which recovers spontaneously. These episodes occur at rest, after exercise or after a night's sleep. Other symptoms include periodic swallowing and breathing weakness. In between episodes patients usually have good strength.

   (c) ECG can be helpful during the acute episodes of the disorder and could be abnormal because of hypokalemia; prolonged PR interval, ST-segment depression, T-wave inversion, and a prominent U wave may be seen.

   (d) Serum electrolytes are helpful during the acute episode and may show a low serum potassium. There are cases of normokalemic periodic paralysis.

   (e) Normal serum potassium does not exclude the disorder because it is self-limited and the potassium level can normalize.

   (f) Glucose administration should probably be limited because hyperglycemia produces an insulin surge, with subsequent intracellular entry of glucose and potassium resulting in hypokalemia.

   (g) I will use a nonglucose containing solution such as normal saline or lactated ringers solution for maintenance fluid therapy.

   (h) It is advisable to avoid muscle relaxants unless necessary for the optimizing surgical exposure.

   (i) Potent volatile agents can potentiate skeletal muscle weakness by suppressing neuromuscular junction function.

5. Spinal Muscular Atrophy (SMA):

   (a) What is the neuroanatomy of the lesion in the spinal muscle atrophies?
   (b) What is the difference between the infantile form (Werdnig–Hoffman disease) and the juvenile form (Kugelberg–Welander disease) as far as your anesthetic management?
   (c) Moebius syndrome, another form of motor nuclear degeneration affecting the VI and VII cranial nerves – does this have specific implications for other anterior horn cell defects?
   (d) How are these similar and different from amyotrophic lateral sclerosis?
   (e) How do these disorders affect your anesthetic care plan?
   (f) Counseling of the patient and the family?
   (g) Choice of agents?

6. You are called to intubate an 18-year old in the ICU, there for a week following a flu shot, with progressive weakness starting with difficulty walking and resulting in difficulty breathing.

   (a) Your differential, and then most likely, diagnosis?
   (b) The patient's NG tube feeding was shut off 1 h ago – should he be intubated awake? He fights you.
   (c) Would you perform a rapid sequence intubation?
   (d) What are the effects of succinylcholine in a patient with Guillain–Barre syndrome?

5. (a) The disease is caused by degeneration of the anterior horn cells.
   (b) The infantile form manifests within the first 3 months of life and is usually a severe form of the disease. Severe muscle weakness is associated with difficulty swallowing, impaired secretion handling, and difficulty breathing. These infants are at risk for aspiration and may require postoperative ventilatory support. Kugelberg–Welander disease is a milder form of the disease and progresses more slowly than the infantile form.
   (c) The Moebius syndrome is associated with hypoplasia or agenesis of the cranial nerve nuclei in the brainstem. The cranial nerves are primarily motor nerves and hence this syndrome is analogous to SMA syndrome because it involves lower motor neuron degeneration.
   (d) Both Moebius syndrome and SMA disorders affect motor neurons. Amyotrophic lateral sclerosis specifically affects the motor cortex, spinal motor neurons, or both. Unlike SMA, amyotrophic lateral sclerosis affects both the upper and lower motor neurons. It may manifest as spastic weakness as opposed to flaccid weakness in SMA syndrome.
   (e) These patients have weak and atrophic muscles of respiration and may require ventilatory support postoperatively. They are at risk for aspiration pneumonitis and postoperative pneumonia due to an inability to cough effectively from their weakened bulbar reflexes. Therefore, these patients are intolerant of CNS depressants such as sedatives, hypnotics, and opioids.
   (f) Genetic counseling of the family is important to determine whether the disorder is a result of mutation or genetic deletion of the Survival Motor Neuron (SMN) which occurs in approximately 90–94% of SMA patients. Counseling is also necessary for prenatal screening with subsequent pregnancy; the screening test has a 98% reliability. This information makes this SMN gene test very useful for the diagnosis of SMA.
   (g) Anesthetic agent choices are made bearing in mind that patients with generalized muscle wasting are unable to protect their airways and have limited respiratory system reserve. Therefore, these patients have increased an sensitivity to nondepolarizing muscle relaxants and are unable to compensate for hypoventilation and decreased central respiratory drive following administration of CNS depressants such as anesthetic agents and opioids administered after surgery.

6. (a) Possible etiologies include postviral syndromes, metabolic, or autoimmune disorders. Following a flu shot, most likely etiology for this adolescent is Guillain–Barre syndrome.
   (b) I will not intubate this patient awake, I will use anesthetic agents such as ketamine or propfol if hemodynamically stable. If hemodynamics are unstable, intubation of the trachea can be achieved with IV midazolam and a low dose of etomidate.
   (c) I will perform a "semi-rapid" sequence induction without the use of a muscle relaxant because the bulbar muscles are either paralyzed or weak enough from the disease to allow adequate rapid intubating conditions.
   (d) Succinylcholine should be avoided because in the acute phase of Guillain–Barre disease there is an active demyelination process that likely predisposes to serious hyperkalemia.

General References

1. Abel M, Eisenkraft JB (2002) Anesthetic implications of myasthenia gravis. Mt Sinai J Med 69:31–37
2. Dillon FX (2004) Anesthesia issues in the perioperative management of myasthenia gravis. Semin Neurol 24:83–94
3. White MC, Stoddart PA (2004) Anesthesia for thymectomy in children with myasthenia gravis. Paediatr Anaesth 14:625–635
4. Driessen JJ (2008) Neuromuscular and mitochondrial disorders: what is relevant to the anaesthesiologist? Curr Opin Anaesthesiol 21:350–355
5. Vercauteren M, Heytens L (2007) Anaesthetic considerations for patients with a pre-existing neurological deficit: are neuraxial techniques safe? Acta Anaesthesiol Scand 51:831–838
6. Ngai J, Kreynin I, Kim JT, Axelrod FB (2006) Anesthesia management of familial dysautonomia. Paediatr Anaesth 16:611–620
7. Klingler W, Lehmann-Horn F, Jurkat-Rott K (2005) Complications of anaesthesia in neuromuscular disorders. Neuromuscul Disord 15:195–206

Chapter 21
Endocrinopathies

An 8-year-old girl, 22 kg, previously healthy, presents with diffuse abdominal pain most pronounced in the right lower quadrant, lethargy, weakness, and recent weight loss. She is mildly febrile (100.7°F), with a blood pressure of 80/60 mmHg, a heart rate of 140 bpm, and a respiratory rate of 46/min. She is nauseous and has vomited twice in the ED and several times at home over the preceding few hours. She has a "strange" odor to her breath. Her urine is dipstick + for glucose and ketones. You are called to the emergency room to evaluate her in preparation for appendectomy.

R.S. Holzman et al., *Pediatric Anesthesiology Review: Clinical Cases for Self-Assessment,*   427
DOI 10.1007/978-1-4419-1617-4_21, © Springer Science+Business Media, LLC 2010

Preoperative Evaluation

1. Is this patient volume depleted? How would you assess her volume status? What factors would you address in correcting her volume status preoperatively? Which intravenous fluid would you choose?

2. What metabolic studies are important to evaluate preoperatively? How will this influence your preparation for surgery? Over what period of time would it be appropriate to delay the start of the case? Is this problem likely to resolve with improvement of her metabolic status? What organ system consequences are there of uncontrolled diabetic ketoacidosis in the acute phase and chronically?

3. If this patient was a known diabetic and had developed an increasing requirement for insulin (e.g., from 8 to 40 units per day) prior to this event, how could this be explained? What is the basis for the Somogyi phenomenon? How can you manage this physiological derangement in the immediate preoperative period?

Preoperative Evaluation

1. It is very likely that this child has a depleted intravascular volume. Her heart rate is elevated more so than would be due to a low-grade fever. In addition, with fever, insensible losses increase and she has been vomiting. Her blood pressure is low but within normal limits for an 8-year-old girl. Since blood pressure is preserved in hypovolemic children until compensation fails, a "normal" measurement is not reassuring. Dehydration is generally classified by percentage decrease in body weight. A child who is 3% dehydrated has a 30 mL/kg deficit and clinically has an increased HR, dry mucous membranes, and concentrated urine. A child with 6% dehydration has a fluid deficit of 60 mL/kg and a significantly increased HR, very dry mucous membranes, and oliguria. In a child with 9% dehydration, the fluid deficit is 90 mL/kg, the blood pressure is decreased, and there is poor capillary refill, Kussmaul breathing, and obtundation. Fluid replacement should be with isotonic solution such as NS or LR and should be given relatively rapidly.

2. Serum electrolytes including phosphorus and calcium, anion gap, glucose, and perhaps blood gases should be evaluated preoperatively [1]. If the child is in diabetic ketoacidosis (DKA), surgery should be delayed at least until intravascular volume has been replenished and control of her DKA is underway. It is entirely possible that her abdominal pain is due to DKA and not any surgical problem [2]. Conversely, acute appendicitis can be the insult that precipitates DKA in a child who has diabetes mellitus but has not yet come to medical attention.

   While a big part of the problem in DKA is dehydration, overly aggressive replenishment can lead, in some cases, to the development of cerebral edema [3]. Cerebral edema has been documented in many patients during DKA but most patients remain asymptomatic. Fluid administration should be kept to <4 L/m^2/day. In addition, insulin infusion should be tailored to keep the decrease in glucose concentration to <100 mg/dL. During therapy for DKA, frequent measurement of serum osmolality is important in preventing a worsening of the cerebral edema.

3. The Somogyi phenomenon has been described as hypoglycemia begetting hyperglycemia. In this situation, the patient's own counter-regulatory hormones are stimulated by hypoglycemia that is due to excessive exogenous insulin administration. If daily insulin doses exceed 2 U/kg and this hypoglycemia/hyperglycemia phenomenon is occurring, the treatment is to carefully reduce the dose of insulin. In the immediate perioperative period, a good choice for management of this problem is to use an infusion of insulin, starting at 0.02–0.1 U/kg/h with frequent checks of serum glucose and electrolytes.

Intraoperative Course

1. What are your monitoring considerations? Does this patient need an arterial line? Should the patient have a central venous catheter? A urinary catheter? How would it help your management? Are there any confounding issues?

2. What agent would you choose to induce general anesthesia? Any advantage for Propofol, Thiopental, Etomidate? What inhalation agent would you choose? Is a regional anesthetic a better choice for the procedure? What effects of the various induction methods are particularly important for diabetic patients?

3. Is succinylcholine safe to give to this patient? What if the pH is 7.25? What is the effect of ketoacidosis on pharmcokinetics of nondepolarizing neuromuscular blockers? Would you administer bicarbonate?

Intraoperative Course

1. The usual monitors are indicated and given the frequency with which serum glucose, electrolytes and pH will be checked, an arterial line is indicated as well. The line will also be very helpful in postoperative management. The case for a central venous catheter is not as strong. If two adequate peripheral IVs and a foley catheter are in place, she can be managed without a CVP. Urine output will not be a good measure of preload since she will have an osmotic diuresis due to glycosuria. However, the quality of the arterial waveform as well as the progress in improvement of her metabolic acidosis are indicators of the adequacy of her intravascular volume. If there is a question of access or she remains unstable despite what is thought to be adequate fluid replacement, a CVP catheter should be placed after the induction of anesthesia.

2. The induction of anesthesia should proceed with the assumption that she is not fully fluid resuscitated. This patient should have an intravenous induction. Given her nausea and vomiting, she should have full stomach precautions. Any IV agent can be used if dosed appropriately. Propofol and thiopental both will lead to hypotension if given in the usual doses to a hypovolemic patient while etomidate will suppress the adrenal cortex in this child with new-onset diabetes mellitus, DKA, and possible appendicitis. The choice of muscle relaxant to facilitate intubation presents difficulties. A nondepolarizing relaxant will take longer to provide intubating conditions in this child who would do better without mask ventilation, while succinylcholine will cause an increase in the serum potassium in a patient who may already have an acidosis-related elevation of that ion.

3. Succinylcholine can be used but there may be problems. In patients with metabolic acidosis and hypovolemia and/or hemorrhage, the administration of succinylcholine has caused a greater increase in serum potassium that it does in healthy patients. If succinylcholine is used and hyperkalemic arrythmias occur, treatment with hyperventilation, calcium chloride, and bicarbonate should be started immediately. Nondepolarizing relaxants are also affected by the presence of metabolic acidosis. Metabolic acidosis may augment the neuromuscular blockade from a nondepolarizing relaxant. The antagonism of blockade is not impaired by metabolic acidosis as it is by respiratory acidosis; however, bicarbonate administration should be reserved for severe acidosis (pH < 7.2). There are several possible adverse outcomes from bicarbonate administration. Alkalosis will increase potassium entry into cells, bicarbonate may worsen the CNS acidosis. HCO_3^- combines with H^+ to form H_2O and CO_2 and CO_2 diffuses rapidly into the CNS while HCO_3^- does not.

4. Blood work during surgery reveals pH=7.22, PaO_2=160 mmHg, $PaCO_2$= 34 mmHg, K=5.5 mEq%, Na=127 mEq%, Cl=97 mEq%, and S_{osm}=320. How should this be managed? What implication does this have for your anesthetic choice and technique? Should this be more of a "stress-free" anesthetic? Can this be accomplished with an inhalation anesthetic, or would a narcotic anesthetic technique be preferable?

Postoperative Care

1. Should this patient go to the ICU postoperatively? What are you particularly concerned about? How frequently should the patient be metabolically monitored postoperatively?

2. You are called to the PACU for a urine output of 7 mL in the first 2 h postoperatively. How do you evaluate? Is a fluid bolus indicated? If so, what type of IV fluid? Is insertion of CVP catheter indicated? Would a urine analysis help understand this situation?

3. Should this patient's pain relief be managed with an epidural or morphine PCA? What are the advantages and disadvantages of each?

4. The ABG shows a metabolic acidosis and respiratory alkalosis. The patient has hyponatremia and at the same time hyperosmolarity. The hyponatremia may only be apparent, not real, if the water content of the plasma is reduced by the presence of excess lipids. Serum osmolality can be calculated from the electrolytes as follows: $(Na + K) \times 2 + glucose/18 + BUN/3$. If we assume the contribution of BUN to osmolality is 10 then the equation reduces to: $320 = (132.5 \text{Å} \sim 2) + glucose/18$. The serum glucose is then 990 mg/dL. The patient's DKA is not being treated effectively at all. Therapy should include further fluid resuscitation, and an additional regular insulin dose of 0.5 U/kg while the insulin infusion continues.

Postoperative Care

1. This patient will be better off in an ICU overnight so that she can have frequent monitoring of her metabolic condition. Even if she had not undergone surgery, her condition was serious enough to warrant an ICU admission. She has arrived with a very large fluid deficit and severe metabolic acidosis. She is at risk for cerebral edema during her resuscitation and the initial signs of raised ICP might easily be missed if she were not in an ICU. This patient should have hourly determinations of serum glucose, potassium, sodium, pH, and HCO_3^-. Her urine output, urine ketones, and glucose also should be monitored very often.

2. Depletion of intravascular volume is a major part of the pathophysiology in DKA. The low urine output noted in the patient in the PACU can likely be attributed to that problem. Assessment of the degree of dehydration in the postoperative period is similar to what was done preoperatively, namely, history (anesthesia and ED records), physical exam (vital signs, skin turgor, and mental status), and laboratory (urinalysis, electrolytes, and glucose). Be aware that an abnormal mental status can be due to hypoglycemia, raised ICP, residual anesthetic medications, and hypovolemia. Urinalysis is also complicated in this situation. Glycosuria will affect the specific gravity determination and will also cause an osmotic diuresis. While a fluid bolus is indicated, care must be taken with the speed of administration given the propensity of these patients to develop cerebral edema [3]. A CVP catheter would be a good guide to fluid administration and help minimize the risk of cerebral edema. Clinically, cerebral edema is not present when the child presents with DKA but develops during therapy for DKA, often as biochemical measures are actually improving.

3. Pain management for this 8-year-old child following an appendectomy incision should be easily accomplished with IV opioids and IV PCA. Generally, these patients begin oral intake within 24 h of surgery and are easily switched to oral analgesics. Regional analgesia offers little additional benefit for the risks, albeit low, involved in placement of an epidural catheter. Provided she has not suffered any damage to her kidneys during her DKA episode, ketorolac can be added to her analgesic regimen.

Additional Topics

1. A 14-year-old male presents with growth failure, increased intracranial pressure, and visual field cuts (binasal hemianopsia). His imaging workup so far is consistent with craniopharyngioma. Are there any endocrinopathies you would suspect in this patient? What if he had short stature? What if he was obese? Was still a Tanner stage 1?

2. An 18-year old with acromegaly presents for saggital split osteotomy to correct mandibular prognathism. Would you expect airway difficulties? Are there any metabolic abnormalities to be prepared for?

3. What is the relationship of U_{osm} to P_{osm} in SIADH? Why? How does furosemide work to correct this problem? Should furosemide be utilized intraoperatively if this diagnosis can be made, or should fluid restriction be the treatment of choice?

4. A 3-month old presents for a cleft lip repair; she has a funny, puffy face, with widely separated fontanelles and a flattened nasal bridge, consistent with congenital hypothyroidism. She breathes through her mouth which has a large, protruding tongue. Her skin is cool to the touch and "marbleized" (cutanea marmorata). What anesthetic concerns does this patient present?

Additional Topics

1. Craniopharyngioma, a benign suprasellar tumor, is one of the most common supratentorial tumors in children. Signs and symptoms are due to the location of the tumor. It may be confined to just the sella turcica or it may extend through the diaphrgma sella and compress the optic nerve with resulting visual field cuts as in this case. Pituitary–hypothalamic involvement leads to short stature and if the tumor extends into the third ventricle, hydrocephalus may result. Most craniopharyngiomas have calcifications and these are visible on plain films or CT. Adrenal and thyroid dysfunction also are possible in these children. The preop evaluation of these patients should include evaluation for the various endocrine abnormalities discussed [4]. Hypothyroidism and/or adrenal insufficiency can cause problems if not managed appropriately. Although DI may be part of the initial presentation, it is more often seen postoperatively [5].

2. Acromegaly is the result of oversecretion of growth hormone in a person with closed epiphyses. If excess GH is due to a pituitary adenoma, it is possible that the tumor growth will compromise other anterior pituitary function. Secretion of gonadotropins, thyrotropin, or corticotropin may be impaired. The airway may be involved in this disorder [6, 7]. In addition to growth of bone, excessive GH secretion causes enlargement of the tongue and epiglottis. Cases of difficult intubation have been reported as has laryngeal stenosis. The patient should be questioned about dyspnea and examined for stridor. Peripheral nerves can become trapped by overgrowth of bone and connective tissue leading to various neuropathies.

3. In SIADH, levels of antidiuretic hormone are inappropriately high for the osmolality of the blood and do not decrease with further dilution of the osmolality. There are many causes of SIADH such as CNS disorders, pneumonia, the use of positive pressure ventilation, and vincristine administration. The signs and symptoms are due to the hyponatremia that results from water intoxication. Urine osmolality > serum osmolality, $U_{osm} > P_{osm}$. In general, treatment of the underlying disorder will correct the problem. In addition, fluid restriction with administration of maintenance sodium often will correct hyponatremia. In severe cases, administration of a diuretic such as furosemide will induce a diuresis and eliminate some of the excess water [8].

4. Congenital hypothyroidism can occur sporadically or in a familial pattern. Newborn screening programs are in place throughout the country and most children with this disorder are detected this way. The overall prevalence is 1:4,000 (1:20,000 in African Americans and 1:2,000 in Hispanics) and it is seen twice as often in females compared with males. Although there are many causes, most are due to thyroid dysgenesis, either aplasia or rudimentary ectopic thyroid tissue. In cases where the diagnosis is missed by the neonatal screen, clinical manifestations may not be evident at birth due to presence of transplacentally acquired maternal thyroxine (T4).

5. A 15-year old presents with a posterior mediastinal mass extending from T3 to T8. What is your differential diagnosis? What would you specifically attempt to evaluate by history in order to differentiate? Preoperative lab work? Radiological studies? The 24-h catecholamines are still pending; as you are placing the epidural in the thoracic space (patient awake, sedated, and comfortable) you notice that the blood pressure is 220/130. What do you do? (You recycle the cuff and it is about the same result.) Should the case be delayed, or can you proceed safely, with your new knowledge?

5. Mediastinal masses can have deleterious cardiovascular effects on affected patients and these effects are significantly worsened during the induction of anesthesia [9]. The differential diagnosis of a mediastinal mass depends upon the location in anterior, middle, or posterior division of the mediastinum.

Anterior mediastinum: lymphoma, llymophangioma, teratoma, and thymoma
Middle mediastinum: bronchogenic cyst, granuloma, lymphoma
Posterior mediastinum: enteric cysts, neuroblastoma, ganglioneuroma

While all locations can cause airway obstruction, anterior mediastinal masses also often decrease cardiac output by impairing filling of the right atrium and right ventricle. Affected children will present with an SVC syndrome in addition to any signs and symptoms of airway compromise [10]. History and physical exam can give the anesthesiologist clues to the degree of airway and cardiovascular impairment. The presence of stridor and/or difficulty breathing in various positions should be reviewed and progression of these complaints over recent time evaluated. Dilated veins on the face and upper extremities may be present. The preoperative laboratory evaluation of children with anterior mediastinal masses should include, in addition to as thorough an evaluation of the airway as possible, a cardiac [11, 12] echocardiogram. Older children with mediastinal masses should undergo imaging studies as well as flow-volume loops [9]. A CT scan of the chest and airway will give important information about tracheal size and/or deviation caused by the mass. Younger children often do not cooperate with the positioning and immobility needed for a CT scan or the more demanding pulmonary function testing. In these cases, the clinical assessment is even more important. General anesthesia for children with anterior mediastinal masses presents many challenges to the entire OR team, anesthesiologists, surgeons, and OR RNs [13].

One of the possible diagnoses for a posterior mediastinal mass is neurogenic tumor including pheochromocytoma. The elevation of blood pressure noted during placement of the epidural may be the result of excess catecholamine release by the pheochromocytoma. Anesthetic care of patients with pheochromocytoma requires careful preoperative evaluation and preparation. Once the diagnosis is confirmed with measurement of metanephrine, a metabolite of norepinephrine in the urine and in plasma, a thorough search for the full extent of the tumor is undertaken. In addition, prior to going to the OR, the patient should be treated with alpha blocking medications until orthostatic blood pressure and heart changes are evident. Only when this is accomplished, can beta blockade be administered. Even once satisfactory alpha and beta blockade has been accomplished, the procedure can be safely undertaken provided the anesthesiologist is prepared for significant vital sign swings. Invasive hemodynamic monitoring is indicated. Induction and maintenance should be planned to minimize the response to surgical stress. Epidural analgesia is a useful adjunct for these patients.

6. An 8-month-old girl with ambiguous genitalia and virilization is scheduled for urological reconstructive surgery. Any metabolic derangements you should expect in the preoperative evaluation? What if her Na^+ was 121 mEq% and K^+ 5.9 mEq%? What problems would you expect? How could this be managed medically? What problems would you expect with surgery? How should her fluids be constituted? Should she be treated with fludrocortisone (Florinef®) and hydrocortisone? Hydrocortisone only?

6. Ambiguous genitalia in females is the result of a defect in the enzymes responsible for synthesis of cortisol. The most common form is due to deficiency of 21-hydroxylase, an enzyme located in the adrenal cortex in the pathway to production of cortisol and aldosterone from cholesterol. The precursor 17-OH-progesterone increases in concentration leading to excessive production of androgen. This is the cause for virilization seen clinically. In addition to impaired cortisol production, aldosterone production is also affected. Decreased levels of aldosterone, another result of the 21-hydroxylase deficiency, lead to hyponatremia and hyperkalemia. One of the clinical variants of 21-hydroxylase deficiency, salt wasting, can present as an Addisonian crisis with severe sodium loss. Perioperative treatment of 21-hydroxylase deficiency patients involves administration of hydrocortisone, 2 mg/kg every 6 h. If salt wasting is present, IV fluid replenishment with NaCl-containing solutions and administration of IV mineralocorticoid such as fludrocortisone is indicated [14, 15].

Annotated References

Connery LE, Coursin DB (2004) Assessment and therapy of selected endocrine disorders. Anesthesiol Clin North America 22:93–123

This review includes discussion of general anesthetic principles of perioperative care, primarily of adult patients, with diabetes mellitus, thyroid disease, adrenal insufficiency, and pheochromocytoma. Even though the discussion includes etiology and pathophysiology for adults with these disorders, many management issues included have some relevance in the care of children.

Rhodes ET, Ferrari LR, Wolfsdorf JI (2005) Perioperative management of pediatric surgical patients with diabetes mellitus. Anesth Analg 101:986–989

This paper reviews the epidemiology of diabetes mellitus, current outpatient management options for children with this condition, the effects of surgery and anesthesia on glycemic control as well as perioperative management of affected children.

Jospe N (2006) Thyroid disease. In: Kliegman RM, Marcdante KJ, Jenson HB, Behrman RE (eds) Nelson essentials of pediatrics, 5th edn. Elsevier Saunders, Philadelphia, pp 805–811

This chapter reviews the embryology and development of the thyroid gland and thyroid diseases common in children such as congenital hypothyroidism, Graves Disease, and acquired hyperthyroidism. Medical and surgical management of hyperthyroidism, thyroid storm, and hypothyroidism is included.

Hack HA (2000) The perioperative management of children with phaeochromocytoma. Paediatr Anaesth 10:463–476

This paper reviews the pathophysioogy of the condition and the associated pharmacology. The specifics of these tumors as they present in children are discussed. Management of the cardiovascular changes expected during surgical removal is also reviewed.

Anghelescu DL, Burgoyne LL, Liu T et al (2007) Clinical and diagnostic imaging findings predict anesthetic complications in children presenting with malignant mediastinal masses. Paediatr Anaesth 17:1090–1098

This retrospective review of the records of 118 pediatric patients with mediastinal masses was undertaken in an effort to identify specific historical, physical exam, and laboratory findings that predict complications when anesthesia is induced. In this series, 11 patients did experience anesthesia-related complications. Orthopnea, upper body edema, great vessel compression, and mainstem bronchus compression were significantly associated with anesthesia-related complications.

References

1. Quiros JA, Marcin JP, Kuppermann N et al (2008) Elevated serum amylase and lipase in pediatric diabetic ketoacidosis. Pediatr Crit Care Med 9:418–422
2. Waseem M, Narasimhan M, Ganti S (2008) A child with abdominal pain and hyperglycemia: is it diabetic ketoacidosis? Pediatr Emerg Care 24:39–40
3. Hom J, Sinert R (2008) Is fluid therapy associated with cerebral edema in children with Diabetic ketoacidosis? Ann Emerg Med 52:69–71
4. Burton CM, Nemergut EC (2006) Anesthetic and critical care management of patients undergoing pituitary surgery. Front Horm Res 34:236–255
5. Karavitaki N, Wass JA (2008) Craniopharyngiomas. Endocrinol Metab Clin North Am 37:173–193
6. Schmitt H, Buchfelder M, Radespiel-Troger M, Fahlbusch R (2000) Difficult intubation in acromegalic patients: incidence and predictability. Anesthesiology 93:110–114
7. Law-Koune JD, Liu N, Szekely B, Fischler M (2004) Using the intubating laryngeal mask airway for ventilation and endotracheal intubation in anesthetized and unparalyzed acromegalic patients. J Neurosurg Anesthesiol 16:11–13
8. Connery LE, Coursin DB (2004) Assessment and therapy of selected endocrine disorders. Anesthesiol Clin North America 22:93–123
9. Anghelescu DL, Burgoyne LL, Liu T et al (2007) Clinical and diagnostic imaging findings predict anesthetic complications in children presenting with malignant mediastinal masses. Paediatr Anaesth 17:1090–1098
10. Northrip DR, Bohman BK, Tsueda K (1986) Total airway occlusion and superior vena cava syndrome in a child with an anterior mediastinal tumor. Anesth Analg 65:1079–1082
11. Redford DT, Kim AS, Barber BJ, Copeland JG (2006) Transesophageal echocardiography for the intraoperative evaluation of a large anterior mediastinal mass. Anesth Analg 103:578–579
12. Keon TP (1981) Death on induction of anesthesia for cervical node biopsy. Anesthesiology 55:471–472
13. Hammer GB (2004) Anaesthetic management for the child with a mediastinal mass. Paediatr Anaesth 14:95–97
14. Guerra-Junior G, Maciel-Guerra AT (2007) The role of the pediatrician in the management of children with genital ambiguities. J Pediatr (Rio J) 83:S184–S191
15. Ghizzoni L, Cesari S, Cremonini G, Melandri L (2007) Prenatal and early postnatal treatment of congenital adrenal hyperplasia. Endocr Dev 11:58–69

Chapter 22
Transplantation

A 14½-year-old female with a diagnosis of Budd–Chiari syndrome presents for liver transplantation. She has developed decreasing mental status, hyponatremia, and a reduction in urine output.

R.S. Holzman et al., *Pediatric Anesthesiology Review: Clinical Cases for Self-Assessment,*   441
DOI 10.1007/978-1-4419-1617-4_22, © Springer Science+Business Media, LLC 2010

Preoperative Evaluation

1. How would liver failure affect pulmonary function? What evaluation of pulmonary function would be helpful for this case? Would bronchodilator therapy be indicated preoperatively?

2. What cardiovascular abnormalities would you expect in this patient?

Preoperative Evaluation

1. Children with liver disease severe enough to be candidates for transplantation nearly always have abnormal pulmonary function [1–3]. Restrictive lung disease is caused by ascites in these children. In addition to the peritoneal space, there may be abnormal transudation of fluid in the pleural space. Pleural effusions will also compromise pulmonary function. Abdominal distention also decreases the FRC. These children are often malnourished and the muscles of respiration, the diaphragm, and intercostals are weakened, leading to a further decrease in the FRC. In addition to restrictive pulmonary pathophysiology, these children have other reasons for hypoxemia. The hepatopulmonary syndrome of hypoxemia and intrapulmonary shunts in these patients contributes to pulmonary morbidity. Intrapulmonary shunting of blood and impaired hypoxic pulmonary vasoconstriction lead to lower hemoglobin saturation. Pulmonary hypertension with increased PVR can affect right ventricular performance. A small subset of patients with severe liver disease will manifest pulmonary hypertension.

2. Children with end-stage liver disease (ESLD) presenting for transplantation have significant derangements of cardiovascular function [4, 5]. These children have an increased cardiac output, increased ejection fraction, and lowered systemic vascular resistance (SVR). Peripheral vasodilatation and arteriovenous shunts account for the lower SVR. The circulating plasma volume is increased. The etiology of the hyperdynamic state of the circulatory system is unclear. Although children with liver failure generally have preserved cardiac function, those with severely advanced disease can exhibit impaired left ventricular performance. SvO_2 is often elevated, probably due to the A–V shunts and to decreased oxygen delivery to the tissues. The RBCs in these patients are depleted of 2,3-DPG and deliver less oxygen to the periphery. These children nearly always have low albumin as part of ESLD. The Child–Pugh classification system includes serum albumin (along with bilirubin, prothrombin time (PT), and degree of encephalopathy) as one of the factors in determining the severity of liver insufficiency.

3. Is this patient exhibiting hepatic encephalopathy? Does she have raised ICP? What treatments should be given for each of these problems?

4. Does the decreased urine output indicate the presence of the hepatorenal syndrome?

5. Is this patient at risk for gastrointestinal hemorrhage? Would the presence of a portosystemic shunt affect the preop evaluation?

3. Patients with severe liver disease often have CNS changes. The cause for hepatic encephalopathy is not known but the severity of the CNS dysfunction does parallel the severity of the liver disease. Possible causes for hepatic encephalopathy are the elevated levels of ammonia and other products of metabolism that accumulate as the liver fails, or the appearance of false neurotransmitters derived from amino acids that had not undergone degradation. The encephalopathy usually improves when appropriate therapy for the liver failure is started. Acute worsening of hepatic encephalopathy is usually an indication that the underlying liver disease has also worsened. In situations where more is demanded of the liver such as GI hemorrhage or increased protein intake, hepatic encephalopathy will worsen. Infections or dehydration will also worsen hepatic encephalopathy. Treatment of hepatic encephalopathy includes restriction of protein intake, enteral lactulose, and neomycin and maintenance of as normal a metabolic state as possible [6–9]. If the patient is in fulminant hepatic failure, raised ICP is likely to be present. The exact etiology of the cerebral edema is not known, but vasogenic and cytotoxic mechanisms are thought to contribute. As the cerebral edema worsens, the ICP increases and the patient becomes more and more encephalopathic. Treatment is supportive and includes the usual measures used in the treatment of raised ICP [10]. These include intubation, sedation, and ventilation to modest hypocarbia, mild hypothermia, and treatment of blood pressure to maintain adequate cerebral perfusion pressure (CPP = MAP – ICP or CVP). Placement of an intracranial pressure monitor is necessary to have an accurate measurement of ICP.

4. Patients with ESLD often also have impaired renal function, either secondary to lowered GFR resulting from dehydration or from having developed the hepatorenal syndrome. Urine sodium concentration is generally low (<10 mEq/L) in both conditions, but in patients with prerenal azotemia, urine output increases and serum BUN and Cr levels decrease following expansion of the intravascular volume. Patients with hepatorenal syndrome have oliguria and increased BUN levels that are generally not responsive to volume administration. Affected individuals also have ascites, and overly aggressive treatment of the ascites with diuretics may play a role in the development of the syndrome. Often dialysis is needed to reverse the pathophysiologic alterations of the hepatorenal syndrome until liver transplantation, which reverses the syndrome, can be accomplished [11, 12].

5. Portal hypertension is often part of liver failure [13]. Bleeding from esophageal and gastric varices are major consequences of portal hypertension. A moderately severe episode of GI hemorrhage may tip a patient in tenuous condition into fulminant hepatic failure. Even if the bleeding is controlled, as the blood in the GI tract is metabolized and absorbed, the encephalopathy will worsen and the episode of hypotension associated with the bleeding episode will worsen the renal ischemia, with the possible development of hepatorenal syndrome. Breakdown of liver glycogen is an important mechanism in the maintenance of normoglycemia. In liver failure, there is diminished breakdown of liver glycogen, making these patients susceptible to episodes of hypoglycemia.

6. What disorders of the hematologic system would be expected in their patient?

7. How should she be evaluated for metabolic abnormalities?

Intraoperative Course

1. What are the effects of liver disease on pharmacokinetics and dynamics of medications?

6. Coagulation abnormalities are quite likely in patients with severe liver insufficiency or failure. In addition, these patients usually are anemic and thrombocytopenic. Fibrinogen, prothrombin, plasminogen, and many other coagulation factors synthesized by the liver are greatly diminished in patients with liver dysfunction/failure. Many patients with liver failure produce an abnormal fibrinogen molecule. In addition, bile salts are needed for absorption of fat-soluble vitamins which includes vitamin K, a cofactor in the production of many coagulation factors. Many interventions by anesthesiologists, such as NG tube placement, intubation, and cannulation of vessels, have the potential to cause bleeding so that correction of coagulation abnormalities often is undertaken prior to the induction of anesthesia. Treatment of the coagulopathy seen in patients with liver failure may require replacement of factors and vitamin K. If platelet dysfunction is evident, DDAVP may be needed.

7. Patients with liver failure have derangements of many serum electrolytes. Common abnormalities are hypoglycemia and hyponatremia. Elevated BUN and Cr as a result of renal dysfunction are present and elevated levels of ammonia are thought to be responsible for the encephalopathy [12].

Intraoperative Course [14, 15]

1. There is a complex set of effects on the action and distribution of medications in patients with liver failure. These patients have a decreased serum albumin, which would lead to an enhanced effect of IV medications given at the usual dose on a mg/kg basis. These patients also have impaired hepatic metabolic function as well as impaired renal function. As a result of these abnormalities, the serum levels of medications will remain high for longer periods of time and will be less bound to protein. In addition, these patients may have depressed cardiovascular and pulmonary function prior to the induction of anesthesia.

2. What preparations should be made with the blood bank and laboratory support for this case? How will rapid transfusion be accomplished? Would you expect to use veno–veno bypass?

3. Describe special consideration for monitoring and vascular access for this patient and procedure.

2. Preparation of the OR should be for a long case in which massive blood loss is expected, temperature maintenance will be problematic, invasive hemodynamic monitoring will be needed and many metabolic derangements will occur. The OR table should be particularly well padded since these cases may last for many hours. Devices for rapid transfusion should be, at the very least, available or fully prepared. In the past, in larger patients, venovenous bypass was used, with the expectation that bowel edema and bleeding would be decreased compared with cases in which the vena cava was simply clamped. This practice is generally no longer used, however, simplifying the intraoperative management of liver transplant patients. The blood bank should be given as much notice as possible in order that the proper amounts and types of blood products are available. As a general guideline, 10 units of PRBCs, 10 units of FFP and 6–10 units of pooled platelets should be immediately available, with the expectation that more may be needed. Of course, these amounts should be adjusted upward or downward based upon the size and condition of the patient. Throughout the case, many ABGs, sets of electrolytes, coagulation profiles, CBCs etc. will be sent. It may be necessary to have additional laboratory personnel to run these frequent and multiple tests.

3. In addition to routine monitors, temperature should be measured in more than one location. Rectal or bladder probes can be used in addition to esophageal. Several large IVs are needed, preferably in the upper extremities. During the anhepatic phase of the procedure, when the IVC is clamped, lower extremity venous return will be limited to collateral veins or the venovenous bypass if it is used. Similar considerations apply to the arterial catheter. In some cases, the aorta will be clamped during the arterial anastamosis. Some centers use two arterial catheters. The direct arterial pressure tracing is unavailable during the frequent sampling and if, because of frequent use, one arterial line fails, the second line will be available. A large, sheath-type central line is used in these cases for monitoring of central venous pressure, administration of vasoactive medications and also administration of fluids and/or blood products. In general, pediatric patients need not be monitored with a pulmonary artery catheter. On occasions when peripheral IV access is difficult two central lines may be used.

4. How will induction be performed? Does this patient have a full stomach? How does ascites affect the induction plan?

5. Describe the conduct of maintenance during the procedure.

6. What problems are expected during the preanhepatic phase?

4. The patient should be comfortably positioned on the padded OR table prior to induction. In the induction of general anesthesia in unintubated patients, full stomach precautions should be observed. Since these patients often have pulmonary dysfunction including a diminished FRC caused by ascites and abdominal distention and hepatopulmonary syndrome, thorough preoxygenation is essential prior to induction. Regardless of the specific IV hypnotic chosen, the dose should be adjusted based on the altered pharmacodynamics previously discussed. There is no specific contraindication to the use of succinylcholine. Often a combination of a hypnotic in a lowered dose and small doses of a benzodiazepine and opioid are used with the goal of rendering the patient unconscious without significant hypotension or heart rate alterations. As in most patients, the use of succinylcholine is associated with an increase in serum potassium of 0.5–0.7 mEq/L. If the patients have significant hyperkalemia prior to induction, the increase in potassium concentration may lead to cardiac arrhythmias. On the other hand, if the patient is compromised with a very small FRC, it is likely that significant hypoxemia will occur in the time required to achieve good intubating conditions using a nondepolarizing relaxant.

5. Although no particular technique has been proven to be advantageous or deleterious to children undergoing liver transplantation, it does seem prudent to avoid high doses of inhaled agents. High doses of inhaled agents have been shown to decrease splanchnic blood flow, possibly placing the graft at risk. A combination of an infusion of relaxant and an opioid with low dose isoflurane or sevoflurane with additional benzodiazepines will likely achieve the goals of maintenance of an anesthetized state in the patient with minimal decrease in cardiac function. Since the procedure will last at least several hours and the child will remain intubated for the first postoperative night, concerns about the prolonged effect of IV medication affecting emergence are unfounded.

6. The preanhepatic phase is the time of greatest blood loss. The surgeons are working to dissect free the failed liver. There may well be adhesions from previous procedures. Of course, during this time, the patient may be hemodynamically unstable, and almost certainly has a coagulopathy. With significant bleeding and the massive transfusion required to maintain hemodynamic and metabolic stability, hyperkalemia, hypocalcemia, hypothermia, and hemolysis may all occur. The use of washed PRBCs or newer PRBCs will decrease the amount of potassium in each unit. Ionized calcium and serum magnesium must be checked frequently during times of rapid transfusion since the citrate in the PRBC units chelates both divalent ions. Even with the administration of warmed blood products and fluids, the child's temperature may decrease during the preanhepatic phase. The abdomen is open and evaporative losses of fluid are significant. During this part of the procedure, ABGs, coagulation profiles and electrolyte determinations should be done as often as every 30 min depending upon the amount of bleeding, transfusion requirements, and the degree of stability or instability of vital signs. In addition to blood loss, hypotension during the dissection phase may be due to either hypocalcemia or torsion of the liver during dissection with sudden decreased venous return.

7. What is important for the anesthesiologist during the anhepatictic phase?

8. What problems are likely to occur during reperfusion?

9. During the neo hepatic/biliary reconstruction phase what problems are expected?

7. The anhepatic stage of the procedure begins when the old liver is removed from the circulation, not with physical removal of the liver. When the infra- and supra-hepatic cavae, portal vein, and hepatic artery are clamped, the child is anhepatic. Vigorous bleeding may still continue at the beginning of the anhepatic phase. In most pediatric liver transplants, femoral-axillary bypass is not used. Children tolerate clamping the vena cava during placement of the graft. While the old liver is out and the new liver not yet in the circulation, the child may demonstrate significant hemodynamic changes. There may be decreases in systemic blood pressure, central venous pressure, and cardiac output. As the child cools, oxygen consumption decreases with a concomitant decrease in carbon dioxide production. Also, during the anhepatic phase, any contribution the failing liver was making to glucose homeostasis is eliminated.

8. Once the vascular connections are complete, circulation is allowed into the new liver. The postreperfusion syndrome will occur in a significant number of patients once this happens. This syndrome includes hypotension and bradycardia, possibly even cardiac arrest. One preventable cause is inadequate flushing of the pre-servative solution from the graft. This solution is hyperkalemic, acidotic, and quite cold. If the graft is not thoroughly flushed, the patient will have profound hemodynamic instability once the preservative enters the circulation. The post-perfusion syndrome can occur even if the graft is completely flushed of the preservative solution, however. Treatment is resuscitation with IV fluids and vasoactive agents. In some cases, only one or two doses of epinephrine are needed to maintain hemodynamic stability but in others infusion of inotropes is needed for several hours after the graft has been open to the circulation. In addition to the postperfusion syndrome, all patients have a rapid increase in end-tidal and arterial carbon dioxide once the IVC is unclamped.

9. As the new liver is connected to the recipient's hepatic veins and artery, coagulation problems begin to diminish. Hepatic artery thrombosis is more of a problem in pediatric liver transplantation, largely due to the smaller size of the vessel. Although no specific management of coagulation in the posttransplantation period has been shown to decrease the incidence of hepatic artery thrombosis, many anesthesiologists do not aggressively pursue complete normalization of PT/PTT as the liver is connected to the circulation unless significant, diffuse bleeding is ongoing. Correction of coagulation abnormalities generally begins as the new liver is connected to the circulation. However, if the patient has hypo-thermia or hypocalcemia, coagulation will be affected. These patients are sent to the ICU postoperatively with plans for mechanical ventilation [16]. Even in cases where the blood loss was not great, for example, less than half a blood volume, extubation should be delayed. The large incision will limit the child's ability to breathe. In addition, after such an extensive procedure, it may take some time to achieve hemodynamic stability.

Additional Questions

1. A 6-year-old s/p cardiac transplant requires inotropic support due to acute rejection.

   (a) What would your choices be to enhance cardiac output?

   (b) Are anticholinergics effective? What are the relative effects of denervation on the adrenergic and cholinergic competency of the transplanted heart?

   (c) Would milrinone be effective in enhancing contractility?

Additional Topics

1. Cardiac transplantation [17, 18]. Cardiac transplant recipients present several challenges to the anesthesiologist. Denervated hearts do not respond normally to input mediated via the autonomic nervous system. Drugs which act through stimulation of the autonomic nervous system may have little or no effect on a denervated heart. The usual bradycardic response to hypertension, mediated through the vagus nerve, occurs rarely if at all in these patients. In general, these patients do not tolerate decreased preload well.

   (a) Pharmacologic enhancement of cardiac output is best accomplished with direct-acting agents such as epinephrine, isoproterenol, or dopamine. A drug such as ephedrine which has both direct and indirect effects in patients with innervated hearts will have only the direct effects on denervated hearts. Catecholamines such as dobutamine, dopamine, epinephrine, and norepinephrine will, via a direct effect on the myocardium, increase cardiac output.

   (b) Atropine or pancuronium, two agents pediatric anesthesiologists rely upon to increase heart rate, will not be effective in cardiac transplant recipients. The alpha agonist phenylephrine, on the other hand, will increase vascular tone but the baroreceptor response of lowered heart rate will not occur in the denervated heart.

   (c) The phosphodiesterase inhibitors such as amrinone have direct effects on myocardial cells; increasing cAMP levels with resulting increased contractility. The systemic effects on preload will also occur but baroreceptor responses to decreased preload will be absent or partially and inconsistently present in patients with denervated hearts.

(d) An adolescent s/p heart transplant for viral cardiomyopathy 6 years ago presents to the emergency room with hypotension, J-point depression on ECG, but without angina. Please explain.

2. Renal transplantation. An adult living related kidney is being transplanted into a 4-year-old recipient.

   (a) What problems should you anticipate with unclamping?

   (b) What is the most common cause of renal failure leading to kidney transplantation in children?

   (c) What age is the greatest risk period for difficulty with perioperative medical management?

(d) Unexplained hypotension in a cardiac transplant recipient may very well be due to myocardial ischemia. These patients often have coronary artery disease after transplant. Rejection remains a major problem limiting survival in heart transplant recipients. The coronary arteries are affected with atherosclerosis when rejection occurs. Coronary artery vasculopathy accounts for approximately 30% of deaths after 1 year in transplant recipients. Angina may not occur in children with coronary artery disease since their hearts are denervated. Evaluation of cardiac transplant recipients for coronary atherosclerosis (vasculopathy) has been done in the cardiac cath lab using angiography. Dobutamine stress echocardiography has been used safely in children as a screen for coronary vasculopathy. Anesthetic management of children with coronary vasculopathy undergoing surgical procedures should be similar to techniques used for adults with coronary artery disease, with particular attention paid to the balance between oxygen supply and demand. The ECG may show ST segment changes with ischemia. Depending upon the procedure, consideration should be given to placement of a CVP or TEE. Children who have had cardiac transplantation who then return to the OR for procedures present several other problems to the anesthesiologist in addition to those outlined above relating to coronary artery disease. The denervated heart will not respond to autonomic input. Medications that affect cardiac rate or contractility via indirect mechanisms will not have those effects on the denervated heart. Direct acting drugs such as epinephrine, norepinephrine, dopamine, and isoproterenol will affect cardiac performance. Baroreceptor responses to blood pressure changes are absent. Heart rate changes in response to decreased intravascular volume occur inconsistently. In addition, vagally mediated slowing of the heart rate will not occur in these patients.

2. Renal transplantation [19–21]

(a) In cases where the kidney to be transplanted is from a person significantly larger than the recipient, significant hemodynamic consequences are likely, particularly when the graft is perfused. Hypotension may result not only from release of graft preservative solution but also from depletion of intravascular volume as the new, large graft is perfused. Prior to opening the vascular clamps the anesthesiologist should have given a generous amount of IV fluids, enough to elevate the CVP. Graft survival is dependent on adequate perfusion. The anesthesiologist must administer additional fluid as needed and/or use inotropes such as dopamine to maintain systemic blood pressure.

(b) Although there are many causes of renal failure, obstructive uropathy, renal dysplasia/hypoloasia, and primary glomerular disease are the most common causes of ESRD in pediatrics.

(c) Younger transplant recipients present greater challenges with regard to perioperative anesthetic management as well as surgical technique. Although renal transplantation offers the best chance for normal growth and development in children with ESRD, nearly all such patients are maintained with either peritoneal or hemodialysis for varying lengths of time prior to renal transplantation.

(d) What long-term effects should you anticipate with immunosuppression postrenal transplantation, and how will it affect your subsequent anesthetic management of patients?

(e) Does anemia resolve postrenal transplantation? Why?

(d) Immunosupression treatment for recipients of renal allografts includes steroids, cyclosporine, and tacrolimus. Cyclosporine is an 11 amino acid peptide that inhibits T cell function by a variety of mechanisms, one of which is inhibition of IL-2 formation and action. Without IL-2, T cell activation is significantly diminished. Cyclosporine is metabolized by the cytochrome P450 system and its metabolism is affected by co-administration of a variety of other medications. This drug has significant side effects. Neurotoxicity, manifested as tremors, paresthesias, headache, confusion, etc., hepatotoxicity, and hypertension and renal toxicity may limit the use of cyclosporine. Tacrolimus (FK506), a macrolide antibiotic similar to streptomycin, has similar immunologic effects as cyclosporine, inhibiting Il-2 and IL-2 receptor expression. Although prednisone has many deleterious side effects, it remains a part of the immunosupression used after renal transplantation. Side effects of importance include hypertension, growth failure, GI bleeding, pancreatitis, and osteoporosis. Posttransplantation lymphoproliferative disease (PTLD) is a very serious complication of immunosupression. This complication occurs in 1–3% of renal transplant recipients and can be seen at almost any time after the transplant. PTLD may result from B cell activation after a viral illness. The proliferation is seen in the GI tract and lymph nodes. The tonsils may be significantly enlarged as part of the presentation. Affected children may present for tonsillectomy/biopsy to confirm the diagnosis.

(e) The anemia seen in patients with ESRD has many causes such as decreased erythropoietin production, inadequate intake of iron and folate, low grade hemolysis, and episodes of bleeding. In many patients the hemoglobin will remain at approximately 6–9 mg/dL. With the administration of erythropeitin, the hemoglobin can be maintained at 10–11 g/dL. Following renal transplantation, most recipients are as anemic as they were preop. Many of the medications used to prevent rejection have deleterious effects on bone marrow production of red cells. For example, calcineurin inhibitors such as cyclosporine or tacrolimus (FK506) and antimetabolites such as azothiaprine have bone marrow toxicity as a side effect. As the medications are adjusted to decrease all side effects, patients' hemoglobin increases but it is not unusual for renal transplant recipients to be treated with erythropoietin (Epo) to increase the red cell mass.

3. Liver transplantation:

    (a) Is flumazenil effective for hepatic encephalopathy?

    (b) What is lactulose, and why is it used?

    (c) What is the importance of a low-protein diet in liver failure?

3. Liver transplantation

(a) There are several possible explanations for the development of hepatic encephalopathy in the setting of liver failure. Ammonia, false neurotransmitters, and GABA are all often elevated significantly in patients with liver failure and hepatic encephalopathy. Although ammonia levels are often elevated in patients with liver failure accompanied by encephalopathy, it is not unusual for an individual patient to exhibit encephalopathy prior to having elevated serum ammonia. GABA (gamma aminobutyric acid) is an inhibitory neurotransmitter thought to play a role in hepatic encephalopathy. It is produced by intestinal bacteria as is ammonia. Both are elevated in patients with liver failure. This molecule binds to CNS benzodiazepine receptors. Evidence in favor of this hypothesis is the fact that administration of flumazenil, a benzodiazepine antagonist, has partially reversed hepatic encephalopathy [7]. False neurotransmitters are also considered a possible cause of hepatic encephalopathy. Specifically, in liver failure the concentration of aromatic amino acids increases. These aromatic amino acids cross the blood brain barrier and participate in the production of neurotransmitters [9]. Management of liver failure includes limiting protein intake as well as therapies to decrease serum ammonia levels [8].

(b) Lactulose converts ammonia in the intestinal lumen into nonabsorbable ammonium.

(c) Minimizing the intake of protein also helps limit the production of ammonia. In addition, if there is less protein breakdown, fewer aromatic amino acids will be produced.

Annotated References

Csete M, Glas K (2006) Anesthesia for organ transplantation. Chap. 53. In: Barash PG, Cullen BF, Stoelting RK (eds) Clinical anesthesia. Lippincot Williams and Wilkins, pp 1358–1376
In this chapter, anesthetic and perioperative considerations for patients undergoing various transplantation procedures are reviewed. Specific types of transplantation discussed are: renal, hepatic, pulmonary, cardiac, pancreatic islet cell, and small bowel/miltivisceral transplantation.
Bishop WP (2006) Liver disease. In: Kliegman RM, Marcdante KJ, Jenson HB, Behrman RE (eds) Nelson essentials of pediatrics, 5th edn. Elsevier Saunders, pp 615–618
This section briefly reviews the clinical presentation of liver failure in children, common etiologies, laboratory evaluation of these patients, and general management considerations.

References

1. Rodriguez-Roisin R, Krowka MJ (2008) Hepatopulmonary syndrome–a liver-induced lung vascular disorder. N Engl J Med 358:2378–2387
2. Tumgor G, Arikan C, Yuksekkaya HA et al (2008) Childhood cirrhosis, hepatopulmonary syndrome and liver transplantation. Pediatr Transplant 12:353–357
3. Palma DT, Philips GM, Arguedas MR et al (2008) Oxygen desaturation during sleep in hepatopulmonary syndrome. Hepatology 47:1257–1263
4. Alqahtani SA, Fouad TR, Lee SS (2008) Cirrhotic cardiomyopathy. Semin Liver Dis 28:59–69
5. Biais M, Nouette-Gaulain K, Cottenceau V et al (2008) Cardiac output measurement in patients undergoing liver transplantation: pulmonary artery catheter versus uncalibrated arterial pressure waveform analysis. Anesth Analg 106:1480–1486, table of contents
6. Morgan MY, Blei A, Grungreiff K et al (2007) The treatment of hepatic encephalopathy. Metab Brain Dis 22:389–405
7. Als-Nielsen B, Gluud LL, Gluud C (2004) Benzodiazepine receptor antagonists for hepatic encephalopathy. Cochrane Database Syst Rev:CD002798
8. Als-Nielsen B, Gluud LL, Gluud C (2004) Nonabsorbable disaccharides for hepatic encephalopathy. Cochrane Database Syst Rev:CD003044
9. Als-Nielsen B, Gluud LL, Gluud C (2004) Dopaminergic agonists for hepatic encephalopathy. Cochrane Database Syst Rev:CD003047
10. Blei AT (2007) Brain edema in acute liver failure: can it be prevented? Can it be treated? J Hepatol 46:564–569
11. Arroyo V, Fernandez J, Gines P (2008) Pathogenesis and treatment of hepatorenal syndrome. Semin Liver Dis 28:81–95
12. Leiva JG, Salgado JM, Estradas J et al (2007) Pathophysiology of ascites and dilutional hyponatremia: contemporary use of aquaretic agents. Ann Hepatol 6:214–221
13. Blei AT (2007) Portal hypertension and its complications. Curr Opin Gastroenterol 23:275–282
14. Bennett J, Bromley P (2006) Perioperative issues in pediatric liver transplantation. Int Anesthesiol Clin 44:125–147
15. Yudkowitz FS, Chietero M (2005) Anesthetic issues in pediatric liver transplantation. Pediatr Transplant 9:666–672
16. Fumagalli R, Ingelmo P, Sperti LR (2006) Postoperative sedation and analgesia after pediatric liver transplantation. Transplant Proc 38:841–843
17. Mahle WT (2008) Heart transplantation: Literature review 2006–2007. Pediatr Transplant 16:630–639
18. Mahle WT (2008) Cardiac retransplantation in children. Pediatr Transplant 12:274–280
19. Giessing M, Muller D, Winkelmann B et al (2007) Kidney transplantation in children and adolescents. Transplant Proc 39:2197–2201
20. Della Rocca G, Costa MG, Bruno K et al (2001) Pediatric renal transplantation: anesthesia and perioperative complications. Pediatr Surg Int 17:175–179
21. Coupe N, O'Brien M, Gibson P, de Lima J (2005) Anesthesia for pediatric renal transplantation with and without epidural analgesia–a review of 7 years experience. Paediatr Anaesth 15:220–228

Chapter 23
Minimally Invasive Surgery

A 2½-year-old, 13-kg female is scheduled for a laparoscopic nephrectomy for a unilateral polycystic kidney. She had a cold 3 weeks ago but is now afebrile and appears well.

R.S. Holzman et al., *Pediatric Anesthesiology Review: Clinical Cases for Self-Assessment,*   463
DOI 10.1007/978-1-4419-1617-4_23, © Springer Science+Business Media, LLC 2010

Preoperative Evaluation

1. What are your anesthetic considerations in differentiating candidates for laparoscopic compared with open approaches for the same surgical procedure?

   (a) Intraoperative considerations?
   (b) Perioperative considerations?
   (c) Is their recovery likely to be different?
   (d) How does this influence your postoperative planning for pain management?

2. What safety issues will you face with regard to intraperitoneal insufflation?

   (a) What is the optimal choice of gas?
   (b) What is the optimal insufflation pressure?

Preoperative Evaluation

1. If the surgical goal is accomplishable by either route, then the decision making will be most influenced by the overall medical condition of the patient. Perioperative recovery will be faster and less painful with the laparoscopic route and it should be anticipated that adequacy of postoperative ventilation will be improved with a minimally invasive approach. Extraperitoneal approaches will affect respiration less than intraperitoneal approaches, and retroperitoneal approaches will probably be most favorable for recovery, particularly in the prone compared with the flank position. Some (relative) contraindications to laparoscopic surgery include respiratory disability, cardiomyopathy, and lower limits of age when surgical instruments of proper size may not be available. The contraindications for these underlying medical conditions are relative rather than absolute because judgment has to be exercised with regard to the benefits of a milder perioperative course vs. potentially more adverse intraoperative effects of the laparoscopic surgery on cardiopulmonary interactions.

2. Intraperitoneal gas insufflation will affect respiratory mechanics and cardiovascular performance as well as impose an exogenous load of the particular insufflating gas [1–4]. The creation of the pneumoperitoneum will increase peak airway pressure and plateau airway pressures. Cardiac output and splanchnic blood flow decrease, and cardiac output decreases while systemic vascular resistance increases, leading to recommendations of peak intraabdominal pressures of 8–12 mmHg. Further influences on the cardiopulmonary system are imposed by positioning of the patient in Trendelenburg position and various lateral tilting maneuvers. While several avenues of gas insufflation have been pursued (air, nitrous oxide, and carbon dioxide), carbon dioxide is most favored because of its increased solubility and lack of support of combustion [5].

Intraoperative Course

1. Routine noninvasive monitors are already planned for this case; does it require anything else?

    (a) Is capnographic monitoring required?
    (b) Are the requirements for capnographic monitoring in children different than for adults? How? Would you select a monitor capable of detecting end-tidal nitrogen? Why?
    (c) What other nonroutine monitors might be required?

2. The patient undergoes a routine mask induction; what would your choice of agent be?

    (a) Any special considerations for the use of sevoflurane, if chosen, with regard to renal dysfunction? Would you choose another agent? Why?
    (b) Use nitrous oxide? Why?
    (c) Following intubation, do any other devices need to be placed?
    (d) Is an oral or nasogastric tube necessary?
    (e) A saphenous vein IV is placed; is this an optimal location or would you choose another if available? Why?

3. Would you use nitrous oxide for maintenance?

    (a) If you started with sevoflurane, would you choose to continue, or would you switch to isoflurane?
    (b) Would you use opioids as an adjunct to this anesthetic? Why? What would your choice be?
    (c) Is the addition of ketorolac a good idea?
    (d) Any special considerations for its use in this patient?

Intraoperative Course

1. Additional monitors are not required unless dictated by the patient's underlying concurrent diseases or anticipated sudden blood loss or hemodynamic instability. In this case, the risk seems small. Capnographic monitoring, on the other hand, is important because of the continuous CO_2 load as well as the restrictions to ventilation imposed by the pneumoperitoneum. Requirements for capnographic monitoring in children are different in that the maximum expiratory flow rate is lower and therefore the sampling rate has to be higher to compensate and produce a more discrete capnographic trace; otherwise, the signal will "blur" resulting in a sine-wave appearance with an elevated baseline and a truncated plateau. Monitoring for end-tidal nitrogen would be important for a suspicion of air embolism (venous or arterial) and if available could certainly be used; however, it would be a rare occurrence and other monitors would suggest clinically significant venous air embolism at the time. In this regard, a precordial Doppler might be useful if concern about a venous air embolism persisted.

2. I would choose sevofllurane + nitrous oxide + oxygen for the mask induction. Although sevoflurane can, in specific circumstances, be associated with elevated markers of renal dysfunction, this has only existed when circuit flows have been low, anesthetic duration is prolonged, and the patient had impaired renal function preoperatively. Even then, elevation of the markers did not have direct bearing on perioperative renal outcome. Nitrous oxide is reasonable to use to get started but I would probably discontinue it after induction of anesthesia because a closed, gas-filled space is going to be created, into which the nitrous oxide could pass. In addition, the use of the nitrous oxide might contribute to postoperative nausea. A gastric tube is necessary to decompress the stomach of any air insufflated during anesthetic induction and make it safer to perform the pneumoperitoneum. Likewise for a bladder catheter. A saphenous vein IV is okay to get started with, but because the procedure is transabdominal and retroperitoneal, there is always the chance that needed medications might not be getting to exactly where they need to go quickly enough. I would replace the IV in an upper extremity, if possible.

3. I would avoid nitrous oxide for the above reasons. I would continue with sevoflurane because of the smoothness of induction, until the IV was in and I had the trachea intubated. Opioids would allow a lower dose of volatile agent to be utilized and also allow for a more rapid and smoother emergence from anesthesia. Ketorolac would be fine as an opioid adjunct but its potential for nephrotoxicity must be borne in mind for this particular case. On the other hand, it would be very efficacious for peritoneally initiated discomfort and would make it possible to decrease the use of opioids.

4. What are your considerations for neuromuscular blockade? Does this patient require it?

5. You note that the patient's temperature has not decreased during the course of surgery, but has rather increased such that by the first 2 h of surgery the temperature is 37.2°C. Over the next hour it has increased to 38.3°C.

   (a) What do you think may be going on?
   (b) How can you figure it out?
   (c) Is there evidence for runaway hypermetabolism? How could you be sure?
   (d) What mechanisms might be at work here?

6. What are your considerations for management of mechanical ventilation?

   (a) What influences your decision?
   (b) What will influence your management of minute ventilation?
   (c) What will influence your management of ventilation mechanics?
   (d) During the course of the case, the patient becomes more difficult to ventilate over a 10-min period; the $ETCO_2$ is decreased and the peak inspiratory pressure is high (changed from 25 to 60 cmH_2O); what are your considerations?
   (e) The SpO_2 is now 88% on 100% O_2 and the blood pressure 60/40 mmHg; how does this influence your analysis? What would you do?
   (f) You listen to the chest and the breath sounds are heard only on the left; your conclusion? Management?

4. There are several compelling reasons to ensure a good level of neuromuscular blockade. First of all, motionlessness is required for initial puncture and subsequent manipulation via the laparoscope. Second, this patient will likely have an increased level of end-tidal CO_2 as a stimulus to breathing. Diaphragmatic movement is at best disturbing to the continuous view through the laparoscope and at worst may cause visceral organ damage while working with these small instruments. Therefore, I would use a muscle relaxant along with neuromuscular blockade monitoring to assess the level of relaxation and ensure reversibility at the end of surgery.

5. The elevation in temperature is not surprising for several reasons. First of all, this is closed cavity surgery, and although cold anhydrous gas is being insufflated, there is no open abdomen to radiate heat. Although the mechanism is unclear, the increase in temperature is common in small children and may be a result of brown fact activation either through the mechanical stimulation of the increased abdominal or retroperitoneal pressure or as a response to the increase in CO_2 load. Even an increase to $38.3°C$ is not disturbing as long as CO_2 production (plus CO_2 load from exogenously administered gas) is manageable by a proportional increase in minute ventilation. If it is unmanageable by an increase in minute ventilation, then the differential diagnosis needs to be broadened to include malignant hyperthermia.

6. Mechanical ventilation has to be tailored to this unique situation; an increase in CO_2 production because of an increase in body temperature plus a fixed amount of exogenous CO_2 load will result in a requirement for increased minute ventilation. At the same time, the restrictive ventilatory defect imposed on the diaphragm by the pneumoperitoneum will usually mean that decreased total airway compliance will require a more modest increase in tidal volume (in comparison with an open abdomen procedure) and an increase in respiratory rate to make up for the increased minute ventilation requirement. A progressive decrease in compliance can result from several issues – (1) plugging of the endotracheal tube (2) movement of the tip of the endotracheal tube closer to the carina or to a mainstem bronchus (as a result of cephalad movement of the diaphragm and the mediastinum) (3) pneumothorax as a result of distending gas dissecting past the diaphragm and into the chest. Progressive V/Q mismatch and hemodynamic compromise would suggest space-occupying gas in the chest. Immediate auscultation may reveal asymmetry of breath sounds suggesting a pneumothorax; immediate intervention would require chest decompression and placement of closed chest drainage either with a catheter or a chest tube. If there is enough time, a chest X-ray would make the diagnosis.

7. Intraoperative leak: Following abdominal insufflation, you note an airleak at the mouth at 6 cm H_2O, and a change in the morphology of the capnographic trace from

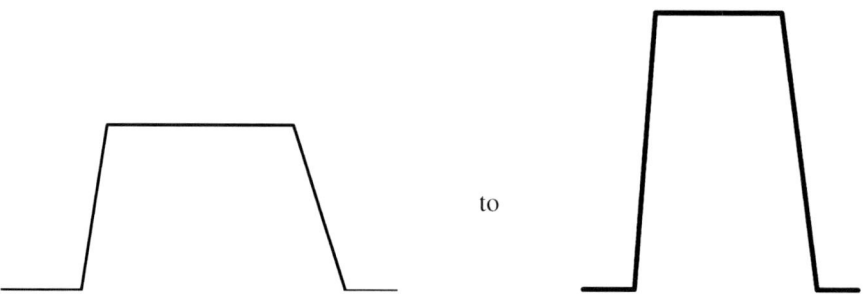

to

(a) Your next move?
(b) Leave things the same?
(c) Change tube (if so, to what)?
(d) Pack throat?

Postoperative Course

1. The patient has now had three episodes of vomiting and continued dry heaves in the first half hour in the PACU; what do you think is going on?

   (a) Is there any increased susceptibility to this with laparoscopic surgery?
   (b) How will you treat?
   (c) You administer metoclopramide, 0.15 mg/kg, and the patient becomes dysarthric and has cogwheel rigidity. What do you think is going on?
   (d) Is she at risk for malignant hyperthermia?
   (e) Anything further diagnostic that can be done?
   (f) Are there any drugs to administer?
   (g) Should the patient be admitted to the ICU overnight?

2. Pain management?

7. The decreased total compliance of the airway is probably the cause of this leak at the same mechanical ventilatory settings. There are several ways to deal with the leak, but it is most important to use this event as a bellwether for the rest of the case, i.e., if compliance is going to get worse as the case goes on, plans have to be made now for providing more effective positive pressure ventilation. The endotracheal tube should be changed for a larger size without a cuff or the same size with a cuff; I would probably opt for the cuffed endotracheal tube as a replacement because what may also follow are changes in position that may increase the risk of reflux as well [6]. Intracuff pressure should be carefully assessed so as not to put too much pressure on the tracheal mucosa and result in subglottic edema in the postoperative period. Placement of a throat pack, while "sealing" (or at least muffling) the leak, will ultimately not be as effective as a more properly sized tube.

Postoperative Course

1. Perioperative nausea and vomiting is not unusual following peritoneal insufflation; maximum medical therapy would include ondansetron, metoclopramide, and dexamethasone. Even with this multimodal therapy, all nausea and vomiting is unlikely to be ablated, only lessened. Metaclopramide, even in this dose range, may produce extrapyramidal side effects which can be alleviated with diphenhydramine. The rigidity is a side effect of the metaclopramide and is not a sign of malignant hyperthermia. The patient will probably not need an ICU admission, although some prolonged observation in the PACU for recurrence would be worthwhile.

2. Pain is difficult to manage following the laparoscopic approach because the peritoneal and diaphragmatic irritation with referred pain to the shoulders seems out of proportion to the small puncture sites that lend themselves so easily to infiltration with local anesthetic. Small doses of titrated opioids are best, along with ketorolac as a NSAID adjunct. In older patients PCA analgesia seems to work well.

Additional Questions

1. A 3-week-old, 31-week postconceptual age infant is coming to the OR for a video-assisted thoracoscopic surgical (VATS) closure of a patent ductus arteriosus. The surgeon visualizes two pulsatile vessels, places the initial clip and within 8 s the patient becomes progressively bradycardic, hypotensive, and then asystolic. What do you think happened? What would you like to do? What should the surgeon do? How can you prevent this from occurring again?

2. A 15-year-old female is scheduled for a laparoscopic cholecystectomy. She has sickle cell disease. What are the relative advantages of the laparoscopic approach with regard to her perioperative care in the setting of this particular disease? Any disadvantages or special risks intraoperatively? What? Why? Would she benefit from a neuraxial anesthetic for postoperative pain control? Are there any risks for her? Her hematologist, pulmonologist, nephrologist, and cardiologist are all waiting to talk to you on the phone. What do you think they want to know, and what are you going to tell them?

Additional Questions

1. The surgeon probably placed the clip around the aorta, which can look just like the ductus, particularly through the thoracoscope. The surgeon should quickly remove the clip while you support the circulation with (1) volume (2) external cardiac massage to circulate the (3) epinephrine. Chances are the patient's cardiac rhythm will be restored almost immediately because this is a "witnessed" arrest. To differentiate the two vascular structures, the surgeon could temporarily occlude the structure he believes to be the ductus and then place a clip on the same structure thereafter. If he accidentally occludes the aorta with his temporary occlusion it should be easily detectable on the pulse oximeter plethysmographic trace.

2. Cholecystectomy in a sickle cell disease teenager is a relatively common procedure. A laparoscopic approach will allow her to have much less pain and a better ability to breathe postoperatively. Compared with a right upper quadrant incision with an open cholecystectomy it will restrict her ventilation far less, improve her ability to maintain her FRC and take deep breaths, and lessen the chance that atelectasis will contribute to postoperative VQ mismatch and hypoxemia. Intraoperatively, one has to be careful to ventilate her with optimal tidal volumes to allow for adequate chest wall expansion and prevention of alveolar collapse. In addition, an adequate minute ventilation should defend her against respiratory acidosis and hypercarbia. It would be good to discuss an epidural with her for postoperative pain relief, but the majority of her pain may be as a result of diaphragmatic irritation with referred shoulder pain, and therefore, a high lumbar or thoracic epidural may not be of more help than a PCA. The various specialists are probably all concerned about the various end-organ effects of sickle cell disease and the kind of anesthetic technique that would minimize such effects. To minimize the chance of further sickling, the patient should have an adequate (or slightly above adequate) volume status, be kept warm and well oxygenated, and have a Hb SC level of less than 30–40% [7]. The prevention of chest crises can best be accomplished by adequate gas exchange intraoperatively and an optimal plan for postoperative pulmonary toilet, which can probably be accomplished with (1) laparoscopic surgery (2) adequate analgesia via the epidural or PCA route and (3) supplemental oxygen to maintain oxygen saturation at reasonable levels. The nephrologist will be concerned about her renal function, particularly in the renal medulla which is susceptible to sickling in a hypoxic environment. Again, adequate volume repletion, warmth, and pain control will help renal blood flow and the maintenance of red cell integrity.

3. An 8-year-old, 27-kg boy, with a right-sided empyema and a respiratory rate of 80 bpm with a SpO_2 of 89% is in the ICU, getting ready to come to the OR for an evacuation and thoracoscopy. The surgeon wants you to use one-lung ventilation to the left lung while he insufflates the pleura to visualize the empyema better. How can you do this?

4. An 18-year old with pansinusitis and cystic fibrosis is scheduled for functional endoscopic sinus surgery (FESS). His preoperative pulmonary function tests indicate a FVC of 80% of predicted prebronchodilator and 87% postbronchodilator and FEV1/FVC of 82 and 85% pre- and postbronchodilator, respectively. He is not wheezing. Any special considerations? He wants to avoid a general anesthetic and wonders if there is a way to do this with sedation and blocks? Any blocks you can suggest?

3. An 8-year-old, 27-kg child is too small for a 28 French double lumen endotracheal tube, so there are several options left to isolate the lungs. A left mainstem intubation can be planned with fiberoptic guidance, allowing the right lung to decompress and not be ventilated. A bronchial blocker could be placed along the side of the endotracheal tube to further isolate the lung. I would, however, favor placement of an Arndt coaxial endobronchial blocker through an in situ endotracheal tube under fiberoptic guidance. The difficulty with this is the inability to passively supply additional oxygen through the endobronchial blocker to take advantage of passive oxygenation in the nonventilated lung, and therefore, one has to be open to the possibility that the patient may require bilateral lung ventilation and the surgeon may have to compress the lung if oxygenation is difficult.

4. These pulmonary function tests are not bad for an 18-year old and should be judged against a history and physical examination, but his level of function is probably pretty good. He does not show dramatic improvement pre- and postbronchodilator PFTs so his medical management is probably close to optimal and will therefore likely tolerate a general anesthetic well. He is curious about the possibility of not going completely to sleep and that is understandable, but should be explored further not only with the patient but also with the surgeon. There is substantial danger to the patient if he moves during the FESS procedure, and many surgeons are also concerned about an awake patient and the possibility of uncontrolled bleeding or ocular damage during the FESS. Theoretically, it should be possible to sedate the patient and provide analgesia through a sphenopalatine block, anesthetizing the ipsilateral palate and maxillary sinus. It may be carried out transorally with injection of local anesthetic through the greater palatine foramen or transnasally at the level of the middle turbinate (which it often is anyway because of the application of local anesthetic by the surgeon prior to instrumentation). However, the intraoperative discomfort likely extends beyond the area that is immediately affected by the sphenopalatine ganglion and because of these concerns as well as bleeding and comfort and control by the surgeon, I would opt for recommending against a local/deep sedation approach.

Specific References

1. Aoki A (1993) Time course of acid-base regulation following intraperitoneal CO_2 administration in man. Jpn J Physiol 43:239–246
2. Bardoczky G, Engelman E, Levarlet M, Simon P (1993) Ventilatory effects of pneumoperitoneum monitored with continuous spirometry. Anaesthesia 48:309–311
3. Kelman G, Swapp G, Smith I, Benzie R, Gordon N (1972) Cardiac output and arterial blood gas tension during laparoscopy. Br J Anaesth 44:1155–1161
4. Pacilli M, Pierro A, Kingsley C, Curry J, Herod J, Eaton S (2006) Absorption of carbon dioxide during laparoscopy in children measured using a novel mass spectrometric technique. Br J Anaesth 97:215–219
5. Neumann G, Sidebotham G, Negoianu E, Bernstein J, Kopman A, Hicks R, West S, Haring L (1993) Laparoscopy explosion hazards with nitrous oxide. Anesthesiology 78:875–879
6. Roberts C, Goodman N (1990) Gastro-oesophageal reflux during elective laparoscopy. Anaesthesia 45:1009–1011
7. Esseltine D, Baxter M, Bevan J (1988) Sickle cell states and the anaesthetist. Can J Anaesth 35:385–403

General Reference

8. Holzman R (1996) Special anesthetic considerations for endourologic procedures and laparoscopy in children. In: Smith A, Badlani G, Bagley D, Clayman R, Jordan G, Kavoussi L, Lingeman J, Preminger G, Segura J (eds) Smith's textbook of endourology. Quality Medical Publishing Inc, St. Louis, pp 1293–1306

Chapter 24
Trauma

A 5-year-old, 22-kg boy, previously healthy, is brought to the emergency room following a terrorist bombing at his school. He was in a remote corner of the gym when the bomb went off, also in the gym. He is writhing in pain in the ER, clutching his stomach, short of breath, and bleeding from his left ear. He has a broad bruise across his chest where he was hit by a volleyball pole. He seems to have difficulty hearing you in between his crying: HR 150 bpm, RR 28/min and crying, BP 75/50 mmHg, Hct 27%. There is a 22 ga. IV in place in the left saphenous vein, and seems to be running well.

R.S. Holzman et al., *Pediatric Anesthesiology Review: Clinical Cases for Self-Assessment*,   477
DOI 10.1007/978-1-4419-1617-4_24, © Springer Science+Business Media, LLC 2010

Preoperative Evaluation/Preparation

1. What systems do these various signs and symptoms point to? Why?

    (a) What is the most important monitor in the ER? Why?
    (b) What are you most worried about?
    (c) Should the patient receive supplemental oxygen en route to the OR?
    (d) Does the patient need a head CT scan as part of his work-up? A body CT scan? A C-spine series? Chest X-ray? EKG? Fundoscopic examination?

2. If he lost consciousness for a period of time, would this influence your work-up and plan? Why?

3. What is the significance of bleeding from the ear?

    (a) What if he had a clear discharge from his nose as well as bleeding from the ear?

Preoperative Evaluation

1. Starting from the top down, you would have to be concerned about any secondary head and cervical spine injuries, although his mental status seems all right [1]. The hearing impairment and bleeding from the ear suggest tympanic membrane rupture from the shock wave injury, which would also rupture other gas containing structures like the lung and bowel [2]. The stomach pain suggests that might be the case with intestinal disruption. The shortness of breath and tachypnea may reflect lung injury, but could also reflect myocardial contusion and impaired myocardial performance as a result of the chest wall trauma [3]. The blood pressure is lower than expected and the heart rate higher than normal, which could represent volume depletion or myocardial impairment. The hematocrit is moderately decreased, but this could also be artifactually high if he was hemoconcentrated. The mental status is probably the most important monitor in the ER, followed by the cardiovascular system. Supplemental oxygen would be advisable; at the very least, it would provide a margin of safety should further interventions be required on an urgent basis. If there is time, a head and body CT scan and C spine series might reveal additional areas of injury, but the yield might be low. A chest X-ray would be helpful for rib fractures, cardiac size, and contour as well as pneumo- or hemothorax. A KUB of the abdomen might also reveal free air, and could be obtained at the same time as the chest X-ray in the ER; this strategy would probably have a higher yield than the CT scan. An ECG is necessary to look for myocardial injury. The fundoscopic examination might reveal retinal hemorrhages, which reflect the severity of the blast injury as well as retinal detachment.

2. A loss of consciousness should prompt more aggressive investigation for closed head injury and the C spine.

3. Bleeding from the ear is highly suggestive of moderately severe blast injury and gas-containing body systems (ear, sinuses, lungs, and bowel) should be carefully examined. A clear discharge from the nose, in the absence of recent symptoms of an URI, should be suspicious for a CSF leak from the skull base.

Intraoperative Care

1. Does this patient need an arterial line? Why/why not? Prior to induction, or after?

    (a) What about stat mode on the noninvasive blood pressure cuff? Is it the same?

    (b) What about a central line?

    (c) The patient's neck veins are distended, and do not appear to be varying with respirations; what is the significance? What is the differential diagnosis; most likely diagnosis?

    (d) Does the patient need a chest tube prior to induction of anesthesia, or can one be placed after rapid sequence induction and intubation?

    (e) What if there was subcutaneous emphysema? Clinical significance and implication for anesthesia plan.

2. Assume no pneumothorax; how would you proceed with induction?

    (a) Would you leave the saphenous vein IV in place, or insert one in a different location prior to induction; just after induction? Why?

3. Does this patient need a rapid sequence induction? With what?

    (a) Why not inhalation induction with halothane or sevoflurane?

    (b) What about use of nitrous oxide? Why/why not?

4. Exploratory laparotomy reveals a large hepatic subcapsular hematoma and a fractured spleen. Unfortunately, the vascular clamp has come off the splenic pedicle, the pedicle has retracted out of reach, and the capsule has ruptured; there is a unit of blood in the belly, the BP is 53/20 and the HR 200. What to do next?

    (a) Get an ABG? Give bicarb?

    (b) Can the surgeons help you at all? How?

    (c) Is the saphenous vein IV of any use? How much?

Intraoperative Care

1. The patient definitely needs an arterial line, which should be anticipated from the number of systems potentially involved as well as the likelihood of postoperative ICU support. He may not require it preinduction (and you may not be able to get one in anyway) but it should be placed as early as possible. Stat mode on an automated blood pressure cuff will work for blood pressure assessment until the line is established, although it provides less information (discontinuous, no waveform analysis). A central line may not be a bad idea, especially if peripheral veins are collapsed, but it is not likely to be necessary, based on the previous information. With distended neck veins, the patient probably has obstruction of venous drainage to the central circulation; likely causes include pericardial tamponade [4], intrathoracic obstruction with impaired venous drainage, or pneumo/hemothorax with mediastinal shifting. While in most circumstances with adults it would be fitting to place a chest tube prior to anesthetic induction, it may be more practical with conscious children to induce anesthesia first and then be prepared to place a chest tube immediately following induction. Subcutaneous emphysema would suggest disruption of the tracheobronchial tree with air leak and it would be unwise to proceed to positive pressure ventilation until the site of the air leak was identified and could be bypassed or repaired.

2. If there were no pneumothorax (or subcutaneous emphysema), then following rapid sequence induction and endotracheal intubation, additional vascular access should be secured, primarily above the level of the diaphragm assuming that a superior vena caval syndrome existed. Again, for practical purposes, insertion of the IV above the diaphragm, assuming that veins were visible, could be done immediately following induction.

3. The patient probably needs a rapid sequence induction because of the risk of recent ingestion along with the stress of the trauma and possible abdominal injury resulting in an ileus. Because the intravascular volume status and myocardial status are unclear, it may be safest to proceed with ketamine or etomidate as the hypnotic agent and succinylcholine for muscle relaxation. The circumstance that would mitigate against this strategy is an uncertain airway or a worsening pneumothorax with subcutaneous emphysema. Nitrous oxide should be avoided because it does not permit an F_iO_2 of 100% and it may accumulate in gas-filled spaces.

4. Vascular access and volume replacement are of the utmost importance. As an immediate measure the surgeons should try to control ongoing blood loss in the field with the use of direct pressure and control of the aorta with a cross clamp until additional access is established. This can be most readily accomplished by the anesthesiologist via the internal jugular or subclavian veins; the surgeons can also insert a catheter in the inferior vena cava and once access is established in another site, close the venotomy with a pursestring suture. The saphenous vein access will not be of much use in this setting until the bleeding site in the abdomen is repaired

5. Following vigorous resuscitation, the patient is now 31.2°C. How did this happen?

   (a) What mechanisms of heat loss are most significant?
   (b) Is it worthwhile putting in a heat and moisture exchanger in the breathing circuit at this time? What advantage is it over a heated humidifier? What are some of the problems with both?
   (c) How can you warm the patient? Is this desirable?
   (d) Should your goal be normothermia?
   (e) You begin to see a widening of the QRS complex; clinical significance?

6. You note ST segment elevation on your lead II monitor; differential? Significance?

   (a) Options available? Insert PA line? Add modified V5 monitor? Start nitroglycerine?
   (b) What if hypotensive as well?
   (c) What if SpO_2 is now 91% on 100% FiO_2? Would physical exam help?
   (d) TEE? What would you expect to find?
   (e) What if pink froth is coming out of the endotracheal tube; etiology?

Postoperative

1. Should this patient remain intubated? Why?

   (a) What are your criteria for extubation in this setting?

2. Would you utilize an epidural if you had to cover exploratory lap pain as well as chest tube pain?

   (a) Should the patient be on PCA because the bowel was not prepped?
   (b) What if a bowel resection was required?

5. With a temperature of 31.2°C, the risk of arrhythmias is increased and the patient must be warmed aggressively. Chances are that the mechanism of the heat loss was primarily radiation, but conduction and convection also come into play here. A heat and moisture exchanger will do very little good at this point. It would be more useful to warm the patient by lowering the fresh gas flow rate to minimal or closed circuit flows, deliver heat calories in the form of a Bair hugger and a warm water blanket, use radiant heat lamps, and consider core warming with warmed saline and peritoneal lavage. The widening of the QRS is a worrisome sign that conduction system delay is occurring; this can worsen cardiac conduction, progressing to heart block, ventricular irritability with fibrillation, and cardiac arrest.

6. ST segment elevation indicates injury and should prompt a more geographically oriented investigation such as a 12 lead ECG; in this setting, one would be suspicious for an anterior wall pattern of injury because of the volleyball pole's path of chest injury. A V5 monitor would aid in looking at the lateral wall, but would probably be of relatively low yield in this age group, with this particular history, which seems more referable to the anterolateral precordium. If the patient was hypotensive it could be due to volume depletion or primary cardiac dysfunction as a result of tamponade. Nitroglycerin is not likely to be of any benefit in this setting and may actually make the patient worse because of the reduction in preload. A low SpO_2 may reflect pulmonary contusion with resultant shunting or myocardial injury with a drop in cardiac output and increased venous admixture with shunting. Physical exam might help with regard to pinning down a cardiac cause. Oxygen desaturation may be accounted for by worsening venous admixure, primary myocardial failure, and pulmonary contusion. Pink froth coming out of the endotracheal tube suggests congestive heart failure (pump failure), volume overload, or pulmonary hypertension.

Postoperative

1. In all likelihood this patient should remain intubated, if for no other reason than to keep the respiratory system in balance during the acute phase of recovery. Mitigating against this would be the need to see the patient awaken to assess mental status. Both, however, can be accomplished. The usual criteria for extubation include adequacy of tidal volume, minute ventilation, and bellows strength. In addition to that, one would have to anticipate the perioperative course; massive transfusion, for example, might influence a conservative approach to weaning and extubation.

2. If it is anticipated that the patient will remain intubated for several days, then continuous infusion opioids would be a reasonable perioperative pain management plan. Early extubation would probably favor a segmental neuraxial block, although that would have to be balanced against the risk of perioperative infection as well as coagulopathy if the patient had been massively transfused. Traumatic bowel injury, therefore, might be a relative contraindication to neuraxial blockade.

Additional Questions

1. A 6-year-old boy was brought into the local ER in Omaha after playing in the corn fields while a crop duster flew by. He is short of breath, bradycardic, pupils are miotic, and he is complaining of intense abdominal cramps. His SpO_2 is 88%. What are your thoughts?

2. A 16-year old went to the store to get milk for his grandmother when he was shot with an automatic weapon in a drive-by. You see an entry wound at the lower left abdomen, no obvious exit wound, and the patient complains of shoulder pain. What is the first thing you should do when he arrives, mostly dressed including his leather jacket, in the OR? Once you disarm him, what should you do next? What are your anesthetic considerations? What is a dumdum bullet, and what is its clinical significance?

3. You are preparing a patient with a chest tube for MedEvac transport via nonpressurized fixed wing aircraft. What are your critical care considerations for this flight? How will you monitor? Does it matter if he is intubated or not? Is it any different for helicopter transport?

4. A knife fight between two gangs results in one member (the lucky one) arriving in your OR with a stiletto in place, piercing his trachea at approximately the level of the cricoid cartilage. He was brought directly to the OR, and skipped the ER entirely. How will you proceed?

Additional Questions

1. The shortness of breath, bradycardia, miosis, increased gastrointestinal motility, and history are all strongly suggestive of organophosphate poisoning, with signs and symptoms of anticholinesterase poisoning [4]. The hypoxia is probably due to a proliferation of airway secretions and worsening of shunt. The patient may also have neuromuscular weakness. Medical treatment with atropine and pralidoxime chloride (2-PAM) is indicated if there is time for a medical intervention, otherwise, he should be intubated, have his airway protected, receive ventilatory support as well as medical intervention.

2. The first thing to do if the victim of violence arrives fully dressed is to disrobe and disarm him and fully assess for entry and exit wounds. The assumption should never be made that an exit wound can be predicted from the trajectory of the entrance wound; many bullets are flattened or carved (dumdum bullet) and therefore their exit wound can be very remote from the point of entry. Anesthetic considerations include stability of the cardiovascular system, volume loss, injury to the lungs with pneumo- or hemothorax, and therefore the need to avoid positive pressure ventilation, recent food intake, and history of intoxication/drug use/and drug intolerance.

3. Nonpressurized aircraft will have a lower ambient cabin pressure and lower atmospheric oxygen tension as they rise in altitude. If chest tubes are clamped as the aircraft leaves the ground, the increase in altitude and lower atmospheric pressure will result in expansion of the pneumothorax and respiratory embarrassment. This will be aggravated by the lower oxygen tension in the cabin atmosphere if the patient is not receiving supplemental oxygen (assuming he is breathing on his own). Respiratory compromise has to be treated by decompressing the clamped chest tube and readjusting it if necessary. Helicopters fly at a lower altitude than fixed wing aircraft.

4. The biggest risk in this scenario is that the knife is physically interfering with the passing of an endotracheal tube, which must be accomplished before the neck can be explored. The knife may also be tamponading any blood vessel through which it has passed, so that the ideal airway management would be an awake intubation, with the surgeon already having prepped the neck for exploration. As the patient is undergoing laryngoscopy and intubation, the surgeon should be prepared to remove the knife and exert pressure for local vascular control until the neck can be incised (following intubation) and the structures identified. This calls for a patient who is cooperative and topically anesthetized – in an ideal circumstance. Otherwise, speed counts, and after the neck is prepped, the patient must be rapidly induced, the trachea intubated and the surgeon prepared immediately to explore the neck. Positive pressure ventilation must be gentle and kept to a minimum in anticipation of accumulating subcutaneous emphysema.

5. What is the difference between a high-velocity missile injury and a low-velocity missile injury? A fragmentation bullet vs. a nonfragmentation bullet?

5. High-velocity missile injury is caused by missiles (bullets or fragments) traveling at a rate >750 m/s [5, 6]. While low velocity missiles, such as .38 caliber, .45 caliber, and 9 mm pistols typically carried by police will result in laceration and crushing of surrounding tissue, high velocity missiles form a temporary cavity due to energy transfer from the missile to the tissue and create a tissue shock wave that compresses tissue in front of the missile. The physics of this phenomenon are such that it is especially destructive against solid tissue. Fragmentation bullets are engineered to break apart after a certain traveling distance following penetration. The bullet fragments penetrate radially from the bullet path for a variable distance, usually of several centimeters. The degree of bullet fragmentation decreases with increasing shooting distance.

Specific References

1. Adelson P (2000) Pediatric trauma made simple. Clin Neurosurg 47:319–335
2. Bowen T, Bellamy R (1988) Blast injuries. In: Bowen T, Bellamy R (eds) Emergency war surgery. Government Printing Office, Washington DC, pp 74–82
3. Mattox K, Flint L, Carrico C (1992) Blunt cardiac injury. J Trauma 33:649–650
4. de Jong R (2003) Nerve gas terrorism: a grim challenge to anesthesiologists. Anesth Analg 96:819–825
5. Bowen T, Bellamy R (1988) Missile-caused wounds. In: Bowen T, Bellamy R (eds) Emergency war surgery. Government Printing Office, Washington DC, pp 13–34
6. Reinhorn M, Kaufman H, Hirsch E (1996) Penetrating thoracic trauma in a pediatric population. Ann Thorac Surg 61:1501–1505

Chapter 25
Trauma II

A 4-year old who fell into an empty swimming pool head first is brought to the hospital for evaluation and treatment. A cervical spine fracture is noted on the X-rays taken in the ED. At the preop visit in the ICU, the child is awake and alert in a hard collar, breathing spontaneously but with slight tracheal retractions. He wiggles his fingers and toes. VS: BP = 100/60 mmHg, HR = 65 bpm, and RR = 22/min. He is scheduled for fixation of his cervical spine fracture.

R.S. Holzman et al., *Pediatric Anesthesiology Review: Clinical Cases for Self-Assessment,*
DOI 10.1007/978-1-4419-1617-4_25, © Springer Science+Business Media, LLC 2010

Preoperative Evaluation

1. Evaluation for other injuries?

Preoperative Evaluation

1. This child should have a head-to-toe evaluation for other injuries. In this case, there is not a neurosurgical emergency necessitating an immediate trip to the OR. There is time to complete a thorough evaluation for other injuries to the child. The hard collar must not be removed but nevertheless a physical exam looking for signs of other injuries can be done. With major pediatric trauma, the head is the most frequently injured body area. The neurologic exam should assign a Glasgow Coma Scale score and evaluate the child for the presence or absence of raised intracranial pressure. The presence of raised ICP will have important impact on the overall management of the child as well as the conduct of an anesthetic [1]. The Glasgow Coma Scale was initially developed to provide an organized, uniform measure to the level of consciousness [2]. Using the scale, CNS injuries are categorized as mild (13–15), moderate (9–12), or severe (≤8). In addition, cranial nerve function should be assessed and focal signs in the motor exam noted. During the evaluation of the cranial nerves, signs of basilar skull fractures such as hemotympanum and "raccoon eyes" should be noted.

Activity	Best response	Score
Eye opening	Spontaneous	4
	To verbal stimuli	3
	To pain	2
	None	1
Verbal	Oriented	5
	Confused	4
	Inappropriate words	3
	Nonspecific sounds	2
	None	1
Motor	Follows commands	6
	Localizes pain	5
	Withdraws from pain	4
	Flexion to pain	3
	Extension to pain	2
	None	1

In addition to the neurologic exam, the child should be evaluated for injuries to the thorax and abdomen. CT has become the primary tool for the evaluation of pediatric trauma patients for abdominal damage. A child who is victim of a major trauma should first have a CT of the head and then, if clinically stable, the scan should include the thorax, abdomen, and pelvis. When deciding about the importance of these scans, the clinician must balance the time needed and the IV and enteral contrast administration required for the scans against the urgency for surgical intervention for other injuries. It is important not to ignore the long bones during the evaluation of a pediatric trauma victim. Fractures of the femur can be associated with significant bleeding in the absence of obvious clinical signs.

2. What is the significance of the neurologic exam?

3. Which laboratory tests are important prior to going to the OR?

4. Is there a role for the immediate administration of steroids?

Intraoperative Care

1. Which monitors and vascular access are necessary for this case?

2. It is encouraging that the child is awake and alert. The GCS score of the child as described would likely be at least 13. (Eye opening: spontaneous: 4, Verbal, oriented: 5, Motor withdraws to pain: 4). With a higher score on the motor portion of the scale, the GCS could be as high as 15. The fact the child is moving his fingers and toes is an indication that there is some neurologic function below the level of the cervical spine fracture but the residual function appears to be incomplete.

3. Additional radiologic studies are indicated unless the child requires emergent surgical intervention. In addition to scans of the head, chest, abdomen, and pelvis, several additional tests are indicated prior to going to the OR. The X-rays taken that showed the spine fracture should be reviewed. It may be that additional studies are needed to rule out additional fractures including a limited CT of the neck. Blood should be sent for a CBC, type and cross, and coagulation studies.

4. A prospective study done in the 1990s demonstrated that spine-injured patients given large doses of methylprednisolone very soon after the injury had a slightly improved neurologic deficit. The study was not designed to assess long-term neurologic function. The doses of methylprednisolone used in the investigation were 30 mg/kg IV followed by 5.4 mg/kg/h for 23 h. There have been three trials of this drug and dose, one conducted in North America (NASCIS), one in Japan, and one in France. A meta-analysis of these trials indicated that significant recovery of motor function occurred when the therapy outline began within 8 h of the injury. A more recent trial showed that continuing the therapy for an additional 24 h led to additional improvement in motor function particularly if the therapy is not begun with the 8-h period. Significant controversy still exists regarding the use of high dose steroids for spinal cord injury [3].

Intraoperative Course

1. Prior to administration of any medication, the child should have at least one well-functioning IV and should have had fluid resuscitation with normal saline. If additional injuries had been uncovered in the workup, IV placement may be affected. If there is also significant abdominal or lower extremity trauma with potential for hemorrhage, IVs should be placed in the upper extremities. The usual ASA monitors should be used. In addition, once induction is completed and the airway secured, a arterial line and central venous pressure line should be placed. If the preoperative evaluation revealed any signs of raised ICP, consideration should be given to placement of an intracranial pressure monitor. Since the child will be in the prone position for the approach to the fractured spine, placement of a precordial doppler and/or monitoring end-tidal nitrogen will be important for detection of venous air emboli.

2. How should general anesthesia be induced? Which muscle relaxant should be used to facilitate laryngoscopy?

3. Are there particular concerns regarding prone positioning for the repair of the cervical spine fracture?

4. Are there particular maintenance agents best suited in cases where neuroprotection is important? What is the optimal BP for this procedure?

2. Given the X-ray findings and clinical exam, it is imperative that the child not move his neck during induction and when the airway is secured. An IV drying agent such as glycopyrrolate should be given prior to any airway manipulations. It should be assumed that the child has a full stomach during the induction even though a complete RSI would not be indicated in this situation. The child has retractions with respirations. If the CXR does not reveal any possible etiology, it is possible that the child has traumatic damage to the airway. The child may have aspirated during the traumatic event and the CXR has not yet shown abnormalities. There could be partial or complete paralysis of the vocal cords or edema or hematoma formation within the airway. Given these considerations, securing the airway with fiberoptic bronchoscopy is a prudent choice. Following administration of a drying agent, the child is gradually anesthetized with an IV agent such as propofol such that spontaneous respiratory effort is maintained. Topical lidocaine, in the proper dose and concentration, is applied to the nasal and pharyngeal mucosa prior to instrumentation of the airway.

3. Once the airway is secured, and if no further neurologic exams are to be performed, the child can be completely anesthetized and muscle relaxants administered. If the vital signs are satisfactory and ventilation adequate, the child can be safely positioned prone for the procedure. The hard collar should be kept in place and the neurosurgeon should be present and control the head during the turn from supine to prone. Fortunately, the child is small so that s/he can be easily lifted and rolled to the prone position. In the prone position, the abdomen should be free to minimize effects on ventilation. With the abdomen free, the loss of FRC is minimized. If the head is above the level of the heart, the risk for venous air embolism is increased but if the head is below the level of the heart, venous congestion of the face, neck, and CNS can become problematic. Visual impairment has been reported in patients who were kept prone for long periods and who also had impaired oxygen delivery to the retina from hypotension, anemia, and/or excessive pressure on the eye, limiting blood flow.

4. Although barbiturates have the reputation for cerebral protection, other commonly used induction and sedative agents such as propofol, etomidate, and benzodiazepines also lower cerebral blood flow (CBF), $CMRO_2$, and ICP while maintaining autoregulation. Ketamine causes an increase in CBF as well as ICP. Opioids have no direct effect on these parameters but, as respiratory depressants, will lead to hypercarbia and the resultant cerebral vasodilation in the spontaneously breathing patient. All inhaled anesthetics, nitrous oxide included, dilate cerebral vessels to varying degrees. This effect is mitigated by hyperventilation. Isoflurane and sevoflurane are both appropriate for neurosurgery. Both do increase CBF to a modest degree. Both decrease $CMRO_2$. Blood pressure management is directed toward maintaining adequate cerebral perfusion pressure (CPP) [4]. Cerebral perfusion pressure is equal to mean arterial pressure minus ICP or CVP, whichever is higher.

$$CPP = MAP - ICP(or\ CVP\ if\ CVP > ICP)$$

Since in this case we do not know the ICP or CVP, the blood pressure should be kept at or within 20% above the BP measured preoperatively.

5. During the procedure, the patient has bradycardia, with HR decreasing to the
   60s. What might be the etiology? Your response?

6. The surgeon expects that the case will be 45–60 min. Would you plan to extubate
   the child at the end of the procedure?

Perioperative

1. Following extubation, the child is hoarse. Possible etiologies? Management?

5. The sudden occurrence of bradycardia in a neurosurgical procedure can be the result of raised ICP or a venous air embolism (VAE) [5, 6, 7]. If associated with VAE, the bradycardia is accompanied by hypotension, the "mill-wheel" murmur from the precordial doppler and lowered $ETCO_2$. Bradycardia cause by raised ICP is part of the Cushing's triad of bradycardia, hypertension, and abnormal respirations. In the anesthetized patient receiving mechanical ventilation, only bradycardia and hypertension will be seen. The treatment of a suspected VAE includes notification of the surgeon, positioning the head below the level of the heart, flooding the operative field with saline, discontinuing N_2O, treatment of the hypotension and bradycardia with epinephrine, and if needed chest compressions. Once the VAE has been pushed through the heart, the vital signs and $ETCO_2$ normalize. Raised ICP severe enough to cause Cushing's response is indicative of imminent herniation and requires immediate treatment. Maneuvers to lower ICP include lowering the $PaCO_2$ with judicious ventilatior management, assuring free venous return from the head, administration of additional sedation, muscle relaxants, raising the head of the bed, and administration of mannitol or hypertonic saline [1, 8, 9]. Decompressive craniectomy may be needed if these maneuvers are not successful in reversing the vital sign abnormalities [10, 11].

6. The length of the procedure is only one of a number of factors that affect the decision to extubate this child. The degree of difficulty with airway management preoperatively is a consideration. In addition, the child is likely to remain in some sort of fixation device postoperatively and will now have just had a stabilization procedure on the cervical spine and might benefit from a period of complete immobility. Also, if during the case the vital sign instability was due to raised ICP, it may be important to continue with intubation until that problem has resolved. If, after consideration of the factors listed above extubation is thought to be in the child's best interest, then it should be done with the child awake and responsive.

Perioperative

1. Hoarseness following intubation has several possible etiologies in the case. Many causes of respiratory distress in this child may also cause hoarseness without necessarily involving edema of the vocal cords themselves. If the endotracheal tube was tight, there may be postintubation edema in the subglottic area, leading to both hoarseness and inspiratory stridor. It is possible that, during the fiberoptic intubation the arytenoid cartilages were damaged or dislocated leading to hoarseness. In the preoperative assessment, some respiratory distress is noted. The cervical fracture itself may have damaged cervical roots that innervate the diaphragm (C2–C4) and the respiratory insufficiency is leading to hoarseness. Spinal cord injury without radiographic abnormality (SCIWRA) is a well-described entity in children. MRI and electrophysiologic testing such as SSEPs are used to determine the presence and extent of this type of spinal cord injury [12]. In addition to hoarseness, neurogenic pulmonary edema may occur.

Additional Topics

1. A previously healthy 16-year-old male arrives in the emergency department 15 min after he was an innocent bystander in a convenience robbery, held hostage, and shot in the mandible with a pistol, type unknown. Are there further studies you would like? Additional concerns? What if the surgeons want to go directly to the operating room? What are your extubation considerations?

2. What are your concerns about the patient with rhabdomyolysis? In what clinical setting does this occur? How would you treat? Specific anesthetic considerations? Why?

Additional Topics

1. Facial trauma of any type is of particular concern since, in addition to the problems that result from hemorrhage, there is significant likelihood of airway compromise. When a child or teenager is brought to the ED for evaluation following a gun shot injury to the jaw, evaluation of airway patency is essential. Radiographic evaluation is a very important part of the initial survey. The gun shot bullet or pellets not only will cause bleeding, but as foreign bodies can lodge anywhere in the airway, inside the skull, orbits, or sinuses.

   If the patient is unstable, an airway must be established immediately and the best option in this case would be a tracheostomy with local anesthesia. If the patient is stable and able to breathe with relative comfort, further evaluation can be done prior securing the airway and inducing anesthesia. A brief survey for other injuries can be done as the patient is prepared for surgery and anesthesia. Portable radiographic studies can be done and if the patient shows no signs of deterioration, an urgent CT scan of the head can be performed. If a CT is done the anesthesiologist and ORL surgeon should accompany the patient to radiology, prepared to intervene with emergency airway support if needed. Additional IV access can be secured and an arterial line placed, a drying agent administered and appropriate analgesic and an anxiolytic administered as the patient is taken to the OR. The airway should be secured with either a tracheostomy or fiberoptic bronchoscopy based on the result of the evaluation and consultation with the surgeons. If it is likely that the jaw will be wired shut postoperatively, this will affect planning for extubation at the conclusion of the case if a tracheostomy was not done. Another consideration that will affect airway management will be the degree of airway edema anticipated in the postoperative period. If extubation is planned, it will be important that the patient be awake and following commands prior to extubation. Antiemetics should be given and the stomach emptied before removing the endotracheal tube.

2. Children who have suffered extensive musculoskeletal injuries are at risk for myoglobinuria. If this occurs, renal dysfunction is possible. The patient should have the urine alkalinized and urine flow maintained with vigorous IV fluid administration and administration of diuretics if necessary. Another complication occasionally seen in children who have had extensive long bone trauma with multiple fractures is fat embolism, although this problem is not generally seen immediately following the injury.

3. How is a triage area organized to effectively deal with trauma? Are there commonly accepted triage categories? Are there special roles for anesthesiologists in triage care? What are they?

3. Organization of the triage area for trauma depends upon the type of patients expected by the facility. Trauma centers are given one of three designations depending upon the medical services available [2]. Trauma centers devoted specifically to children were first created in the 1970s at several major pediatric medical centers. The organization of a triage area at a particular center will depend upon the resources available at that location. Level I trauma centers have the largest range of services and medical personnel available while Level III centers provide stabilization of trauma victims prior to transport to centers with more extensive resources.

Level I: These centers have immediate availability of trauma surgeons, anesthesiologists, nurses, physician specialists, and resuscitation equipment. These centers treat 240 major trauma patients/year.

Level II: These have similar requirements for the availability of personnel as Level I Trauma Centers but there are no requirements for the number of cases/year.

Level III: These centers can evaluate and stabilize trauma patients prior to transfer to level I or II centers. Emergency surgery is available.

Trauma centers for children have been characterized in the University of Michigan Pediatric Trauma Classification System into three levels:

Level I: These centers treat children with single or multisystem injuries, unstable VS and respiratory distress shock, neurologic injury, or gunshot wounds or burns.

Level II: These centers treat children with multisystem injuries and stable VS such as children with open fractures, less severe burns, or less severe neurologic injuries with stable GCS.

Level III: These centers treat children who are conscious with an isolated injury and low potential for multisystem injury.

Individuals are assigned to triage categories as follows, in decreasing order of urgency:

Urgent.   Life-saving intervention is indicated if death is to be prevented. If initial resuscitative interventions are successful and some degree of stability is achieved, then the urgent casualty may revert to a lower priority.

Immediate.   Severe, life-threatening wounds that require procedures of moderately short duration; high likelihood of survival. They remain temporarily stable while undergoing replacement therapy and further evaluation.

Delayed.   Able to be supported and evacuated. May go unoperated for several hours, after which there will be a direct relationship between time lapse and complications.

Minimal or Ambulatory.   Superficial wounds requiring no more than cleansing, minimal debridement under local anesthesia, tetanus toxoid, and first-aid type of dressings.

4. Advantages/disadvantages of various locations for vascular access?

Expectant. Little chance for survival with or without surgical intervention; even if they were the sole casualty and had the benefit of optimal medical resource application, their survival would still be very unlikely.

An alternate classification scheme is used in Advanced Trauma Life Support (ATLS):

T1: Requiring immediate life-saving intervention

T2: Requiring early intervention

T3: Requiring late intervention

T4: Hopeless prognosis, no active intervention

And yet another in hospitals of the International Committee of the Red Cross (ICRC):

Category I.   Those patients for whom urgent surgery is required and for whom there is a good chance of reasonable survival.
Category II. Those patients who do not require surgery (includes patients with wounds so slight that they do not need surgery and those who are severely injured and for whom reasonable survival is unlikely).
Category III. Those who require surgery but not on an urgent basis.

4. Vascular access is always an important consideration in trauma patients but particularly so in pediatric trauma victims [2]. Central access is important in patients who have suffered more severe trauma. In children, the internal jugular or subclavian veins are not good choices for a variety of reasons. Pediatric trauma victims are generally in cervical collars, limiting access to these sites. Even if the cervical spine was not involved in the accident and there is no worry about its stability, there remains a significant risk of pneumothorax or hemothorax from placement of CVLs into the internal jugular or subclavian veins. Cannulation of a femoral vein is a good option for central access in pediatric trauma patients. However, the risks of delay in establishing access in the unstable patient are real. Intraosseus lines can be readily placed even in very small trauma victims. The safest location is the medial surface of the proximal tibia. There are a variety of needles in different sizes for placement in all ages of children.

Annotated References

Tasker RC (2008) Head and spinal cord trauma. Chap. 56. In: Nichols DG (ed) Rogers' textbook of pediatric intensive care. Wolters Kluwer Lippincott Williams and Wilkins, Philadelphia, pp 887–911
This chapter reviews the epidemiology and pathophysiology of various types of CNS traumatic injury such as blunt and sharp trauma and compression injury. Also included is a discussion of clinical, laboratory, and imaging assessment of patients

with CNS trauma, management of raised ICP and spinal injury, and review of the available outcome data.

Baird JS, Cooper A (2008) Multiple trauma. Chap. 27. In: Nichols DG (ed) Rogers' textbook of pediatric intensive care. Wolters Kluwer Lippincott Williams and Wilkins, Philadelphia, pp 384–407

This chapter is a good survey of trauma in children with emphasis on the initial assessment and stabilization of trauma victims. The emphasis is on nonneurologic injuries.

References

1. Orliaguet GA, Meyer PG, Baugnon T (2008) Management of critically ill children with traumatic brain injury. Paediatr Anaesth 18(6):455–461
2. Holzman R (2008) Trauma and casualty management. In: Holzman R, Mancuso TJ, Polaner DM (eds) A practical approach to pediatric anesthesia, 1st edn. Wolters Kluwer/Lippincott Williams and Wilkins, Philadelphia, pp 636–654
3. Nesathurai S (1998) Steroids and spinal cord injury: revisiting the NASCIS 2 and NASCIS 3 trials. J Trauma 45(6):1088–1093
4. Grinkeviciute DE, Kevalas R, Matukevicius A, Ragaisis V, Tamasauskas A (2008) Significance of intracranial pressure and cerebral perfusion pressure in severe pediatric traumatic brain injury. Medicina (Kaunas) 44(2):119–125
5. Agrawal A, Timothy J, Cincu R, Agarwal T, Waghmare LB (2008) Bradycardia in neurosurgery. Clin Neurol Neurosurg 110(4):321–327
6. Harris MM, Yemen TA, Davidson A et al (1987) Venous embolism during craniectomy in supine infants. Anesthesiology 67(5):816–819
7. Albin MS, Carroll RG, Maroon JC (1978) Clinical considerations concerning detection of venous air embolism. Neurosurgery 3(3):380–384
8. Wakai A, Roberts I, Schierhout G (2007) Mannitol for acute traumatic brain injury. Cochrane Database Syst Rev (1):CD001049
9. Taplu A, Gokmen N, Erbayraktar S et al (2003) Effects of pressure- and volume-controlled inverse ratio ventilation on haemodynamic variables, intracranial pressure and cerebral perfusion pressure in rabbits: a model of subarachnoid haemorrhage under isoflurane anaesthesia. Eur J Anaesthesiol 20(9):690–696
10. Kan P, Amini A, Hansen K et al (2006) Outcomes after decompressive craniectomy for severe traumatic brain injury in children. J Neurosurg 105(5 Suppl):337–342
11. Hutchinson P, Timofeev I, Kirkpatrick P (2007) Surgery for brain edema. Neurosurg Focus 22(5):E14
12. Pang D (2004) Spinal cord injury without radiographic abnormality in children, 2 decades later. Neurosurgery 55(6):1325–1342, discussion 1342–3

Chapter 26
Regional Anesthesia

R.S. Holzman et al., *Pediatric Anesthesiology Review: Clinical Cases for Self-Assessment*,
DOI 10.1007/978-1-4419-1617-4_26, © Springer Science+Business Media, LLC 2010

Case 1

You are the only physician on a Boy Scout training sailboat, 2 days from the closest hospital. One of the Scouts stepped on a sharp, serrated fishhook which implanted itself deep in the mid plantar area of the right foot. You must excise the fishhook immediately to prevent infection. You have various syringes and needles along with one 20 mL bottle of 1% plain lidocaine in your medicine cabinet; what techniques could you use to eliminate pain during the painful excision of this fishhook?

Case 2

A 17-year old underwent a prolonged penile reconstruction under epidural anesthesia. Today he complains of bilateral foot drop. His only medical history is that of a 2-year use of hydrodiuril for swollen ankles. What is the differential for foot drop? What do you do to rule out epidural hematoma? The patient's serum K^+ is 2.5 mEq%. What is your management?

Case 1

I will perform an ankle block and specifically anesthetize the posterior tibial nerve that supplies the innervation to the plantar aspect of the foot. The tibial nerve runs behind the medial malleolus, under the flexor retinaculum, and lies posterior to the pulsation of the posterior tibial artery. With the patient supine in bed, the knee is flexed and the medial malleolus area is cleansed with soap and water. A skin wheal is made with a 25-gauge needle behind the pulsation of the posterior tibial artery and the needle is advanced behind the pulsation until a paresthesia is elicited when contact is made with the tibial nerve or contact is made with the malleolus bone. The needle is slightly withdrawn until no paresthesia is felt or the needle is off the bone. After negative aspiration for blood a total of 4 mL of the lidocaine 1% solution is injected, provided there is no resistance to injection.

Case 2

Bilateral foot drop could result from either an epidural hematoma, direct trauma to the spinal cord, or compression neuropathy related to intraoperative lithotomy positioning. The occurrence of an epidural hematoma is less likely in healthy patients who are not anticoagulated in whom the placement of the epidural catheter was atraumatic. The presence of an arteriovenous malformation of the epidural vessels may pose a risk for epidural hematoma. Needle or catheter trauma of an epidural vein can result in excessive bleeding and the development of a hematoma that may compress the spinal cord and cause a neurological deficit.

If an epidural hematoma is suspected the epidural infusion should be stopped to allow complete sensory and motor recovery to allow neurological examination. If neurologic impairment persists an MRI should be obtained immediately because the epidural hematoma should be decompressed within 6–12 h to avoid permanent neurological deficit. MRI is also useful to rule out direct spinal cord trauma. Prolonged intraoperative positioning in lithotomy may predispose to stretch of the lumbo-sacral plexus resulting in a neuropathy particularly in obese and very slender patients, or in the presence of subcutaneous edema. Foot drop following surgery in the lithotomy position can also occur from the compression of the common peroneal nerves against the heads of the fibula due to abnormal positioning of the legs in stirrups rather than straps. The presence of bilateral foot drop with the preservation of perineal sensation and sphincter function favors the "distal" diagnosis of bilateral common peroneal nerve palsy. Bilateral foot drop associated with urinary and fecal incontinence results from either lumbo-sacral plexus stretch neuropathy, cord trauma or cord compression from hematoma, resulting in a cauda equina syndrome.

Case 3

A 15-year old with vasculopathy and some type of autoimmune process broke her right forearm 1 year ago. She now has reflex sympathetic dystrophy for which you have been asked to give the first of a series of stellate ganglion blocks. Three minutes after your injection of 10 mL of 0.25% bupivacaine with epinephrine she complains of shortness of breath. How do you do a stellate block? What is the differential for her SOB? How do you manage the problem?

Case 4

You are asked to consult on the management of a 14-year-old male with severe frostbite of both hands. What can you contribute to his management? Give details of the stellate ganglion block that could be performed. How do you assess the adequacy of blockade? What are the complications?

Case 3

The block is performed with the patient supine and the neck slightly extended. The C6 transverse process tubercle (Chassaignac's tubercle) is identified with the index and middle fingers of the nondominant hand placed at the level of the cricoid ring between the trachea and the sternocleidomastoid muscle. A short-beveled 25-gauge needle is introduced perpendicular to the skin and advanced until the needle tip makes contact with the C6 transverse process. The needle is withdrawn a few millimeters and immobilized. After negative aspiration for blood and CSF a total of 8–10 mL of a local anesthetic is injected incrementally and without resistance.

The complaint of shortness of breath after stellate ganglion block could be due to the feeling of a lump in the throat as result of blockade of the recurrent laryngeal nerve, intradural (epidural/intrathecal) injection of local anesthetics, paresis or paralysis of the phrenic nerve, and pneumothorax. The SOB due to recurrent laryngeal paralysis is best managed by reassurance and offering supplemental oxygen. SOB due to subdural injection, if severe, may require ventilatory support and sedation. The management of pneumothorax depends on severity; usually a pneumothorax of 10% or less does not require specific treatment other than reassurance. More severe pneumothorax may require monitoring in the hospital or placement of a chest tube.

Case 4

Cervicothoracic sympathetic block can improve circulatory insufficiency and pain associated with frostbite. Stellate ganglion block is confirmed by observing sympathetic dennervation to the ipsilateral half of the face described by Horner's syndrome: facial and conjunctival flushing, dry face, nasal congestion, ptosis, miosis, enophthalmos, and a rise in the hand temperature. Potential complications with stellate ganglion block are transient hoarseness due to recurrent laryngeal nerve block, local hematoma, pressure produced by injection of a large volume of local anesthetic, and neuralgia of the chest wall and upper arm. Serious complications are accidental injection of a local anesthetic into vertebral artery leading to seizures and epidural or subarachnoid injection. Less common complications are neural blockade of the brachial plexus and phrenic nerve, pneumothorax, and osteitis of the C6 transverse process.

Case 5

You have just administered a Bier block to a 16-year old having plastic surgery to her left hand. Within a minute of injecting 30 mL of 0.5% lidocaine into a vein on the dorsum of her left hand you notice a dramatic wheal and flare reaction with swelling of the entire extremity distal to the tourniquet. What do you think is going on? What is your management?

Case 5

The observed manifestation is consistent with a local allergic reaction to either lidocaine or less likely due to latex gloves. IgE-mediated sensitivity has also been reported to parabens or metabisulfite, two preservatives often used in local anesthetics. In either case all latex-containing products should be disposed of. Secure large-bore intravenous access. The tourniquet should not be released until after prophylactic measures are taken which consist of the administration of adequate IV volume replacement, diphenhydramine, and epinephrine just prior to tourniquet release. The tourniquet should be deflated gradually and intermittently to avoid severe systemic anaphylaxis and allow effective antagonism of systemically released antigens.

General References

1. Warner MA, Warner DO, Harper CM, Schroeder DR, Maxson PM (2000) Lower extremity neuropathies associated with lithotomy positions. Anesthesiology 93:938–942
2. Erol O, Ozcakar L, Kaymak B (2004) Bilateral peroneal neuropathy after surgery in the lithotomy position. Aesthetic Plast Surg 28:254–255
3. Janik JE, Hoeft MA, Ajar AH, Alsofrom GF, Borrello MT, Rathmell JP (2008) Variable osteology of the sixth cervical vertebra in relation to stellate ganglion block. Reg Anesth Pain Med 33:102–108
4. Tran D, Clemente A, Finlayson RJ (2007) A review of approaches and techniques for lower extremity nerve blocks. Can J Anaesth 54:922–934

Chapter 27
Pain Management

A 16-year-old, 48 kg, female gymnast with a history of reflex sympathetic dystrophy in the right foot is scheduled for a left ACL reconstruction. Pulse rate 95 bpm, BP 108/70 mmHg, and RR 16/min.

R.S. Holzman et al., *Pediatric Anesthesiology Review: Clinical Cases for Self-Assessment*, DOI 10.1007/978-1-4419-1617-4_27, © Springer Science+Business Media, LLC 2010

Preoperative Evaluation

(a) What is reflex sympathetic dystrophy?

(b) The patient is taking amitriptylline, 75 mg QHS. What are the anesthetic implications?

(c) Are there any maneuvers/anesthetic techniques which can reduce her chance of further neuropathic pain?

Preoperative Evaluation

(a) Reflex sympathetic dystrophy is a painful syndrome of unclear etiology and pathophysiology. It is presumably due to dysfunction of small fibers of the skin and deeper tissues associated with regional sympathetic nerve dysfunction that manifests with increased cutaneous sensitivity (allodynia & hyperalgesia), skin discoloration, and impaired or excessive sweating, and vasomotor tone. The condition commonly affects distal parts of the limbs in a stocking distribution (nondermatomal) and is more frequent in females. Some patients may experience motor dysfunction, weakness, and myoclonus. In advanced conditions, the muscles, bone, and skin are wasted and the joints become stiff with resultant loss of limb function.

(b) Amitriptyline is a tricylic drug that inhibits norepinephrine and serotonin reuptake at second order neurons. It has a strong anticholinergic effect and may cause delayed atrioventricular conduction or AV block, prolonged QRS and QT syndrome, torsades de pointes, lowering of the threshold for seizures, urinary retention, hyperthermia, increased intraocular pressure, extrapyramidal syndrome, and anticholinergic psychosis. Its atropine-like effect may cause sinus tachycardia and premature ventricular contractions particularly when combined with other anticholinergic or sympathomimetic drugs such as atropine, glycopyrrolate, pancuronium, meperidine, succinylcholine, halothane, isoflurane, etc.

(c) A predominant theory of chronic neuropathic pain syndrome is the hyperexcitability of the second-order neuron (i.e., central sensitization) in the dorsal horn caused by the injured nerve. It is reasonable to assume that the use of spinal or epidural anesthesia with local anesthetics in this patient could block the nociceptive impulses generated at the surgical site from reaching the dorsal horn neurons and hence minimize the acute excitation trigger of the dorsal horn neurons and reduce the potential for flare-up of the RSD pain postoperatively.

Intraoperative Course

(a) How would you induce anesthesia in this patient?

(b) How would you maintain anesthesia in this patient?

(c) After induction blood pressure drops to 75/45. How do you treat this?

(d) The patient develops ventricular tachycardia. How do you treat this?

(e) Is emergence from anesthesia expected to be slower or faster than expected compared with healthy children?

Postoperative Course

How will you manage the patient's pain postoperatively? What monitoring is required?

Intraoperative Course

(a) I will premedicate the patient with small doses of midazolam and fentanyl, and induce anesthesia with intravenous sodium pentothal, vecuronium, and fentanyl.

(b) I will maintain the anesthesia with nitrous oxide, oxygen, fentanyl, a propofol infusion, and a low dose of isoflurane, as tolerated.

(c) Chronic use of amitriptyline can deplete norepinephrine. The blunting of central sympathetic drive by anesthetic agents can result in hypotension. The hypotension is best treated with intravenous volume, and if ineffective, then low incremental doses of norepinephrine (1–2 mcg/kg IV) may be necessary to maintain adequate vascular tone and blood pressure.

(d) The ventricular tachycardia usually occurs due to augmentation of anticholinergic effects of amitriptyline. It is best treated by slow and incremental intravenous administration of cholinergic drugs such as edrophonium 0.5–1 mg or physostigmine 0.25–0.5 mg. A major side effect of these drugs is bradycardia.

(e) Emergence from anesthesia can be slow in patients on chronic tricyclic agents due to depletion of central catecholamines. Amitriptyline, like other tricyclic agents, produces sedation that could be enhanced by concurrent administration of opioids and other sedative-hypnotics in the perioperative period.

Postoperative Course

I will continue the epidural analgesia to control the postoperative pain. Alternatively, intravenous morphine and other opioid analgesics can be provided via patient-controlled analgesia (PCA) but opioids are less effective in controlling neuropathic pain including that of RSD. The patient should be monitored for excessive sedation, mouth dryness, and paralytic ileus due to enhancement of the antcholinergic effect of amitriptyline by opioids. I would avoid the concurrent use of anticholinergic drugs such as diphenhydramine and hydroxyzine for the treatment of pruritus.

Additional Questions

(a) How do you perform a stellate block? What set-up should you have before
    starting the block?

(b) You wish to perform an interscalene block with the patient asleep. How will
    you localize the nerves? What settings will you use on the nerve stimulator?
    What do you look for?

(c) A patient with prostate cancer has metastases to the spinal cord. What options
    do you have in managing his pain if he sees you as an outpatient? If he is increas-
    ingly debilitated and has just entered hospice care? If he is at the end of life?

Additional Questions

(a) A stellate ganglion block should be performed in a setting where resuscitation equipment and drugs as well as personnel trained in cardiopulmonary resuscitation are readily available. The block is performed with the patient supine and the neck slightly extended. The C6 transverse process tubercle (Chassaignac's tubercle) is identified and the index and middle fingers are placed at the level of the cricoid ring between trachea and sternocleidomastoid muscle. A short beveled 25-gauge needle is introduced perpendicular to the skin and advanced until the needle tip makes contact with the C6 transverse process. The needle is withdrawn a few millimeters and immobilized. After negative aspiration for blood or CSF a total of 8–10 mL of local anesthetic is injected incrementally. Anxious adolescents and younger children may require general anesthesia to avoid movement during the performance of the block. The patient is anesthetized with an inhalation agent via mask and is allowed to breathe spontaneously to monitor accidental epidural or intrathecal injection. This technique is suitable for monitoring cessation of breathing or seizure activity in the event of an accidental intrathecal or intravascular injection of local anesthetic.

(b) Nerve injury can be minimized by the use of nontraumatic needles (blunt pencil tip needle), an insulated needle for precise localization of the nerves, and a nerve stimulator. The block needle tip is placed in the fascial plane encompassing the brachial plexus, as guided by the topological landmarks and/or ultrasound and the feel of tissue resistance of the brachial plexus sheath through which the needle passes. An initial current of 1–1.5 mA at 1 or 2 Hz is used to identify proximity to the nerve(s) as the needle is advanced. After identifying the appropriate motor response to the stimulated nerve(s) distal to elbow, the stimulating current is gradually decreased as the needle is advanced until a maximum motor response is maintained at a current between 0.2 and 0.5 mA, indicating that the needle tip is within 1–2 mm of the target nerves.

(c) Surgery followed by radiation is the most effective treatment for spinal cord compression caused by metastatic cancer. The addition of surgery allows most patients to remain more mobile and to retain bladder control. If the metastatic prostate cancer is not amenable to anticancer therapy, the goal of hospice care is to improve the quality of life by providing pain and symptom relief. Oral and/or intravenous opioids and adjuvant antineuropathic pain agents are administered to manage the pain. If the pain is not adequately controlled or unacceptable side effects occur then intrathecal opioids and/or local anesthetics should be considered. At the end of life, pain and distressing symptoms could be alleviated by incremental large doses of opioids, adjuvant drugs, and sedatives.

(d) An internist refers a 22-year-old male to you for a lumbar sympathetic block as treatment of reflex sympathetic dystrophy. He injured his left leg in a lawn mower accident 8 months ago, suffering superficial lacerations that healed in 2 weeks. He has had debilitating pain since and now walks only short distances. How would you proceed?

(e) You are called to see a 19-year old for placement of an epidural catheter for labor pain. She fell and sprained her ankle several days ago and has been taking NSAIDs for pain. How will you proceed? During placement of the catheter a dural puncture occurs. What would you do?

(d) The patient should be evaluated for underlying causes of RSD (chronic regional pain syndrome type 1 (CRPS type 1) and causalgia (CRPS type 2), nerve entrapment, neuroma, and phantom pain. RSD and causalgia are not distinguishable by their clinical presentation. Unlike RSD, in causalgia a defined injured nerve is identifiable. When the diagnosis of RSD is established, a single diagnostic lumbar sympathetic blockade is performed. If the blockade relieves pain it can be repeated at intervals of days to weeks based on the patient's response. Alternatively, a lumbar paravertebral or epidural indwelling catheter can be placed for continuous infusion of a local anesthetic to facilitate aggressive physical therapy and mobilization of the painful limb. In addition to the above medical management, psychological counseling should be encouraged to manage the emotional distress associated with chronic pain and disability.

(e) If sufficient time is available, a bleeding time should be obtained to assess the effect of the NSAID agent on platelet function. If the bleeding test cannot be performed with sufficient speed, I will assess the patient for clinical evidence of bleeding tendencies such as a history of bruising with minor bumps and nosebleed. In the absence of clinical evidence of bleeding, I will proceed with the placement of an epidural catheter. If the patient develops a postdural puncture headache, the NSAID drug should be discontinued for at least 48 h while treating the PDPH conservatively. After 48 h the effect of a short-acting NSAID should dissipate and an epidural blood patch can be performed effectively if conservative therapy is unsuccessful.

General References

1. Rowbotham MC (2006) Pharmacologic management of complex regional pain syndrome. Clin J Pain 22:425–429
2. Schwartzman RJ, Alexander GM, Grothusen J (2006) Pathophysiology of complex regional pain syndrome. Expert Rev Neurother 6:669–681

Chapter 28
Burns

A 3-year old is rescued from a burning apartment after hiding under the bed. He has a 55% burn, primarily below the knees and above the waist, including the face, and around the chest. He is short of breath, tachypneic, with a blood pressure of 130/90, a heart rate of 160, and a temperature of 39.4°C. He has a headache, is restless, and somewhat confused. You are his ICU doctor.

R.S. Holzman et al., *Pediatric Anesthesiology Review: Clinical Cases for Self-Assessment*,
DOI 10.1007/978-1-4419-1617-4_28, © Springer Science+Business Media, LLC 2010

Initial Evaluation

1. How do you determine whether this patient should be intubated? Are there physical signs that would help in this evaluation? Chest X-ray? Arterial blood gas? Would steroids be of any help in decreasing airway edema?

2. What toxic products of combustion would you be concerned about? How can you evaluate the clinical significance? What will you do? Would prophylactic antibiotics be of any help? Why/why not? What about steroids? Why/why not? What are the important considerations for management of carbon monoxide poisoning?

Initial Evaluation

1. Because the child was burned in an enclosed environment and sustained a facial burn, has shortness of breath and is tachypneic, the child probably is suffering from thermal injury to the airways and alveoli from smoke, noxious gases, and hot air inhalation. This child's trachea should be intubated prophylactically in anticipation of rapid swelling of the upper airways and respiratory tract that can make glottic access for subsequent tracheal intubation impossible. Chest X-ray may not be very helpful in the early stages of the pulmonary thermal injury. Arterial blood gas analysis may show lactic and respiratory acidosis. It will not be useful in diagnosing carbon monoxide poisoning because it measures dissolved oxygen and thus overestimates the true oxygen saturation of hemoglobin. Similarly, a standard pulse oximeter overestimates the true oxygen because it cannot differentiate normal oxyhemoglobin from carbon monoxyhemoglobin, although there are more sophisticated pulse oximeters that can do so. Clinically, carbon monoxide poisoning is suspected in burn victims when CNS symptoms of headache, dizziness, restlessness, and confusion are present. This clinical diagnosis is confirmed with a co-oximeter or a handheld breath analyzer capable of carbon monoxide analysis. Steroids are not helpful with the massive inflammatory process and may increase the risk of infection.

2. Carbon monoxide gas is of most concern because it is colorless and odorless and is produced in large quantities during incomplete combustion of carbon or carbon products and fuels. The clinical significance is that carbon monoxide poisoning can produce severe hypoxemia and long-term neurological impairment. Carbon monoxide gas has 200–250 times the binding affinity for hemoglobin to form carboxy-hemoglobin and shifts the oxyhemoglobin curve to the left. As a result oxygen delivery to tissues is seriously impaired. The primary treatment of carbon monoxide toxicity is the administration of 100% oxygen by a nonrebreathing system and in severe cases (carboxyhemoglobin >30%) via positive pressure ventilation or hyperbaric oxygen. Prophylactic antibiotics can be helpful to treat opportunistic infection. Steroids are not helpful to treat respiratory tract massive edema resulting from thermal burns.

3. What are your initial considerations in volume support? Why is this patient hyperdynamic? Is it safe to give so much fluid initially? What formula would you use? Why? Is there ever a need to modify this? Is it likely that this hemodynamic picture will change? Over what period of time? Why? Is it likely to change back again? What is your initial critical care management?

Supportive Management

1. What special considerations do you have for mechanical ventilation of this patient? Metabolic basis? Mechanical basis?

2. What are the nutritional needs of a burn patient? When should hyperalimentation begin? Should it be central, peripheral, or enteral? Why choose one?

3. What are the consequences of a 55% total body burn on thermoregulation? Of what importance is that in your ICU management? How do you compensate for increased thermogenesis and increased heat loss? Will occlusive dressings or raised ambient temperature alter this caloric loss? Why/why not? How do you compensate for increased free water loss? To what extent is electrolyte loss a component? How do you compensate for that?

3. This patient should be cared for in the intensive care unit from the beginning because large volume resuscitation is necessary initially and can be guided by either the Parkland formula [crystalloid 4 mL/kg×percent burn×wt (kg)] or the Brooke formula [crystalloid 0.5 mL/kg+colloid 1.5 mL/kg×percent burn×wt (kg)]. These formulas are useful guides for the replacement of massive fluid loss but the overall requirement is determined by clinical monitoring of the patient's mental status, hemodynamic parameters, acid–base balance, and urine output. Nevertheless, these formulas may underestimate fluid requirement in infants under 10 kg. Some burn centers use hypertonic saline or colloids, particularly in the very young and elderly to minimize edema but controlled trials have not demonstrated differences in outcome and mortality among the different types of solutions. Usually the fluid losses via inflamed surfaces continue for days to weeks depending on the extent and severity of the burns. The hyperdynamic circulation is due to loss of extracellular fluid (in the "third space") and the hypermetabolic state and circulatory effects resulting from thermal injury-induced cytokines and endotoxins.

Supportive Management

1. The mechanical ventilation parameters are set at higher settings to eliminate the increased carbon dioxide production and meet the increased oxygen demand resulting from the hypermetabolic state. High positive end expiratory and inspiratory pressures may be necessary for effective oxygenation in the presence of pulmonary edema from thermal burn of the alveoli and airway passages.

2. The hypermetabolic state is associated with increased utilization of glucose, fat, and protein and that in turn leads to greater oxygen demand and increased carbon dioxide production. Hyperalimentation is started soon after the initial fluid resuscitation and stabilization of the hemodynamics. The hyperalimentaion fluid is administered via a central line. It is difficult to secure peripheral venous access for a prolonged infusion time if all extremities are involved in the burn injury. Patients with severe burns develop gastric stress ulcers and ileus and as a result enteral absorption is ineffective and insufficient for the increased nutritional requirement.

3. A 55% skin burn produces extensive destruction of the body surface and results in significant loss of body heat leading to serious hypothermia. To prevent hypothermia, it is crucial to cover the patient's body, elevate the ambient temperature, use radiant warmers, and warm the inspired gases. Occlusive dressings and insulating blankets are more effective in preserving heat, minimizing evaporative losses, and reducing caloric requirements. In contrast, nursing of open wounds in a raised ambient temperature will enhance evaporative water and electrolytes loss.

4. If you were a nephron, how would your physiology be altered as a result of a burn injury? Why? What is the effect of decreased cardiac output, increased endogenous catecholamine activity, decreased splanchnic blood flow on renal sodium conservation? Why? Are there any consequences to antidiuretic hormone elaboration? What are they? How do they affect renal function?

5. Twelve hours after admission the patient develops diffuse petechiae associated with bleeding at line sites. How would you evaluate? Why do you get this picture? Would fibrin split products analysis be of any help? You do a factor analysis and factors V and VIII are actually elevated – does that matter? Why/why not? What kind of support is necessary in this circumstance? Would whole blood help?

Anesthesia Consultation

1. When called to intubate this patient, an anesthesia resident asks you if he should do a rapid sequence induction – your answer? Why? What about using rocuronium? Any special considerations for burn patients with regard to nondepolarizing neuromuscular blocking agents? What if this is the first day post burn and the patient is going for escharotomy?

4. Nephron function is adversely affected immediately after the burn due to hypovolemia, hypotension, hypoxemia, myoglobinuria, and hemoglobinuria leading to acute tubular necrosis. Other contributing factors are stress-related release of catecholamines, angiotensin, vasopressin, aldosterone, and endothelin-1 which cause systemic vasoconstriction, hypertension, and impairment of renal function. Therefore, fluid retention occurs during the first 5–7 days after the burn injury; diuresis occurs thereafter.

5. DIC is the presumptive diagnosis of the diffuse spontaneous bleeding until proven otherwise. Extensive tissue burns and intravascular hemolysis can introduce tissue phospholipids into the bloodstream resulting in activation of the extrinsic clotting system. To confirm this possible diagnosis, I will send a sample of the patient's blood for prothrombin time (PT) (>15 s), fibrinogen concentration less than 160 mg/dL, and a platelet count less than 150,000 mm³. Platelet consumption is the most sensitive indicator of DIC. The presence of high circulating levels of fibrin split products and D-dimer concentration is a reflection of a secondary fibrinolytic process that accompanies the thrombosis during disseminated intravascular coagulation. Initially, factors V and VIII could be elevated in response to burn stress. The most important component of therapy is to maintain an adequate circulating volume. Since the primary cause of the DIC cannot be reversed, the consumed coagulation factors (factors V, VIII, fibrinogen, and others) should be replaced by transfusion of cryoprecipitate, fresh frozen plasma, and platelets. The use of whole blood depends on its shelf life. Unrefrigerated fresh whole blood is useful but usually does not contain adequate levels of coagulation factors and platelets to replace the elevated requirement during DIC.

Anesthesia Consultation

1. I will discourage the resident from performing rapid sequence induction without assessing the airways. The inhalation of smoke and toxic fumes may cause severe swelling of the oral mucosa, tongue, and glottis that can make intubation very difficult if not impossible. Although succinylcholine is safe to use within the first 24 h after the burns, even a small acute rise of serum potassium in burn patients can produce serious arrhythmias and cardiac arrest because the skeletal muscle burns and intravascular hemolysis produce a rapid rise of serum potassium. Rocuronium is safe to use provided there is no evidence of direct oral and respiratory tract burns, e.g., inhalation of steam. It is well recognized, for reasons not well understood, that burn victims are resistant to nondepolarizing muscle relaxants, hence larger doses must be used to achieve adequate intubation conditions. The onset of neuromuscular blockade with rocuronium is longer compared with succinylcholine. From 24 h after the burn until the wounds are completely healed, succinylcholine should not be used because of upregulation of the cholinergic receptors at the neuromuscular junction and at extrajunctional sites on the skeletal muscle membrane. The admin-

istration of succinylcholine may produce exaggerated muscle contractions and a rapid rise in serum potassium, to serious and even lethal concentrations.

2. How can you keep a burn patient warm in the OR? Any special considerations, different from a nonburned patient?

Additional Questions

1. An electrical worker reached for a capacitor and it shorted through his arm. Other than excruciating pain, he actually looks like he only has a little, superficial puncture wound. The surgeon is very worried and wants to rush him to the OR for exploration, fasciotomy, angiography, and debridement. Why is he making such a big deal out of it? Is deep tissue destruction more likely with an extremity electrical burn than superficial tissue? Why?

2. A 14-year-old boy was standing in a corn field in Nebraska imitating a cow when he was struck by lightning, suffering a cardiac arrest which he fortunately was resuscitated from successfully because an EMT was right there next to him. What kind of burn injury is he likely to suffer? Why? How is this

different than the previous case of electrical conduction through the arm of the victim? Why does this tend to be a superficial rather than deep burn? Which is more lethal?

2. Burn victims tend to develop hypothermia in the OR because of the hypermetabolic state as well as rapid evaporative fluid losses from exposed burn surfaces. To minimize heat loss in the OR, the room should be heated to 28–30°C, intravenous solutions should be warmed and the inhaled anesthetic gases should be humidified and heated.

Additional Questions

1. Electrical injuries produce minimal skin injury but massive internal tissue injury. The current spreads through the neurovascular bundles and produces extensive depolarization and thermal burn of nervous tissue, cardiac and skeletal muscles, and all soft tissue in general. As a result, there is a massive fluid shift, myonecrosis (rhabdomyolysis, compartment syndrome), and hemolysis (vascular spasms, thrombosis). The electricity involves the flow of energy (electrons) along the path of least resistance toward a natural ground. All tissues are either resistors (skin and bone) or conductors (neurovascular bundles, soft tissue). Therefore, deeper soft tissues such as the nervous system, cardiac and skeletal muscles, GI and vascular system are at high risk for electrically induced depolarization and thermal burns.

2. Lighting may cause complete cardiac arrest by inducing asystole or central apnea. Extensive depolarization of the heart muscles leads to asystole and massive depolarization of the brain can result in apnea. Therefore, lightning injury is

more detrimental than standard household current. This patient may have had transient asystole, which may account for the prompt response to resuscitation. Unlike the previous case, lightning involves a single massive current pulse that is approximately equivalent to a DC burst of 2,000–2 billion volts of extremely short duration of 0.1–1 ms.

3. You are moonlighting in the University walk-in clinic when a chemistry major student is brought in with burns on his arms from white phosphorus powder; he was playing in the lab. How do you treat this chemical burn? Any special precautions? What is your general approach to chemical burns? How do you assess when the airway is of significant concern?

3. I will remove the patient's clothes and footwear to avoid further contact with white phosphorus, and irrigate or apply saline-soaked or water-soaked pads to the affected skin to wash off the offending agent and stop further oxidation of the phosphorus. Phosphorus is a lipophilic agent and tends to bind to fatty tissue. Upon oxidation it produces an exothermic reaction resulting in second and third degree burn injury. I will avoid the use of any greasy solutions to irrigate and cleanse the affected area because it will enhance binding to the tissue. Contact with the patient's clothes contaminated with white phosphorus must be avoided because it is ignitable and can cause chemical burn injury to the patient or the healthcare provider. Lacerated, devitalized, or contaminated tissue must be debrided. Visualization of phosphorus is aided with a Wood's lamp (ultraviolet light) by fluorescing the white phosphorus.

The general approach to all chemical injuries is to remove the offending agent because the injury becomes progressively more severe as long as the offending agent is in contact with the skin. Individuals who are affected must promptly have their clothing and footwear removed, they must have the dry chemical brushed away, and water lavage to dilute and remove the chemical must be provided.

Some chemicals are insoluble in water, and other chemicals create exothermic reactions when combined with water. For example, dry lime contains calcium oxide, which reacts with water to form calcium hydroxide, an injurious alkali. Therefore, dry lime should be dusted off the skin prior to washing with water. Phenol is water insoluble, and it should be wiped off the skin with sponges soaked in a 50% concentration of polyethylene glycol. Concentrated sulfuric acid often causes an exothermic reaction when combined with water, therefore, soap or lime should be used first to neutralize the agents. The use of neutralizing agents is the exception to the rule because the key to effective treatment is dilution. Some antidotes may produce exothermic reactions and thereby increase toxicity. Some have advocated use of turpentine for white phosphorus burns.

General References

1. Beushausen T, Mucke K (1997) Anesthesia and pain management in pediatric burn patients. Pediatr Surg Int 12:327–333
2. MacLennan N, Heimbach DM, Cullen BF (1998) Anesthesia for major thermal injury. Anesthesiology 89:749–770
3. Young CJ, Moss J (1989) Smoke inhalation: diagnosis and treatment. J Clin Anesth 1:377–386
4. Gueugniaud PY, Carsin H, Bertin-Maghit M, Petit P (2000) Current advances in the initial management of major thermal burns. Intensive Care Med 26:848–856

5. Opara KO, Chukwuanukwu TO, Ogbonnaya IS, Nwadinigwe CU (2006) Pattern of severe electrical injuries in a Nigerian regional burn centre. Niger J Clin Pract 9:124–127
6. Dokov W (2008) Assessment of risk factors for death in electrical injury. Burns 35:114–117
7. Ogilvie MP, Panthaki ZJ (2008) Electrical burns of the upper extremity in the pediatric population. J Craniofac Surg 19:1040–1046
8. Weissman BA, Raveh L (2008) Therapy against organophosphate poisoning: the importance of anticholinergic drugs with antiglutamatergic properties. Toxicol Appl Pharmacol 232:351–358

Chapter 29
Anesthesia Outside the Operating Room

An 18-month-old, 18-kg boy is scheduled for an MRI of the brain to evaluate new onset grand mal seizures, photophobia, and increasing irritability. He has been well previously. He is currently on phenobarbital and dilantin.

R.S. Holzman et al., *Pediatric Anesthesiology Review: Clinical Cases for Self-Assessment*,
DOI 10.1007/978-1-4419-1617-4_29, © Springer Science+Business Media, LLC 2010

Preprocedural Evaluation

1. What would you like to know about his current anticonvulsant regimen? Is it important to know levels? Why? Would you insist on this information prior to anesthetizing him? Why or why not? If he is poorly controlled on this multi-modal regimen, would you cancel the case in favor of adding another medication to hopefully improve his seizure control? Is he not likely to improve and will require the diagnostic procedure anyway?

2. Is he at any increased risk for perioperative morbidity from seizures? Why?

3. Would you insist on an IV prior to induction or is it okay for him to undergo a mask induction with a volatile agent? Is a parent-present induction all right, or is this "too high a risk?"

Preprocedural Evaluation

1. The efficacy of his anticonvulsant therapy has to be questioned first of all, because he is on two medications. This may relate to the frequency and duration of his seizures. Grand mal seizures of the tonic–clonic variety are usually the easiest to control, particularly if they originate in a single seizure focus, but generalized tonic–clonic seizures associated with a progressive metabolic disease or complex partial seizures are more difficult to control. Multimodal therapy is often required in these circumstances. The history is important here; he may be optimally (although poorly) controlled with this regimen, and yet require a diagnostic study to determine whether there is a specific focus that needs mapping, particularly in anticipation of surgical resection. Blood levels are important to obtain for a baseline, but often, pediatric patients may be optimally controlled with levels either below or above recommended ranges. In this regard, communication with the neurologist is critical because it can add to the historical perspective of the child's treatment.

2. Seizure thresholds may be affected by the administration of or the withdrawal from a general anesthetic, in the first case raising the threshold and in the second case lowering it. Therefore, during emergence, the patient maybe at increased risk for a seizure. All of the general inhalation anesthetics as well as the majority of intravenous hypnotic agents are anticonvulsant. Some inhalation agents produce myoclonus or promote seizure activity in association with hyperventilation (enflurane, sevoflurane) but can also act as anticonvulsants. Methohexital, particularly in association with hyperventilation, can act as a proconvulsant medication, but thiopental is anticonvulsant. Given the multiple attempts at intravenous access, the increased stress of the patient and the likelihood that much air has been swallowed during the attempts, a parent-present inhalation induction may produce a calmer child. In a sitting to partially upright position, with the application of gentle cricoid pressure, a completely asleep child will be a much better candidate for IV placement and the completion of this induction intravenously with the use of a muscle relaxant if placement of an endotracheal tube is considered. Rather than dealing with insistence one way or the other with the parents, it is probably wiser to educate them about the various options. I would be inclined to proceed with a mask induction as outlined above, but if there were other considerations supervening, then another individual could attempt intravenous access and continue with a rapid sequence induction if, for example, active reflux was a consideration.

3. I would not insist on an IV prior to induction. While there is always some risk to a mask induction in this age group it usually revolves around fear of separation and fear of the unknown. The separation can be dealt with by a parent-present induction and the fear of the unknown with a preinduction medication strategy of either a rectally administered barbiturate such as thiopental (not methohexital because of its seizure-lowering potential). If crying and struggling are minimized, then the patients' risk of preinduction seizure is lowered because of less stress and the risk of aspiration lowered because of less aerophagia.

4. What are the relevant equipment issues related to the MRI environment?

Intraoperative Course

1. The patient is crying, screaming, and fussing with the placement of routine non-invasive monitors; is it all right to go ahead without them? Does he need any additional monitors?

2. What anesthetic technique will you choose? The nurses have already tried X3 to place an IV; the patient is now crying, sweaty, and terrified? The parents insist on a mask induction; would you go ahead or cancel the case?

4. Ferrous-containing elements of the anesthetic equipment have to be eliminated for the sake of patient safety as well as the test results. Iron-containing materials become missiles in the MRI scanner, depending on iron content and mass, but magnetic attraction obeys the inverse square law such that the closer it gets to the bore of the magnetic the greater the attraction becomes, and therefore, with greater mass, can easily become a projectile. Oxygen tanks, tables, and anesthesia machines have been "sucked into" the bore of the magnet and attest to the risks of not considering these issues with regard to patient safety. For the provider, anything in pockets which contain iron can become projectiles as well, such as stethoscopes, scissors, etc. In addition, personal identification cards such as hospital ID cards and credit cards can have their information rendered useless; beepers and telephones will have their radiofrequency chips scrambled to the point of uselessness.

Intraoperative Course

1. This becomes a matter of risk/benefit ratio while dealing with a fearful toddler. What often happens is despite being surrounded by several adults, the toddler will succeed in pulling off the monitors at a rate faster than that which the adults can place them, all the while being terrified and swallowing more and more air. I would opt for placement of a pulse oximeter to begin with, and then rapidly progressing to either an intravenous or inhalation induction in a sitting or semi-sitting position and application of cricoid pressure after the loss of consciousness. Additional monitors can be placed by others when the patient will no longer resist their placement.

2. As outlined above, the smoothest anesthetic technique would probably be the best for the patient. If this involved a rectal or p.o. preinduction medication, I would probably choose thiopental rectally (rather than methohexital because of its proconvulsant properties) or p.o. midazolam, if the patient was terrified of the experience. Depending on my assessment of the potential ease of intravenous access, it might lead me to choose IV placement first followed by propofol as an induction dose and then continuous infusion with a natural airway, or alternatively, a mask induction with sevoflurane, oxygen and nitrous oxide, and then continuation either with an LMA and sevoflurane or continuous infusion with propofol.

3. Every time the patient is positioned in the head holder he begins to cough and obstruct his airway; what is your next move? Would you deepen the anesthetic (whether infusion or inhalation)? Should an LMA be placed? Endotracheal tube?

Postoperative Course

1. As the patient is emerging, he develops rhythmic tonic–clonic movements which begin in one arm and progress to generalized tonic–clonic activity. What to do next? Why did this happen? What if the anesthetic technique was continuous infusion propofol without an endotracheal tube? What are his risks of aspiration? What would you do to treat the seizure? How long would you keep the patient in the PACU? Should he be admitted? If not, how will you counsel the parents?

2. When would you restart his phenobarbital and dilantin? Should he receive a supplemental dose intravenously in the PACU? Why or why not?

3. Because the study requires a motionless patient, at some point, the anesthesiologist will have to produce this condition, no matter what the technique. It would be worthwhile trying to deepen the patient with incrementally larger doses of propofol according to the usual depth-assessment criteria, but if it turns out that the patient is intolerant of this approach for any reason (breath holding, coughing, impaired pharyngeal competence, or a partially obstructed airway because of positioning considerations) then an airway device would be indicated. The LMA could be used if the patient could be deepened sufficiently to tolerate the LMA, breathe spontaneously, and remain motionless otherwise. If this approach fails, then the patient should probably be relaxed and intubated so the study can be accomplished.

Postoperative Course

1. This situation is not very surprising; the emergence from a general anesthetic produces an abrupt change in the patients anticonvulsant status, and this shift can especially make a more poorly controlled patient have an increased incidence of seizures. Preparation is the key to treating this problem. If the airway is protected with an endotracheal tube then the seizure can be treated with small intravenous doses of thiopental or a benzodiazepine. If the airway is unprotected or if an LMA is in place, then the risk/benefit ratio of leaving it in or protecting the patient's airway has to be decided upon. If there have been no preceding difficulties with the airway, incremental doses as described above can be given with the patient receiving supplemental oxygen. If it seems that the patient may progress on to regurgitation then he will be at increased risk of aspiration because the gag reflex will undoubtedly be less competent during the ictal and immediately postictal phase following the seizure. The duration of PACU stay will depend on how many seizures the patient ordinarily has per day, the competence of the parents in dealing with these seizures, and to some extent the risks of driving home (e.g., distance home, distance to closest hospital, etc). I would probably keep the patient for 4–6 seizure-free hours in the PACU, with the resumption of his previous p.o. medications, consultation with his neurologist, and postoperative blood levels, which should be easy to obtain.

2. I would restart his anticonvulsants following the scan. The half-lives are drawn out enough and the onset is long enough that his level will neither decline nor be increased dramatically if he resumes his usually p.o. schedule a few hours later. It will probably be unnecessary to give him any intravenous equivalent doses of his phenobarbital or dilantin.

Additional Questions

1. A 6-year-old status post a CVA 1 month ago is scheduled to undergo cerebral angiography to rule out Moya Moya disease. What is Moya Moya disease? Why does he need cerebral angiography? Would it be sufficient to do magnetic resonance angiography? Any difference in the anesthetic considerations? What are the anesthetic considerations? Anything you should especially consider with regard to volume status? Blood pressure? Depth of anesthesia? Mechanical ventilation? Control of CO_2 tension?

2. A 15-month old is scheduled to undergo sclerotherapy for a vascular malformation. Is it important to differentiate whether the vascular malformation is arteriovenous, venous, or lymphatic? How does this diagnosis influence the anesthetic technique? What are the anesthetic issues if alcohol embolization is planned? Is there a difference between the use of alcohol and Sotrecol as a sclerosing agent? What are the risks of using platinum coils? How does it affect your anesthetic management? How painful will this procedure be in the perioperative period and how will it influence your postoperative management in the PACU?

Additional Questions

1. Cerebral angiography requires motionlessness and exquisite control of ventilation. Additional considerations specific to Moya Moya Disease include strict control of blood pressure, depth of anesthesia, and CO_2 tension to control cerebral blood flow [1]. The same considerations apply to Moya Moya Disease as those for cerebral vascular insufficiency, such as a patient with high-grade carotid disease, because the impairment of blood flow is due to a congenital absence of the middle cerebral artery and in its place, exceedingly small vessels giving the appearance on angiography of a "puff of smoke," which is what Moya Moya means in Japanese. Patients should be adequately volume replete, compensating for NPO deficits, have a mean arterial pressure within 10% of baseline (should not be too low because of inadequate perfusion and should not be too high because of the chance of intracranial bleed), and have their CO_2 tension controlled from normal to slight hypercarbia (e.g., end-tidal CO_2 concentration from 38 to 45 mmHg). An arterial line may facilitate close monitoring for unstable patients, but is not ordinarily required. Adequate depth of anesthesia will help with control of blood pressure.

2. The various kinds of vascular malformations have different transit times for sclerosing agents, and therefore, the anesthesiologist must consider those strategies which influence intravascular volume, hemodynamics, and blood flow at the local level. Very often, high-flow lesions are not autoregulated and therefore hyperventilation, while acting to vasoconstrict blood vessels in general, may actually enhance imaging of nonautoregulated vessels. Adequate intravascular volume and depth of anesthesia as well as preservation of cardiac output is necessary to provide sufficient perfusion pressure and transit time to the intended area of embolization. The embolization material is important as well; while various types of coils have been used (which may result in paradoxical or misplaced embolization), alcohol or Sotrecol is now more commonly utilized, which may have systemic effects (particularly in the pulmonary circulation, with elevation of pulmonary artery pressures) and may also affect emergence because of alcohol intoxication. Alcohol is nephrotoxic, so enhanced urine output is particularly important. Alcohol may produce a coagulum of blood and endothelial necrosis, leading to emboli distant from the intended area of intervention. In addition, perioperative care of the patient may require the participation of an anesthesiologist because exquisite pain crises are often experienced after alcohol embolization which only improve after days to weeks as the acute inflammatory process diminishes.

3. A 7-year-old boy is scheduled to undergo esophagogastroduodenoscopy (EGD) for symptomatic reflux disease. He would like a mask induction because of his fear of needles – what do you think? Is there a safe way to administer nitrous oxide or some other sedative strategy or must he just have an IV placed? Is a rapid sequence induction with succinylcholine necessary? After EGD, biopsies and much air insufflation the endoscopist declares he is done and ready for you to wake the patient up. Your considerations? Is all the air EVER out of the upper GI tract? The patient is now light, bucking on the tube, and eructating – what is your next move? Is a deep extubation preferable?

4. A 3 year is receiving weekly intrathecal methotrexate for a brain tumor. His oncologist requires motionlessness and his parents require lack of recall and comfort. What will your approach be? What does it depend upon? If he has a pansinusitis from his immune suppression (assume his oncologist and parents feel strongly that his treatment must go on), how does this influence your anesthetic choices?

5. A patient with a prior history of hives following contrast injection for IV pyelography is returning for a repeat pyelogram with "anesthesia standby." What is his risk of subsequent reaction? How can he be treated to lower this risk? Why does this occur? How should you be prepared?

3. Chances are a 7-year old will not be particularly enthusiastic about having an IV prior to induction, but unless this is an insurmountable problem, good preparation will probably enable you to place the IV. EMLA cream, the use of local anesthetic (once the EMLA has taken effect), and possibly an oral premed are all reasonable for this child, while carefully explaining to the parents that a mask induction may not be the best strategy. That is not to say that it cannot be done, however, and the risk/benefit ratio has to be evaluated. If it were necessary to go ahead with a mask, then I would have him sit up or be placed in an antireflux position, with cricoid pressure, and then place an IV as soon as practicable. With the amount of insufflation typically necessary for EGD I would have the patient wake up completely rather than consider a deep extubation.

4. Much would depend on the underlying disease being treated and the patient's current medical state. He may be quite debilitated from chronic chemotherapy or doing relatively well, and therefore, this will influence the anesthetic approach. Most 3-year olds (and their doctors) will require motionlessness, and if the patient has an indwelling central line, I would probably start a propofol infusion and slowly let the patient drift off to sleep, then turn him on his side for the bone marrow and lumbar puncture, and encourage the use of liberal amounts of local anesthetic. An intercurrent infection would not be too surprising, and this situation arises frequently because children with prolonged hospitalizations will often acquire various opportunistic infections or even URIs from other patients or visitors. Most of the time this does not interfere with the progression of anticancer therapy because of the urgency involved, unless the patient is significantly symptomatic, showing high fevers, constitutional lethargy, or other signs and symptoms that may make it worthwhile to wait for 24–48 h (but hardly longer because of the context).

5. Approximately 5% of radiological exams with radiocontrast media (RCM) are complicated by adverse reactions, with 1/3 of these being severe and requiring immediate treatment. Reactions occur most commonly in patients between 20 and 50 years of age and are relatively rare in children. With a history of atopy or allergy the risk of a reaction is increased from 1.5 to 10 fold. Reactions may be mild, subjective sensations of restlessness, nausea, and vomiting to a rapidly evolving, angioedema-like picture. Low osmolar RCM are relatively safe with regard to life-threatening reactions. The treatment of severe allergic reactions, whether anaphylactoid or anaphylactic, is no different than for any other allergic reaction. Epinephrine, aminophylline, atropine, diphenhydramine, and steroids have all been employed to control varying degrees of adverse reactions. A patient who requires RCM administration and who has had a previous reaction to RCM has an increased (35–60%) risk for a reaction on reexposure. Pretreatment of these high risk patients with prednisone and diphenhydramine 1 h before RCM administration reduces the risk of reactions to 9%; the addition of ephedrine 1 h before RCM administration further reduces the rate to 3.1% [2].

Specific References

1. Soriano S, Sethna N, Scott R (1993) Anesthetic management of children with moyamoya syndrome.Find more like this. Anesth Analg 77:1066–1070
2. Holzman R (2008) Anaphylactic reactions and anesthesia. In: Longnecker D, Brown D, Newman M, Zapol W (eds) Anesthesiology. McGraw Hill, New York, pp 1947–1963

General References

3. Kanal E, Barkovich A, Bell C, Borgstede J, Bradley W, Froelich J, Gilk T, Gimbel J, Gosbee J, Kuhni-Kaminski E, Lester JW, Nyenhuis J, Parag Y, Schaefer D, Sebek-Scoumis E, Weinreb J, Zaremba L, Wilcox P, Lucey L, Sass N (2007) ACR guidance document for safe MR practices: 2007. AJR 188:1–27
4. Kanal E, Borgstede J, Barkovich A, Bell C, Bradley W, Felmlee J, Froelich J, Kaminski E, Keeler E, Lester J, Scoumis E, Zaremba L, Zinninger M (2002) American college of radiology white paper on MR safety. AJR 178:1335–1347
5. Mason K, Zgleszewski S, Holzman R (2006) Anesthesia and sedation for procedures outside the operating room. In: Motoyama E, Davis P (eds) Smith's anesthesia for infants and children. Philadelphia, Mosby Elsevier, pp 839–855

Chapter 30
Equipment and Monitoring

A 2-month-old, 5-kg baby, born at term without apparent complications, is scheduled to come to the OR emergently for evacuation of a subdural hematoma and repair of depressed skull fracture as a consequence of presumed child abuse. VS: HR 130 bpm, RR 22/min and crying, BP 75/50 mmHg, and Hct 30%. There is a 22 ga. IV in place in the left saphenous vein, and it seems to be running well.

R.S. Holzman et al., *Pediatric Anesthesiology Review: Clinical Cases for Self-Assessment*,   547
DOI 10.1007/978-1-4419-1617-4_30, © Springer Science+Business Media, LLC 2010

Preoperative Evaluation/Preparation

1. Should this baby be monitored en route to the OR? How?

   (a) What is the most important monitor? Why?
   (b) What are you most worried about?
   (c) Receive supplemental oxygen en route?
   (d) How will you check out the oxygen tank prior to transport?
   (e) What if it said 1/4 full; how much time would you have left?

2. You set up the room. How do you do an anesthesia machine checkout?

   (a) Is this the same as the FDA anesthesia machine checkout?
   (b) Is your checkout at the start of the day for the first case the same or different than for subsequent cases? In which way?

3. What circuit will you choose? Why?

   (a) What are the advantages and disadvantages of the various circuits?
   (b) Is there a difference in F_A/F_I with the different circuits? Dead space? Compression volume?
   (c) Is there a difference between a Bain circuit and a Mapleson D?
   (d) Are there different types of Bain circuits?
   (e) What is Pethick's test? Can you use it for a Mapleson D?

Preoperative Evaluation

1. The short answer to the monitoring question is yes, because of the risk of elevated intracranial pressure resulting in a Cushing's triad and herniation. The most important monitor, because of its sensitivity, is the mental status, and any alteration of the sensorium or the development of focal findings should prompt major concern. Monitoring of oxygen saturation and heart rate (by pulse oximetry or ECG) is worthwhile for respiratory and cardiac status as well as intracranial pressure because of the significance of bradycardia. Supplemental oxygen does not hurt and may help provide a greater margin of safety. The oxygen tank should be as full as possible, depending on the horizontal and vertical distance involved. A standard D cylinder of oxygen will be pressurized at 1,900 psig with 660 L oxygen when full. Because oxygen in the cylinder is nonliquiefied, it will show a steady decline in pressure and will have a steady decline in oxygen volume until discharged. The duration of oxygen supply, obviously, will therefore depend on the minute oxygen flow. If it said 1/4 full, there should be 165 L in the tank, and at a total fresh gas flow of 5 L/min, should be expected to last 33 min.

2. The standard FDA checkout of the anesthesia machine addresses the following areas: (1) checkout of emergency ventilation equipment, (2) checkout of the high-pressure system, (3) checkout of the low-pressure system including a low-pressure leak check and flowmeter function, (4) checkout of the scavenging system, (5) checkout of the breathing system including calibration of the oxygen monitor and a leak check, (6) checkout of the manual and automatic ventilation systems, including verification of the unidirectional valves, (7) checkout of all monitors, and (8) final readiness of the machine. Some of these steps can be eliminated for the same user on the same day, such as the emergency ventilation equipment, high- and low-pressure system check and the scavenging system check.

3. A circle system or a Mapleson D (Jackson Rees modification or Bain circuit) can be chosen for a patient this age. I would choose a circle system because it enables you to use a lower total fresh gas flow, although in a 2-month old, this does not make a significant difference. However, it is readily available and does not involve changing over equipment or modifying existing equipment with adapters. If one is routinely used to dealing with Mapleson D systems with infants and is more familiar with that anesthetic circuit in this setting, then the Mapleson D is probably the one to choose. The advantages and disadvantages of the valved/CO_2 absorption circuits vs. the nonvalved systems are as follows:

4. How warm should the room be prior to arrival?

   (a) How long will it take to warm to this temperature?
   (b) Should heat lamps be used? How far away? What difference does it make?
   (c) What is a thermal neutral environment? What temperature range are we talking about?
   (d) Should a blanket warmer be used? If so, should it go underneath the patient, or over the patient?
   (e) What about a Bair Hugger – should that be set up?
   (f) Is this patient at risk for hypothermia?

Bain circuits and Jackson Rees circuits are variations on the same theme; they are both Mapleson D types of systems, with the Jackson Rees circuit having a doubly open breathing bag (a Bain circuit can have one as well) and a fresh gas flow hose residing outside of the exhalation hose. The Bain circuit has the fresh gas flow hose residing within the exhalation hose, a coaxial type of breathing system. Pethick's test evaluates the integrity of the inner fresh gas flow hose of a Bain circuit by creating a Venturi effect designed to collapse the rebreathing bag. It is not foolproof, however, because the creation of turbulent fresh with too high a fresh gas flow during the test will interfere with the proper collapse of the rebreathing bag. The angulation of the fresh gas flow hose of a Mapleson D will interfere with creation of a Venturi effect.

4. The room should be sufficiently warm to allow reasonable maintenance of a thermal neutral environment during the time the patient is not anesthetized. Probably the first action to be taken in the room will be undressing the patient and applying monitors; this will result in significant radiant heat loss. Other considerations for heat loss include convection and conduction heat loss. Warming up the room temperature and applying heat lamps at the appropriate distance (about 2.5–3 m) will also allow for maintenance of a thermal neutral environment and ultimately guard against heat loss from the infant to the environment. The thermal neutral environment is that environmental temperature that minimizes the temperature gradient from the patient to the environment resulting in shivering and heat loss to the environment with the resultant thermal stress to the patient. A blanket warmer will specifically address conduction heat loss when applied under the patient, but will address convection and radiation heat loss (the majority of heat loss) when applied over the patient. A Bair hugger, or forced warm air warmer, will also address convection and radiation loss when placed above the patient and is also a good idea.

Intraoperative Care

1. Does this patient need an arterial line? Why/why not?

   (a) Can you get the same information from a pulse oximeter + end-tidal CO_2 analysis? What is the difference?

   (b) Is HbF a consideration for the accuracy of pulse oximeter monitoring? Why/why not?

   (c) How does the pulse oximeter work?

   (d) Is ETCO2 equivalent to PaCO2?

   (e) Under what circumstances is it different in a 5 kg baby?

   (f) What does the accuracy of ETCO2 depend upon in a 5 kg baby?

   (g) Where should the gas sample be taken from in the breathing circuit?

   (h) What alternatives are available?

   (i) How does a transducer work?

   (j) Would you need a precordial Doppler to do this case? How does a Doppler work?

   (k) Does this patient need a TEE? What size can you use in a 5 kg baby?

   (l) Is a spirometer more accurate when placed on the inspiratory limb, expiratory limb, or the elbow of a breathing circuit?

   (m) What problems arise as a result?

Intraoperative Care

1. The patient needs an arterial line for careful monitoring of blood pressure and blood gases. Although a pulse oximeter and $ETCO_2$ analysis will provide excellent feedback about the quality of oxygenation, ventilation and circulation, dynamic changes in the circulation as a result of intracranial reflexes and blood loss as well as air embolism will require rapid recognition, intervention and monitoring for therapeutic intervention, and an arterial line would be best. Hemoglobin F at this age should not significantly influence the accuracy of SpO_2 analysis; in fact, most pulse oximeters are not significantly affected by the presence of HbF. A pulse oximeter measures the ratio of the concentration of oxyhemoglobin to the combined concentration of oxy plus deoxyhemoglobin. The $ETCO_2$ is not the equivalent of $PaCO_2$ because it reflects the ratio of dead space to tidal volume, with a typical difference of 5–7 mmHg. In small infants and children, the accuracy of the $ETCO_2$ depends on the percent of the exhaled breath actually measured (which can vary because of the use of uncuffed endotracheal tubes) and the maximum expiratory flow rate of the patient relative to the sampling rate of the capnograph (the greater the patient's MEFR and the more rapid the sampling rate, the more accurate the $ETCO_2$ due to minimal "slurring" of the end-tidal trace). The gas sample should be taken as close to the patient's airway as possible; ideally, it should be sampled from within the endotracheal tube, but most typically, it is sampled from the elbow connector. A sampling "straw" which can be threaded from the luer-lock of the elbow connector into the endotracheal tube is available. Most modern pressure transducers at this point work by altering resistance across a Wheatstone bridge thereby altering voltage output and resulting in an electrical pattern in proportion to the pressure changes. A precordial Doppler might be useful for this case because the head in infants is proportionally larger than the rest of the body, therefore, the risk of the head being above the level of the right atrium is greater, although not tremendously so. There are other means of evaluating clinically significant pulmonary embolism such as the end-tidal CO_2, end-tidal nitrogen when available, and alterations in vital signs as well as the presence of a mill-wheel murmur by precordial stethoscopy. A Doppler measures the frequency changes of ultrasonic energy as a result of moving structures, which is why anatomic structures can be imaged by ultrasound. Because air is an excellent reflector of ultrasound energy, air within moving structures can be readily imaged. A TEE, while very sensitive for air embolism detection, is probably not necessary for this case. A 5 kg baby can accommodate a small TEE probe but probably not an adult TEE probe, which is about 12 mm. Spirometers are more accurate the closer they are to the patient because of compression volume considerations of the breathing circuit. Noncompliant tubing will help, but the compliance of anesthesia tubing is not insignificant; therefore, spirometers within the breathing circuit, while good for trend analysis, are not ideal for precise diagnostic work with lung volumes. The practical aspect of placing the spirometer at the level of the Y piece has to do with the amount of drag on the breathing circuit, because of the weight of the spirometer, potentially kinking the circuit or displacing the endotracheal tube unless it is well supported.

2. Can a rebreathing circuit be used for this patient? Why/why not?
   (a) How would you use one? Which would you choose?
   (b) How do you set rebreathing fresh gas flows?
   (c) What if the PaCO$_2$ is 40 at the settings you have chosen…how would you adjust?

3. The patient arrives with intravenous fluids on a continuous infusion syringe pump. The IV is obviously infiltrated. How did this happen?

   (a) Are there not there high-pressure alarms that would notify early?
   (b) Is there any mechanism that is safer?
   (c) What about a flow controller type of mechanism? A cassette pump?

4. You are using a semiclosed circle absorption system with pediatric tubing, and your ETCO$_2$ waveform looks like a sine wave with an elevated baseline. Interpretation? Differential?

   (a) How could you determine if this was a machine problem or a patient problem?
   (b) Do you need an arterial blood gas?
   (c) What effect does respiratory rate have on this capnogram?
   (d) How will you adjust your ventilator accordingly?
   (e) What determines descent of the bellows in an ascending bellows ventilator?
   (f) Where does this gas come from?
   (g) What effect does it rely upon to power the bellows through a ventilatory cycle?

2. A rebreathing circuit, such as some form of a Mapleson D (Jackson-Rees modification or Bain circuit) can be used taking into account the total fresh gas flow and minute ventilation necessary to produce hypocapnea. It does not really matter which is chosen because they work the same way. Rebreathing flows can be set by multiplying the body surface area by 2,500 mL/min for controlled ventilation and then delivering 2.5 times the fresh gas flow as minute ventilation. If the $PaCO_2$ is higher than you want, both the fresh gas flow and the minute ventilation have to be increased because they are dynamically related to each other in a partial rebreathing circuit. If the $PaCO_2$ is 40 mmHg and you want to decrease it to 30, it would be reasonable to multiply the fresh gas flow rate by 40/30 and then increase the minute ventilation accordingly.

3. A continuous infusion syringe pump is designed to continue pumping even as tissue resistance increases because of an infiltrate, unlike a freely dripping IV, which will not continue infusing once tissue resistance is elevated because of the infiltrate. The pressure alarm on a continuous infusion pump has a higher set point than that of a drip pump. The safest method of infusion with regard to an ongoing IV infiltrate is a gravity drip chamber on IV tubing. A flow controller pump typically has a lower alarm point, because it is basically a drip chamber with an "eye" for reading the volume infused. A cassette pump works in a fashion similar to a continuous infusion syringe pump, and is also pressurized and alarmed.

4. An elevated baseline with an inspired CO_2 concentration is often accompanied by more gradual upsloping and downsloping of the tracing; this usually reflects an increase in mechanical deadspace and is not surprising during mask ventilation. It is usually corrected after endotracheal intubation when the excess deadspace is eliminated. In smaller patients, the elbow connector as well as the volume of deadspace in the Y piece can represent a significant volume of mechanical deadspace and therefore a divided Y piece and elimination of the elbow connector may correct the problem. Also, the CO_2 sample can be obtained from within the endotracheal tube by passing a straw sampler through the luer lock of the Y piece. The more rapid the respiratory rate the greater the tendency to slur the capnographic trace; therefore, decreasing the respiratory rate may enhance the mixing and emptying of the lungs of CO_2 and therefore improve the accuracy of the waveform. Descent of the bellows in an ascending bellows ventilator is determined by gravity, airway leak, the total fresh gas flow, and the volume returned by the patient.

5. About 1 h into the case, after skin incision, dissection of the calvarium and elevation of the bone flap, the ETCO$_2$ suddenly drops, concomitant with the onset of
   bradycardia and hypotension.

   (a) What do you think is going on?
   (b) What would you need to confirm the diagnosis?
   (c) What if this occurred just when the table turned, but there was no skin inci-
       sion yet?

6. The patient is now 33.8°C.

   (a) How did this happen?
   (b) Where did it happen?
   (c) What mechanisms of heat loss are most significant?
   (d) Efficient at replacing lost heat?
   (e) Is monitoring of temperature a standard of practice?
   (f) Is it worthwhile putting in a heat and moisture exchanger in the breathing
       circuit at this time?
   (g) Earlier?
   (h) What advantage over heated humidifier?
   (i) What are some of the problems with both?

7. You decide to transfuse, and the nurse brings you cold blood from the refrigerator,
   which she checks with you to your satisfaction.

   (a) Now what? How to warm? Why?
   (b) What different methods are available?
   (c) What about filters? How large? What particles? How important?
   (d) How does a countercurrent blood warmer work?
   (e) Is there a warmer available on the rapid infusion system?
   (f) What is a dry heat warmer?

5. Venous air embolism with a right ventricular airlock and impairment of the pulmonary circulation is high on the list of suspicions. The diagnosis can be confirmed by TEE but it would probably be faster to confirm the physiology of a pulmonary embolism (high Vd/Vt) by drawing an arterial blood gas and looking for a wide discrepancy between the $PaCO_2$ (elevated because of impaired gas exchange) and the $ETCO_2$ (decreased because of the drop in CO_2 delivery to the pulmonary circulation, as well as the drop in cardiac output). If this occurred prior to incision, you would have to suspect an air embolism from another source, such as the IV tubing from an unprimed IV line.

6. It is relatively easy to lose track of temperature loss in infants; just in the induction, prep and drape (which can often take 45 min) the patient's temperature may drift down significantly. Radiation heat loss is probably the culprit in most cases. In well-ventilated rooms, and particularly laminar flow rooms, convection losses may play a significant role, as well as conduction heat losses to the operating room equipment such as the mattress pad. While monitoring of temperature is not a standard of practice (for adults) and is only required on an "availability basis", it is good to monitor the temperature of all children in the operating room. A passive heat and moisture exchanger will conserve water vapor loss from the tracheobronchial tree (and therefore provides a small advantage with regard to temperature conservation because of the defense against the expenditure of calories for the latent heat of vaporization of water), it will not help very much when the patient is already at $33.8°C$. The heated humidifier, on the other hand, will provide a high relative humidity plus calories to the patient; there is a danger of airway burns with the "cascade" type of humidifier.

7. Refrigerated blood should be warmed prior to administration because it can lower body temperature significantly (storage temperature of blood is $4°C$). The most common method of warming blood is to pass it through a blood warmer in a diluted (with normal saline) or undiluted state. Not diluting the blood will result in a slower infusion time because of rheological factors. The same factors will be improved if the blood is diluted with normal saline and then run through a blood warmer. Clot and microaggregates tend to increase with the duration of blood storage and a standard 170-μ blood filter on infusion sets does not effectively filter some of these particles. Micropore filters (40μ) may be useful if massive transfusion is anticipated, but their use is still unproven; to the extent that they interfere with rapid transfusion during massive blood loss, they may be more of a hindrance than help in some circumstances. Countercurrent blood warmers work by using a continuous flow of warmed water in a coaxial tube external to the sterile blood path, running against the direction of flow. There is a warmer available on the rapid infusion system. A dry heat warmer consists of two hot plates that are applied to tubing running between them to warm the blood infused.

Postoperative

1. The infant is active, crying, and moving all extremities, but is so vigorous that the pulse oximeter is not obtaining a reading. The PACU nurses are concerned that this may represent hypoxia.

   (a) Even if you do not think is clinically likely, how can you get the pulse oximeter to read?
   (b) What are the advantages and disadvantages of the signal-to-noise ratio algorithms designed to improve the performance of a pulse oximeter placed on an active child?
   (c) Would it be worthwhile to change the operating mode of the pulse oximeter, and if so, for a longer or shorter averaging time?
   (d) Is residual hemoglobin F a significant consideration at this age? What if the infant was 2 weeks old?
   (e) If the baby is sedated but is so cool and peripherally vasoconstricted that the signal for the pulse oximeter is weak, what could you as an anesthesiologist do to improve the situation?

2. The PACU nurse attaches an automated oscillometric blood pressure cuff to the baby but again has difficulty obtaining consistent readings.

   (a) Why is this so?
   (b) What can you do to make it better?
   (c) How do you select the appropriate sized cuff?

Postoperative

1. A pulse oximeter rarely functions well when it is placed on an active child. Algorithms for improving the signal-to-noise ratio are built into most pulse oximeters, but they interfere with the response time and accuracy. The operating mode can be changed to increase accuracy of reading with different levels of patient activity. This works by changing the averaging time; a 5–7 s averaging time is typical for an inactive patient, while a 2–3 s averaging time is useful for sleep studies but is more affected by patient motion. Lengthening the averaging time up 10–15 s will enhance accuracy during patient movement. Most pulse oximeters are not affected by the presence of fetal hemoglobin, nor by the color of the skin or the bilirubin level (important for hyperbilirubinemia during infancy). To improve the signal of a poorly perfused patient, local warmth can be applied, a digital nerve block, or vasodilating cream. For arterial vasospasm, intraarterial vasodilators may be administered.

2. Automated oscillometric blood pressure cuffs rely on incremental reductions in the pressure in the cuff and require at least two cardiac cycles for their measurements. Patient movement, irregularities of cardiac rhythm or external influences such as someone pressing on the cuff can affect the accuracy of the reading, and successive cardiac cycles will continue to be compared (and the blood pressure determination will be prolonged) until two comparable cycles are recorded at a given cuff pressure. This prolonged cycling duration may cause a great deal of discomfort for awake children and prolong the cycle even more. Sometimes repositioning the cuff to a lower extremity is a successful strategy. Other times, supplemental sedation or analgesia to relieve the surgical pain will ultimately make it easier to monitor the patient during their PACU stay. The proper width for the bladder of the blood pressure cuff should be 0.4–0.5 times the circumference, or 140% of the diameter, of the extremity. The length of the cuff's bladder should be twice the width of the extremity.

Additional Questions

1. What methods exist to compensate for the loss of energy when a liquid is vaporized? What happens to the vapor pressure as the temperature of the liquid decreases?

2. How does a Clark polarographic oxygen electrode work? Given a choice of where you could place it in the breathing system, where would that be? For what purpose?

3. How can you safely perform surgery in a patient with an implanted cardioverter defibrillator (ICD)?

Additional Questions

1. As the temperature of the liquid decreases due to heat energy being lost, the vapor pressure decreases as well. A constant vapor output can be maintained only by compensating for this heat loss. One method is by altering the splitting ratio so that the percent of carrier gas coursing through the vaporizing chamber is changed via thermal compensation, either mechanically by a bimetallic strip that responds to changes in temperature or electronically. As an alternative, heat can be supplied to the vaporizer by an electric heater.

2. A polarographic electrode works by displaying the percent concentration of oxygen detected as a change in current across a gas permeable membrane on one side of which is an anode and the other side a cathode, as well as electrolyte solution. There is also a power source to induce a potential difference between the anode and the cathode. When oxygen molecules diffuse across the membrane and the electrolyte, the oxygen molecules are reduced to hydroxide ions. The probe may basically be positioned on the inspiratory or expiratory limb of the circuit. The advantage of positioning the probe on the inspiratory limb is that it serves to verify the inspired oxygen concentration, is not subject to moisture as it would be on the expiratory limb (where the moisture can effect the membrane permeability and electrolyte solution stability therefore rendering the reading less reliable) and is not subject to any carbon dioxide (which can also affect the electrolyte solution and potential difference, therefore the accuracy of the reading).

3. The danger with the ICD is that the current from the electrocautery may be detected as a tachyarrhythmia and actuate the device causing shocks. The tachyarrhythmia detection should be deactivated before the procedure and then reactivated at the conclusion of the procedure. In addition, the grounding pad should be positioned in such a way as to minimize the flow of current through the ICD, which may damage the electrodes of the ICD. For ICDs that also function as pacemakers, they are more sensitive to electromagnetic interference, resulting in inhibition of the pacing function. A temporary pacing electrode should be placed for external transthoracic pacing. Finally, bipolar as opposed to monopolar cautery should be used whenever possible, and this should be discussed with the surgical team beforehand. If not possible, then the current should be limited to short bursts with long (10 s) intervals at the lowest effective cutting or coagulation settings possible [1].

Specific References

1. Pinski S (2000) Emergencies related to implantable cardioverter-defibrillators. Crit Care Med 28:N174–180

General References

2. Dorsch J, Dorsch S (2007) Understanding anesthesia equipment, 5th edn. Lippincott Williams & Wilkins, Philadelphia
3. Holzman R (1997) Equipment for pediatric anesthesia. In: Sosis M (ed) The anesthesia equipment manual. Philadelphia, Lippincott-Raven, pp 195–217

Chapter 31
Post Anesthesia Care Unit (PACU)

R.S. Holzman et al., *Pediatric Anesthesiology Review: Clinical Cases for Self-Assessment,*
DOI 10.1007/978-1-4419-1617-4_31, © Springer Science+Business Media, LLC 2010

Pain Management

A healthy 4-year old has just undergone open reduction internal fixation of a mid-shaft femur fracture under general endotracheal anesthesia with an epidural in place which appeared to be functioning well during surgery. You are called to the bedside because he is in excruciating pain, clenching his teeth, crying, and he and his parents are wild.

1. How will you manage his pain?

2. How can you confirm your epidural placement? How long would you wait?

3. You test it, and it does not appear to be working. The parents say that their other child received "shots" at another hospital, and did not have *any* of these problems. The patient does not have any relief after 20 min. What other treatment is appropriate?

Pain Management

1. It is important to determine, with as much certainly as possible, that the child's distress is due to surgical pain, not nausea, a full urinary bladder, emergence delirium, anxiety, an NG tube or the tightness of the cast. It may not be possible to accomplish this at the moment at the bedside, however, and the assumption should always be that the child is indeed experiencing surgical pain until proven otherwise. The pain can be treated with IV opioids or the administration of an appropriate dose of a rapid-onset local anesthetic via the epidural catheter. If the epidural infusion used during the anesthetic in the OR contained an opioid, it is important to note the type and amount of narcotic given during the surgical procedure. If the choice is to administer IV opioids, it makes sense not to expose the child to another narcotic. Dosing must be done carefully, however, in view of the possibility of synergy between the neuraxial opioid and intravenous opioid leading to excessive depression of respiratory drive. Once the child is comfortable, the utility of the epidural catheter should be assessed as described below. This will be complicated by the age of the child and the fact the child now has adequate analgesia.

2. If the child's discomfort is such that the few minutes needed for rapid-onset epidural local anesthetics to provide comfort would not cause excessive distress, the catheter position can be tested. Epidural analgesia is a safe and effective analgesic regimen for children [1–3]. Administration of lidocaine will provide a solid sensory block in a relatively short period of time. When administering lidocaine, it is important to consider the dose of local anesthetic that has already been given via the epidural catheter. Local anesthetic toxicity is additive so that a maximum dose of lidocaine given to a child who has been receiving an infusion of local anesthetic will result in that child receiving a total dose above the safe limit. An alternative to assess the epidural catheter is to use 3-chloroprocaine, a drug with an even quicker onset and also a very short duration and better safety profile. In addition, the blockade achieved will be both sensory and motor, perhaps allowing a more accurate assessment of the effectiveness of the epidural catheter.

3. If it appears that the child is receiving no analgesia from the drugs given into the epidural space, that technique must be abandoned and another modality begun as soon as possible. If, after administration of appropriate doses of IV opioid, the child still is uncomfortable, additional doses should be given, titrated to respiratory rate. In addition, adjuncts should be considered. These include oral or rectal acetaminophen or parenteral ketorolac, an effective nonsteroidal analgesic. Although, there is some evidence that ketorolac may affect formation of new bone, it seems to be much more of a problem following spinal fusions, and when many doses are used. Many orthopedic surgeons agree with the use of ketorolac for 24–36 h in the treatment of pain associated with long bone fractures. However, it is important to discuss this therapy with the operative orthopedist prior to administration of ketorolac. In addition to other analgesics, antiemetics and/or anxiolytics should be considered for this child. If benzodiazepines are used, the clinician must be aware of the synergistic effect on respiratory drive these drugs have with opioids.

4. He pulled out his IV in the meantime; should he receive IM morphine before you attempt to reinsert the IV?

Postoperative Nausea and Vomiting

A 15-year-old girl has just undergone laparoscopy for endometriosis. She had a general endotracheal anesthetic. You are called to the bedside because she feels continuously nauseous, has retched a few times, and now has bile-tinged vomitus. She received 4 mg of ondansetron and 10 mg of metoclopramide as part of her anesthetic management.

1. Is there anything else you can offer? Should she have a nasogastric tube placed? You note that one was not passed in the OR – does this make a difference in perioperative nausea and vomiting? Why?

2. Should droperidol be added at this point?

4. If the child now has no IV, venous access should be reestablished as quickly as possible, but it is not an emergency. There is likely time for application of EMLA or, alternatively, the use of other topical analgesics prior to placement of an IV. An IV will be needed for fluid and medication administration. IM medication should be used only as a last resort. Opioid administration to children via PCA/NCA is a good option [4, 5].

Postoperative Nausea and Vomiting

Postoperative nausea and vomiting (PONV) is a complex phenomenon. The young lady in this case has several risk factors for PONV. She is female, has undergone abdominal surgery, and has had general anesthesia with endotracheal intubation. She was given appropriate prophylaxis with a serotonin antagonist and metoclopramide, a medication that stimulates gastric peristalsis through the blockade of dopaminergic receptors. It is used clinically as an antiemetic and as an aid to gastric emptying in conditions with delayed gastric emptying. In the PACU, the OR course should be carefully reviewed. Prophylaxis for PONV can be accomplished with the administration of a serotonin antagonist, dexamethasone or droperidol (at doses <1 mg). Metoclopramide, used in standard clinical doses, has not been effective in prevention of PONV [6, 7].

1. Since prophylaxis with a serotonin antagonist has failed, further treatment with a drug in the same class is not likely to yield good results. Another class of medication, such as promethazine or droperidol can be given. Promethazine (Phenergan®) is a phenothiazine derivative with antiemetic, antihistaminic, anticholinergic, and sedative effects. Although emptying the stomach might have helped decrease this girl's PONV, the trauma of NG tube placement puts that particular intervention lower on the list. Inadequate fluid resuscitation can contribute to PONV and if there is any indication that she has not received sufficient IV fluid, this should be corrected. Dexamethasone is another treatment shown to be effective in prevention of PONV [8, 9].

2. Droperidol is a major tranquilizer belonging to the group of drugs known as butyrophenone antipsychotics. It has antiemetic and sedative effects. In 2001, the FDA issued a black box warning about the use of this drug, describing cases of prolonged QT interval and torsades de pointes in patients given droperidol at or below the recommended doses. Performance of a 12-lead ECG to check for prolonged QTc (>440 ms for females, >450 ms for males) prior to administration of droperidol is recommended. In addition, ECG monitoring for 2–3 h following administration of droperidol is recommended. This report is based on ten cases collected over many years. No case of prolonged QTc or arrthymia has been reported after administration of the small doses of droperidol used to treat PONV [10, 11].

3. On which limb of the emetogenic response does each of the typically utilized antiemetics work?

4. Are some anesthetic techniques better than others for perioperative emesis control?

5. Are some operations more emetogenic than others?

6. What about total intravenous anesthesia with propofol and avoidance of nitrous oxide? How does that work?

7. Is it safe to discharge this patient home? What are you concerned about?

8. What are the optimal times to administer antiemetics?

3. Vomiting is mediated via the vomiting center and the chemoreceptor trigger zone (CTZ) located in the brainstem. The vomiting center is in the reticular formation and the CTZ is located in the floor of the fourth ventricle. The vomiting center is activated directly by visceral afferent impulses from the pharynx, peritoneum, bile ducts, coronary vessels, and the cortex. The CTZ is located on the blood side of the blood–brain barrier and cannot cause vomiting without an intact vomiting center. The exact pathways that cause nausea are not known for certain but it is assumed that they are the same as the pathways described that cause vomiting. Stimuli associated with nausea include pain and memories as well as labyrinthine stimulation.

4. Various alterations in anesthetic technique have been shown to reduce the incidence of PONV. Patients who receive regional anesthesia are at much lower risk for PONV compared to those who are given general anesthesia. When general anesthesia is administered, avoiding or minimizing the use of nitrous oxide has a similar effect in decreasing the incidence of PONV. When propofol is used as the intravenous anesthetic agent, its use is associated with a lower incidence of PONV compared with the potent inhaled vapors. Reversal of neuromuscular blockade with neostigmine is also associated with a higher incidence of PONV. Opioids are well known to be associated with nausea and vomiting [12].

5. Certain surgical procedures are associated with higher incidence of vomiting, although the reasons are not always obvious. Some of these procedures are laparoscopy, laparotomy, ENT procedures, breast surgery, and strabismus surgery [8, 10, 13].

6. In large survey reviews of postanesthetic nausea and vomiting, risk factors identified include the use of nitrous oxide, neostigmine reversal of NMB, and opioids [12]. The potent inhaled agents, although also considered medications that increase the incidence of PONV, are not as clearly identified with this problem. Total intravenous anesthesia (TIVA) with propofol, oxygen, regional analgesia or peripheral nerve blocks, nonopioid analgesia if not contraindicated by the specifics of the surgical procedure or anesthetic requirements can be recommended for patients with a history of severe PONV.

7. In this patient, concerns with discharge include the possibility of dehydration due to continued emesis without PO intake and also bleeding or other surgical complication from repeated forceful contraction of the abdominal muscles. A trial of 2–3 h IV hydration and administration of another antiemetic of a different class than serotonin antagonists might improve the situation. If the girl is then able to tolerate PO clear liquids, she may be safely discharged home.

8. There is no consensus regarding prophylactic vs. rescue treatment of PONV [14]. While it is true that many patients must be given prophylactic treatment to prevent one case of clinically significant PONV, the administration of a serotonin receptor antagonist is very safe. Prophylactic treatment for patients with moderate to high risk for PONV seems a sensible course [15].

Cardiovascular System

You arrive in the intensive care unit with a 13-year-old girl after just finishing a posterior spinal fusion from T6 to L5 with an estimated blood loss of 3,000 mL and a volume replacement of three autologous units of packed red blood cells, 500 mL of cell saver blood, and a reasonable (2 L) amount of crystalloid. She looks pasty on arrival, BP = 50/20 mmHg and a heart rate of 76 bpm.

1. What do you think is going on? Why?

2. Why did these findings become apparent now, and not earlier?

3. Why do you think she is not tachycardic? Could this be anything else? What?

4. She seems sleepy when you try to awaken. her? What are you concerned about? What can you do?

Cardiovascular System

1. This patient has deficient intravascular volume. Significant blood loss is an expected part of scoliosis surgery [16–18]. If we assume that the patient's weight preoperatively was 50 kg, her calculated blood volume would be 3,500 mL. Her EBL, therefore, is approximately one blood volume. The volume she has been transfused is approximately 800 mL autologous PRBC, 500 mL cell-saver, and 2,000 mL crystalloid. If we assume a one-to-one replacement of blood lost with PRBC and cell saver, those products have "replaced" approximately 1,300 mL of her 3,500 mL blood loss with approximately 2,200–2,500 mL of crystalloid. Replenishment of intravascular volume lost from intraoperative bleeding with crystalloid is generally at a 3:1 ratio. In this case, then, adequate IV fluid replacement for the blood loss would be in the neighborhood of 6,000 mL, not the 2,000 given in the OR. The likely explanation for the pasty appearance and hypotension is inadequate preload.

2. Once the surgery had been completed, there was much less stimulation and the sympathetic tone that had been partially responsible (presumably) for BP maintenance has now greatly diminished.

3. The hypotension is not accompanied by tachycardia as would be expected. There are several possible explanations for the low heart rate. The anesthetic may have included high dose fentanyl, or, if induced hypotension was part of the technique, beta-blockers may have been given. Alternatively, it may be that, during the procedure, there was significant spinal cord ischemia that has led to loss of sympathetic tone as well as loss of the cardio-accelerator innervation of the heart. If there were abnormalities in the SSEP tracings during the case, this possibility should be given careful consideration [19]. In any case the lack of a heart rate response to the inadequate preload is only worsening the clinical picture here and increasing the importance of rapid expansion of the intravascular volume [20].

4. An ABG taken at this point would likely show a metabolic acidosis. This is an urgent situation. The child may be at the limit of her ability to sustain an inadequate intravascular volume without suffering a cardiac or respiratory arrest. The ABG obtained will include a hemoglobin measurement and that number will guide IV fluid therapy. Fluid resuscitation should begin immediately with available crystalloid. Once a hemoglobin is available and colloid has become available the specific fluid given can be tailored to the situation. Consideration should be given to measurement of central venous pressure if there is not a rapid improvement in the blood pressure once intravascular volume has been even partially replenished. Sleepiness can also be the result of intraoperative medications, specifically opioids. Opioid effects include somnolence and depression of respiratory drive. If the ABG shows elevated $PaCO_2$, opioid-induced depression of her respiratory drive must be considered. Whether or not to treat this with a reversal agent like naloxone depends upon the degree of hypercarbia. Naloxone administration in this setting must be undertaken carefully, starting with low doses. The starting dose of naloxone for respiratory depression in this case should be 1 mcg/kg IV with additional doses given as needed.

Respiratory Failure

An 18-month old underwent uneventful tonsillectomy/adenoidectomy for peripheral and central sleep apnea, received 3 mcg/kg fentanyl with a sevoflurane/oxygen/nitrous oxide anesthetic. He awakened in the OR, but now you are called to the bedside for periodic breathing, breath holding, and an O_2 saturation of 86%.

1. What do you think is going on? Is this simply hypoventilation? Could it be anything else?

2. What effect would his underlying disease have on the pulmonary circulation that might be contributing to this picture?

3. What if he had laryngospasm at the end of the case – would this change the differential diagnosis? Why?

4. You obtain an ABG and his pH 7.24, $pCO_2 = 48$ mmHg and $pO_2 = 56$ mmHg. What now? What do you think is wrong? Should he be reintubated?

Respiratory Failure

1. This is an urgent situation. As the delivered FiO_2 is increased, the child must be quickly evaluated and the cause determined. Hypoxemia in the PACU can be, and often is, the result of hypoventilation. If the child had been receiving supplemental oxygen and still developed hypoxemia, s/he must have had significant hypoventilation to result in an SpO_2 in the mid 80s. Alternatively, there may be another cause for the hypoxemia. The child may have a decreased functional residual capacity (FRC) due to atelectaisis or extra-vascular lung water that has led to the hypoxemia on the basis of V/Q mismatch. It is important to treat the oximeter reading as accurate and begin therapy and evaluation. However, it is possible that the reading of 86% does not represent the true arterial saturation. If the child is breatholding, it is possible that the valsalva maneuver that accompanies breatholding has "arterialized" the blood the oximeter light is passing through and the reading of 86% does not represent the true arterial saturation. The pulse oximeter calculates SpO_2 using an algorithm based on the differential absorption of red and infrared light by HbO_2 and Hb. HbO_2 absorbs less light in the red wavelength and more in the infrared wavelength. Absorption of light of 800 nm wavelength is identical by both HbO_2 and Hb. In cases of probe malposition or movement artifact, the algorithm may calculate an inaccurate SPO_2 and when this happens the monitor reads an SPO_2 of 85–86%.

2. In addition to hypoventilation, other possible causes of this situation include shunt or V/Q mismatch. If this child has reactive pulmonary vasculature and elevated pulmonary vascular resistance as a result of longstanding obstructive sleep apnea, a brief period of hypoxemia may lead to a longer period of pulmonary artery hypertension with a resulting shunt at the atrial level across a patent foramen ovale. It is possible that longstanding elevated pulmonary artery pressure has resulted in right heart failure (cor pulmonale).

3. If the child had laryngospasm following extubation at the end of the case, another cause for the hypoxemia would be pulmonary edema. Occasionally, after laryngospasm, vigorous inspiration against a closed glottis can lead to the rapid development of negative pressure pulmonary edema. This can be diagnosed on the basis of typical findings on both physical exam and plain CXR.

4. The ABG shows a mixed respiratory and metabolic acidosis. There is moderate hypercarbia and a more severe acidosis than would be caused by the $PaCO_2$ alone. It can be assumed that the child has not had chronic hypercarbia and this can be confirmed by measurement of the bicarbonate. Hypoxemia is also present but the degree cannot be ascertained without knowledge of the FiO_2. The hypoxemia is concerning but if the ABG were done while the child's FiO_2 was low, then intubation and distending airway pressure may not be indicated. The decision whether or not to reintubate should be made on the entire picture, the condition of the child and the expected course he will take over the next 30–60 min.

Postintubation Croup

A 3-month old just underwent direct laryngoscopy/bronchoscopy for stridor evaluation. He has subglottic stenosis as a result of intubation as a neonate, and received some decadron in the OR. In the PACU, the baby is crying, working very hard to breathe, is retracting intensely, and the nurses are unable to obtain a sat reading, but appears pink although in distress.

1. What might be going on?

2. What is a croup score?

Postintubation Croup

1. The baby likely has postintubation stridor. Postoperative, postintubation stridor occurs in approximately 1% of children, particularly in children <4 years of age [21, 22]. The syndrome is the result of edema of the tracheal wall below the level of the vocal cords. The mucosa in this area is not as tightly joined to the submucosa so that when edema develops there, the lumen is compromised to a greater degree than it would be if the mucosa and submucosa were tightly adherent to each other. Resistance to airflow in the trachea is inversely proportional to the radius taken to the fourth power for laminar flow and to the fifth power for turbulent flow. With subglottic edema and increased respiratory rate and effort the gas flow will be turbulent. In this situation, the flow is now inversely proportional to the radius to the fifth power. Therefore, the smaller the tracheal lumen prior to the development of subglottic edema, the more likely it is that any edema will lead to clinical symptoms.

    The Poiselle equation describes the relationship among the variables described above:

$$P = \frac{8Q\mu L}{\pi R^4}$$

where Q is the volumetric flow rate, in.^{3}/s, μ is the viscosity, lb·s/in.^{2}, L is the tube length, in., and R is the tube radius, in.

Some risk factors have been identified for the development of this problem. Tight-fitting endotracheal tubes, movement of the head and neck while intubated, intubation for ≥ 1 h and the presence of a URI may predispose the child to the development of postintubation croup [21, 23, 24]. Stridor usually develops soon after extubation and can worsen for several hours after it first is clinically apparent. In this case, the airway manipulations, including rigid bronchoscopy, are the causes of the stridor. In the situation where the SPO_2 is not reading, it is important to administer a high FiO_2. Without a reliable SPO_2 measurement, one must rely on the clinical picture in evaluating the patient.

2. Downes and Raphley developed the Croup Score as an aid to the clinical evaluation of children with this syndrome, either due to infection or postintubation [25]. The score does not include the SPO_2 measurement and uses clinical parameters to assign a score that reflects the severity of respiratory embarrassment. A score of 0–3 is given for each of five aspects of respiration: stridor, retractions, air entry, color (normal of cyanotic) and level of consciousness, and a score derived (below). The higher the score, the more severe the respiratory compromise. While the determination of a croup score does help the clinician apply a more rigorous assessment to the child with stridor, the variables assessed are not independent. As the condition worsens, all variables will worsen together.

3. How does decadron work to prevent postintubation edema? Is it effective if administered post hoc what will you do?

4. Will sedation help? Does cool mist help? In what way?

5. Would administration of nebulized racemic epinephrine help the child? How much would you give? How would you administer it?

6. Should this baby be reintubated? Why? What size tube would you choose?

Hyperthermia

You are called to the bedside of a 10-month old who has just undergone a cleft palate repair. He has a temperature of 41.2°C.

1. What might have happened that his temperature got to this point?

Criteria	0	1	2	3
Stridor	None	With agitation	Mild	Severe
Retractions	None	Mild	Moderate	Severe
Air entry	Normal	Mild decrease	Moderate decr.	Severe decr.
Color	Normal	N/A	N/A	Cyanotic
LOC	Normal	Restless	Restless	Lethargic

3. Treatment of postintubation stridor includes the administration of dexamethasone (decadron), a potent, longer acting glucocorticoid. This medication will act to limit the degree of inflammation and the severity of the subglottic edema. Decadron administration will not decrease edema already present, however [26, 27].

4. Sedation should be avoided. Depression of respiratory drive is dangerous in this situation. Nebulized racemic epinephrine may help by actually decreasing the degree of subglottic edema. The duration of the effect is generally 1 h or less.

5. Nebulized racemic epinephrine will act to decrease the subglottic edema. Once racemic epinephrine has been administered to a child with postintubation croup, the child should be admitted for observation with the expectation that subsequent doses will be needed. The usual dose of racemic epinephrine is 0.5 mL of the 2.25% solution diluted into 3–5 mL of NS and administered via a nebulizer. The mask is held near the child's face with 100% oxygen used to nebulized the solution.

6. In the event that reintubation is necessary, a smaller than normal endotracheal tube should be used. Intubating conditions should be as good as possible in order that the intubation not cause additional trauma. The narrowed part of the airway, the subglottis, will not be visible to the laryngoscopist but if the tube meets resistance once the tip is beyond the vocal cords, a smaller diameter tube should be used.

Hyperthermia

1. Postoperative hyperthermia usually is the result of excessive warming and is more common in pediatric patients than adult patients. In cases such as repair of cleft palate, the child is well covered by surgical drapes. If warming is undertaken during the case with devices such as forced hot air mattresses, warming blankets, humidification, and warming of inspired gases, the child's core body temperature could easily rise to the level noted in the cases here. Hyperthermia in the PACU that is the result of excessive warming in the OR generally dissipates rather quickly once the sources of additional heat are removed. If the elevated temperature persists, other causes must be sought.

2. Could this represent malignant hyperthermia? Why/why not?

2. It is possible that the temperature elevation is part of a response to systemic infection. Of course, any case of temperature elevation should bring the possibility of malignant hyperthermia to mind. The anesthetic record should be reviewed to learn the time course of the temperature elevation and to review the medications administered during the anesthetic. It is likely that the child would have been exposed to potent inhaled agents during the anesthetic. The presentation described here would be quite unusual for malignant hyperthermia. Most cases of malignant hyperthermia develop within the first few hours of an anesthetic, but there are reports of MH occurring well after the conclusion of a case. It is also unusual for fever to be the presenting sign of an episode of MH. Often tachycardia, hypertension and tachypnea are noted first. If the child in this case were developing MH, mottled skin and muscle rigidity would be expected. The most consistent laboratory finding in cases of MH is a combined respiratory and metabolic acidosis. If MH is being considered in this child, laboratory evaluation should be done prior to instituting any therapy [28, 29].

Annotated References

Desparmet JF, Hardart RA, Yaster M (2002) Central blocks in children and adolescents. Chap. 20. In: Pain in infants children and adolescents, 2nd edn. Lippincott Williams & Wilkins, Philadelphia, pp 339–362

The authors, leaders in the field of pediatric pain treatment, review all central neuraxial blocks in children. Relevant anatomy and physiology is discussed first followed by review of the technical aspects and medications used in caudals, epidurals, and spinals in that order.

Yaster M, Kost-Byerly S, Maxwell, LG (2002) Opioid agonists and antagonists. Chap. 12. In: Pain in infants children and adolescents, 2nd edn. Lippincott Williams & Wilkins, Philadelphia, pp 181–224

In this chapter, the authors undertake a thorough review of opioid receptor physiology, structure and functional differences and similarities among the commonly used opioids. In addition, dosing regimens, schedules, and various routes for administration are discussed. Tolerance, addiction, and physical dependence are defined and contrasted.

Gan TJ, Meyer TA, Apfel CC et al (2007) Society for ambulatory anesthesia guidelines for the management of postoperative nausea and vomiting. Anesth Analg 105:1615–1628

The present guidelines were compiled by a multidisciplinary international panel of individuals with interest and expertise in postoperative nausea and vomiting (PONV). These guidelines identify risk factors for PONV in adults and children; recommend approaches for reducing baseline risks for PONV; identify the most effective antiemetic monotherapy and combination therapy regimens for PONV prophylaxis; recommend approaches for treatment of PONV when it occurs; and provide an algorithm for the management of individuals at increased risk for PONV.

References

1. Llewellyn N, Moriarty A (2007) The national pediatric epidural audit. Paediatr Anaesth 17:520–533
2. Adams HA, Saatweber P, Schmitz CS, Hecker H (2002) Postoperative pain management in orthopaedic patients: no differences in pain score, but improved stress control by epidural anaesthesia. Eur J Anaesthesiol 19:658–665
3. Jorgensen H, Wetterslev J, Moiniche S, Dahl JB (2000) Epidural local anaesthetics versus opioid-based analgesic regimens on postoperative gastrointestinal paralysis, PONV and pain after abdominal surgery. Cochrane Database Syst Rev 2000:CD001893.
4. Monitto CL, Greenberg RS, Kost-Byerly S et al (2000) The safety and efficacy of parent-/ nurse-controlled analgesia in patients less than six years of age. Anesth Analg 91:573–579
5. Anghelescu DL, Burgoyne LL, Oakes LL, Wallace DA (2005) The safety of patient-controlled analgesia by proxy in pediatric oncology patients. Anesth Analg 101:1623–1627
6. Gan TJ, Meyer T, Apfel CC et al (2003) Consensus guidelines for managing postoperative nausea and vomiting. Anesth Analg 97:62–71
7. Gan TJ, Meyer TA, Apfel CC et al (2007) Society for ambulatory anesthesia guidelines for the management of postoperative nausea and vomiting. Anesth Analg 105:1615–1628
8. Subramaniam B, Madan R, Sadhasivam S et al (2001) Dexamethasone is a cost-effective alternative to ondansetron in preventing PONV after paediatric strabismus repair. Br J Anaesth 86:84–89
9. Gunter JB, McAuliffe JJ, Beckman EC et al (2006) A factorial study of ondansetron, metoclopramide, and dexamethasone for emesis prophylaxis after adenotonsillectomy in children. Paediatr Anaesth 16:1153–1165
10. Stead SW, Beatie CD, Keyes MA, Isenberg SJ (2004) Effects of droperidol dosage on postoperative emetic symptoms following pediatric strabismus surgery. J Clin Anesth 16:34–39
11. Domino KB, Anderson EA, Polissar NL, Posner KL (1999) Comparative efficacy and safety of ondansetron, droperidol, and metoclopramide for preventing postoperative nausea and vomiting: a meta-analysis. Anesth Analg 88:1370–1379
12. Visser K, Hassink EA, Bonsel GJ et al (2001) Randomized controlled trial of total intravenous anesthesia with propofol versus inhalation anesthesia with isoflurane-nitrous oxide: postoperative nausea with vomiting and economic analysis. Anesthesiology 95:616–626
13. Broadman LM, Ceruzzi W, Patane PS et al (1990) Metoclopramide reduces the incidence of vomiting following strabismus surgery in children. Anesthesiology 72:245–248
14. Tang J, Wang B, White PF et al (1998) The effect of timing of ondansetron administration on its efficacy, cost-effectiveness, and cost-benefit as a prophylactic antiemetic in the ambulatory setting. Anesth Analg 86:274–282
15. Apfel CC, Korttila K, Abdalla M et al (2004) A factorial trial of six interventions for the prevention of postoperative nausea and vomiting. N Engl J Med 350:2441–2451
16. Meert KL, Kannan S, Mooney JF (2002) Predictors of red cell transfusion in children and adolescents undergoing spinal fusion surgery. Spine 27:2137–2142
17. Edler A, Murray DJ, Forbes RB (2003) Blood loss during posterior spinal fusion surgery in patients with neuromuscular disease: is there an increased risk? Paediatr Anaesth 13:818–822
18. Hedequist D, Emans J (2007) Congenital scoliosis: a review and update. J Pediatr Orthop 27:106–116
19. Nuwer MR, Dawson EG, Carlson LG et al (1995) Somatosensory evoked potential spinal cord monitoring reduces neurologic deficits after scoliosis surgery: results of a large multicenter survey. Electroencephalogr Clin Neurophysiol 96:6–11
20. Cervellati S, Bettini N, Bianco T, Parisini P (1996) Neurological complications in segmental spinal instrumentation: analysis of 750 patients. Eur Spine J 5:161–166
21. Koka BV, Jeon IS, Andre JM et al (1977) Postintubation croup in children. Anesth Analg 56:501–505

22. Galante D, Pellico G, Federico A et al (2007) Postextubation adverse events in children undergoing general anesthesia. Paediatr Anaesth 17:192, author reply 3
23. Khalil SN, Mankarious R, Campos C et al (1998) Absence or presence of a leak around tracheal tube may not affect postoperative croup in children. Paediatr Anaesth 8:393–396
24. Murat I (2001) Cuffed tubes in children: a 3-year experience in a single institution. Paediatr Anaesth 11:748–749
25. Downes JJ, Raphaely RC (1975) Pediatric intensive care. Anesthesiology 43:238–250
26. Anene O, Meert KL, Uy H et al (1996) Dexamethasone for the prevention of postextubation airway obstruction: a prospective, randomized, double-blind, placebo-controlled trial. Crit Care Med 24:1666–1669
27. Markovitz BP, Randolph AG, Khemani RG (2008) Corticosteroids for the prevention and treatment of post-extubation stridor in neonates, children and adults. Cochrane Database Syst Rev 2008:CD001000.
28. Brandom B (2006) Malignant hyperthermia. In: Davis M (ed) Smith's anesthesia for infants and children, 7th edn. Mosby/Elsevier, Philadelphia, pp 1015–1031
29. Mancuso T (2008) Neuromuscular disorders. In: Holzman RS, Polaner M, (ed). Practical aspects of pediatric anesthesia. Wolters Kluwer/Lippincott Williams & Wilkins, Philadelphia, 547–549

Chapter 32
Critical Care

R.S. Holzman et al., *Pediatric Anesthesiology Review: Clinical Cases for Self-Assessment*,
DOI 10.1007/978-1-4419-1617-4_32, © Springer Science+Business Media, LLC 2010

Acute Respiratory Distress Syndrome (ARDS)

A 4-year old with gram-negative sepsis develops increasing respiratory distress concomitant with antibiotic treatment and her admission to the ICU. What do you think is going on? Why? How does endotoxin release promote ARDS? What are some of the vasoactive mediators involved? How does the release of leukotrienes, tumor necrosis factor (TNF), and prostaglandins involve the pulmonary circulation in ARDS? What implications are there for you as a critical care anesthesiologist? Why? Is there a role for surfactant instillation in such patients? Does surfactant work normally in patients with ARDS? Why/why not? What can you do about it? Will PEEP help? Why? What are the adverse effects of high ranges of PEEP? How can these effects be minimized? Under what circumstances would you consider extracorporeal membrane oxygenation (ECMO)? What about extracorporeal CO_2 removal ($ECCO_2R$)? What effects does ARDS have on shunt (venous admixture)? Are there any effects on Vd/Vt? What are they? At what phase of the disease process? What, if anything, can you do about it?

Acute Respiratory Distress Syndrome (ARDS)

This child may be developing ARDS, Acute Respiratory Distress Syndrome [3, 4]. ARDS is characterized by the following:

1. Acute onset of symptoms
2. Severe respiratory failure with PaO_2/FiO_2 $\leq$200 mmHg regardless of PEEP levels
3. CXR that shows bilateral infiltrates
4. Lack of clinical evidence that LV failure is the etiology of the respiratory distress

In addition, the deterioration of pulmonary function often is associated with a nonpulmonary clinical insult [5]. In pediatrics, the more commonly associated conditions are shock, sepsis, or drowning. Other associated conditions include massive transfusion, smoke inhalation, burns, or trauma [6]. Since sepsis is associated with the development of ARDS, endotoxins released by bacteria, mediators released by inflammatory cells, and other compounds such as complement, products of DIC, prostaglandins, and leukotrienes have all been evaluated for their role in the development of this clinical syndrome. Although the effects of these many mediators are interconnected, endotoxin has been shown to have several effects itself.

Lipopolysaccharide from gram-negative bacteria has been shown to directly affect the integrity of the endothelium and also to stimulate macrophages to release TNF and IL-1 [7]. One source of endotoxin in patients with sepsis and hypotension is thought to be the pulmonary capillary endothelium that is damaged. This damage is caused by the release of many of the mediators mentioned above. Once the integrity of the alveolar-capillary membrane is disrupted, a proteinaceous, hemorrhagic fluid enters the alveolar space. Another effect of some of these mediators, particularly products of arachidonic acid metabolism such as the leukotrienes and prostaglandins, is to contribute to the development of pulmonary hypertension. A cycle of pathology ensues. As hypoxia worsens, the pulmonary artery pressure rises further and with continued release of the various mediators, pulmonary edema worsens and reactivity of the pulmonary vessels to hypoxia also worsens. Although the role(s) of mediators in ARDS is being more and more well characterized, therapy directed toward these compounds is still investigational. Studies of the use of steroids have been disappointing. Steroid administration has not reversed the pathophysiology nor decreased mortality in ARDS [8, 9]. In ARDS many of the pathophysiologic abnormalities are due to diminished activity of surfactant. FRC is reduced and lung compliance is decreased. Surfactant acts to stabilize alveoli. Surfactant keeps surface tension proportional to surface area, allowing smaller alveoli to remain inflated at the same transpulmonary pressure as larger alveoli. Without surfactant, smaller alveoli would empty into larger ones resulting in areas of collapse. In the lab, it has been shown that the surface activity of phospholipids from patients with ARDS is poor. Surfactant administration to preterm newborns with RDS, while not curative, has had some salutary effects on the course of the disease such as decreased mortality, decreased incidence of air leak, and improved oxygenation [6]. Unfortunately, administration of surfactant to patients with ARDS has not affected mortality.

The goal of therapy for patients with ARDS is to maintain adequate oxygen delivery while minimizing the harm of the therapy directed toward achieving that oxygen delivery [10]. Loss of FRC is an important part of the pathophysiology in ARDS. Application of PEEP increases the FRC. The likely mechanism for the increase in FRC is recruitment of previously collapsed terminal alveoli. PEEP also improves the static compliance of the lung. The pulmonary effects of PEEP in patients with ARDS, then, are increased FRC and improved compliance resulting in increased PaO_2 and decreased shunt (Qs/Qt). The improved oxygenation is the result of better blood flow to ventilated alveoli. PEEP may also decrease cardiac output, however, primarily by decreasing venous return. At modest levels of PEEP, increasing intravascular volume may compensate for these deleterious cardiovascular effects. At some point, excessive PEEP will actually decrease oxygen delivery since the fall in cardiac output will exceed the increased oxygen content of the blood. Another deleterious effect of PEEP is the development of pulmonary edema. PEEP lowers pulmonary interstitial pressure, increasing the pressure gradient for an increase in extravascular lung water (EVLW).

Nitric oxide, an inhaled pulmonary vasodilator (iNO), has been administered to patients with ARDS. Since pulmonary arterial hypertension is a large part of the pathophysiology of the syndrome, iNO could be an effective treatment. Because it would only be delivered to well-ventilated parts of the lung, iNO in theory could improve V/Q matching while it lowered PAP. In adult studies, iNO has indeed been shown to decrease PAP and Qs/Qt. There is an emerging experience with iNO administration to children with ARDS but no controlled studies have documented improved survival.

Fluid therapy for children with ARDS can have a significant effect on the course of the illness. While both crystalloid and colloid will increase the intravascular volume initially and both will eventually leak in to the alveoli, there are differences. In general, less colloid will leak into the alveoli. The amount of colloid that leaks into the alveoli depends on the molecular weight of the colloid. Pentastarch leakage into alveoli was less than hetastarch in an animal model of septic shock. Blood administration has many advantages in these patients. Oxygen delivery is increased immediately and cardiac output is increased as preload is augmented. In addition, the PRBCs are much less likely to leave the vascular space in significant amounts compared with colloid molecules or the ions in crystalloid.

While ECMO does not appear to offer advantages in the care of adults with ARDS, it may be of benefit to children with this syndrome. The criteria for institution of this therapy (ECMO is not a treatment) have changed over time but some underlying considerations remain. Among the considerations for determining the suitability of a patient for ECMO are the severity of the lung disease, the reversibility of the lung disease, and the involvement of other organ systems. The severity can be judged using a variety of measures such as the oxygenation index (OI), the A-a gradient, and Qs/Qt. The OI ($MAP \times FiO_2 \times 100/PaO_2$) has been used to evaluate possible ECMO candidates for some time. An OI > 40 was believed to represent >90% risk for mortality. Extracorporeal removal of CO_2 ($ECCO_2R$) has not been shown to benefit adults with ARDS and has not been used much at all in the care of children with ARDS.

Shock/Multiorgan System Failure

A 15-year-old girl is admitted to the ICU with a presumptive diagnosis of toxic shock syndrome. Her blood pressure is 64/20 mmHg, heart rate 142 bpm; she is intubated and mechanically ventilated. After arterial line placement, her arterial blood gas ($FiO_2 = 1.0$) is pH $= 7.12$, $paO_2 = 97$ mmHg, and $paCO_2 = 32$ mmHg. How will you proceed? What do you think is going on? She has no urine output; foley catheter is in place. You place a pulmonary artery line; pulmonary capillary wedge pressure (PCW) is 3 mmHg, PA pressures are elevated at 42/22 mmHg. What now? Should you give sodium bicarbonate? Why not? Will it make the dopamine work better? How does that happen?

Shock/Multiorgan System Failure

This patient's condition meets the criteria for shock. She has evidence of circulatory failure and inadequate tissue perfusion [11]. The clinical diagnosis of shock is supported by the following: tachycardia, hypotension, poor capillary refill, oliguria, decreased pulse pressure, and tachypnea. The shock is probably due to both hypovolemia and maldistribution of the circulating blood volume. Abnormal vasomotor tone will exacerbate the effects of preexisting hypovolemia. She may have inadequate preload due to a variety of factors: recent poor PO intake during the prodrome of the illness and loss of intravascular volume through capillary leak. The distributive aspect to shock in this case results from the endotoxins released in the syndrome of toxic shock. These mediators diminish sympathetic tone and the resulting lowered systemic blood pressure contributes to impaired perfusion of organs. The patient is responding to decreased stroke volume with an increased heart rate but with the low systemic blood pressure, perfusion will be inadequate. The first priority in this situation is to improve cardiac output [7]. Increasing preload should be done first. A rapid infusion of isotonic IV fluid, 20 mL/kg, should begin the improvement. If the patient's perfusion still is inadequate after 40–60 mL/kg of isotonic IV fluid, placement of a CVL should be considered to monitor preload more directly and also to support cardiac function.

The ABG shows a metabolic acidosis, severe hypoxemia, and slight hyperventilation. The patient has an A-a gradient of >500. The $P_A O_2$, the alveolar partial pressure of oxygen, can be calculated with the formula:

$$P_A O_2 = (Fi O_2 \times (760 - 47)) - P_a CO_2 / 0.8$$

$$\text{A-a gradient} = P_A O_2 - P_a O_2$$

For this child, the calculation is:

$$P_A O_2 = (1.0 \times (713)) - (32 / 0.8)$$
$$= 713 - 40$$
$$= 673$$

$$\text{A-a gradient} = P_A O_2 - P_a O_2$$
$$= 673 - 97$$
$$= 576$$

As preload is replenished and cardiac contractility is improved, there should be improvement in PaO_2. If the patient's A-a gradient does not improve as the circulatory disturbances are corrected, the ventilator setting should be adjusted. The patient may have better oxygenation with increased peak inspiratory pressures, a higher PEEP or a change in the I/E ratio. Increases in mean airway pressure will generally increase oxygenation but will also affect venous return. As ventilator settings are adjusted, the cardiovascular parameters must be carefully observed for deterioration.

Neurologic Intensive Care

A 5-year old is admitted to the ICU with a small epidural hematoma and closed head injury. The neurosurgeon wants to observe him, and only go to the OR for evidence of acute deterioration. Do you agree with this? What is the basis for observing a patient with an epidural hematoma? The patient arrives from the ER with an IV of D5 1/2NS. Would you change it? Why? Under what circumstances would you reconstitute the IV fluids? The nurse asks you what position you would like the head of the bed to be in Your answer? Why? What are the considerations in your answer? What is the optimal positioning for a patient with a space occupying lesion and possible elevated intracranial pressure? During the night, the patient becomes whiny and combative, and the parents ask if he can be sedated; do you agree? What may be going on? How would you evaluate? What would you be looking for in the physical exam while awaiting the CT scan? He has a seizure 1 h after eating dinner. How would you treat? Would you use a barbiturate? benzodiazepine? Is phenytoin indicated? Would you use phenytoin or phosphenytoin? Should the patient be intubated? What about using succinylcholine in this setting? Would you? What is your differential diagnosis for the cause of the seizure? Assuming the patient is intubated, how will you prevent rises of intracranial pressure during suctioning and noxious procedures? Why is this important? What is the optimal drug regimen to use in order to blunt the elevation of ICP? He begins to develop "raccoon eyes" and discoloration of the eyelids. Now what do you think? He becomes increasingly difficult to ventilate, with O_2 saturations that are slowly but progressively decreasing and coarse sounding breath sounds, reminiscent of rales. Next step? Diagnostic or therapeutic?

The acidosis is most likely due to impaired delivery of oxygen and substrates to the tissues, the pathophysiologic abnormality in shock states. Correction of the circulatory disturbances will lead to correction of the metabolic acidosis. If severe, acidosis will affect function of many enzymatic systems, including those responsible for myocardial performance. In cases of severe acidosis, drugs such as dopamine that enhance cardiac contractility have severely diminished effectiveness. With a pH seen in the ABG, dopamine is likely to have some effect and improve contractility.

The PCWP reflects left atrial pressure, which, in turn, reflects LV end-diastolic pressure or preload. A PCWP of 3 mmHg in this case indicates a relatively low preload. The PA pressure of 42/2 mmHg is elevated. These numbers together indicate a lower preload with PA hypertension and increased RV afterload. Further treatment will be guided by the child's clinical response to fluid therapy and dopamine, urine output, ABGs, and mixed venous blood gas analysis. If the patient continues to exhibit clinical signs of shock and continues with a base deficit of >6 mEq/L, administration of bicarbonate is indicated. Initial dosing of bicarbonate can be estimated with the formula:

$$mEq\ NaHCO_3 = 0.3 \times (wt\ in\ kg) \times (base\ deficit)$$

Neurologic Intensive Care

Although most epidural hematomas, collection of blood between the skull and the dura, are treated with emergency craniotomy and evacuation of the blood/clot, stable patients with this problem can be managed conservatively [12]. Epidural hematomas are not as common in children as adults, possibly because the dura is adherent to the inner table of the skull, especially at the suture lines. Children with an epidural hematoma have had head injuries severe enough to separate the dura from the skull [13]. The collection of blood is often stopped at a suture unless there is an associated skull fracture that crosses the suture line. Children with epidural hematomas who are managed conservatively must be very carefully monitored. The child should have a repeat CT if any neurologic deterioration is noted [14]. Epidural hematomas that result from venous bleeding may continue to enlarge for up to 24 h. Clinical outcome in children with epidural hematomas is related to the speed of evacuation when there is clinical deterioration. If the child is kept in the PICU and carefully monitored and CT is immediately available, s/he may recover without having to undergo a craniotomy.

Isotonic fluid should be used in children with neurologic injuries [15, 16]. Glucose should be avoided except when it is needed to treat symptomatic hypoglycemia. Glucose administered IV can quickly enter the brain and increase water content and hypotonic IV fluid administration can also increase brain water content. In this child with an intracranial mass, therapy should be directed to minimizing the volume of the intracranial contents. The patient's optimal head position would be head up, at 30° and in the midline. This position allows the best cerebral venous drainage, keeping the cerebral blood volume low. If mechanical ventilation

is instituted, airway pressures used should be kept low since elevated airway pressures decrease cerebral venous drainage [17].

A change in the patient's condition, particularly his mental status, is cause for alarm. He should not be sedated. While a CT is arranged, he should be evaluated for signs of increased intracranial pressure. If the epidural hematoma is enlarging and the intracranial pressure is rising, the child will exhibit altered mental status, hyperventilation, and systemic hypertension [15]. Cranial nerve signs may be noted as well. Palsy of the third nerve may occur as it is pressed between the falx and the expanding brain leading to asymmetry of the pupils.

Posttraumatic seizures occur regularly in children who experience head trauma [18, 19]. The more severe the trauma, the greater the incidence. Following severe trauma, up to 30% of children will have seizures. Children who have hematomas or depressed skull fractures are at higher risk for the development of seizures. Seizures should be treated quickly and effectively. Oxygen consumption is greatly increased during seizures as is ICP. IV benzodiazepines will stop most seizures. An alternative would be an administration of IV barbiturates. In treating the seizures, respiratory drive may be impaired. It may be prudent to protect the patient's airway and begin mechanical ventilation. Another reason to intubate the patient and begin ventilation is that the child will likely soon be taken to the OR. The seizures may indicate that the hematoma has enlarged and even if it has remained the same size, surgery and evacuation may be indicated. Intubation of this patient presents several problems. He has a full stomach and raised ICP. Even if he had not recently eaten, he should be treated as though he has a full stomach since he had suffered head trauma earlier and that event would have resulted in delayed gastric emptying. During laryngoscopy and intubation, every effort should be made to minimize, if not eliminate, hemodynamic perturbations. Intracranial pressure will increase if blood pressure increases, if $PaCO_2$ increases, or if PaO_2 decreases. The use of an appropriate dose of hypnotic is essential to prevent hypertension and tachycardia. Thiopental offers a good combination of decreasing ICP and $CMRO_2$. The use of succinylcholine as the muscle relaxant to facilitate intubation is controversial. This relaxant can increase ICP in patients with reduced intracranial compliance. The mechanism is most likely a reflex increase in cerebral blood flow resulting from increased afferent muscle spindle activity. The increase in ICP caused by succinylcholine can be blunted by prior administration of a defasciculating dose of a nondepolarizing relaxant. Hyperkalemia has been seen after administration of succinylcholine in patients with various CNS problems including closed head injury. Although the exact period of vulnerability is unknown, it does not begin until at least 24–48 h after the injury. The advantage of the use of succinylcholine in this situation is its very rapid onset that minimizes the chance for aspiration of gastric contents or the development of hypoxemia/hypercarbia. Once the child is intubated, it is important to provide the brain with adequate cerebral perfusion pressure (CPP=CVP or ICP–MAP). This is done by maintaining systemic arterial pressure and minimizing intracranial pressure. Often, these patients are best cared for sedated and relaxed. An arterial line is needed and often an intracranial pressure monitor as well. In the absence of an ICP monitor, the patients should be kept in the 30° head-up midline position and any signs of excess activity of the sympathetic nervous system treated with IV sedatives, opioids, or barbiturates. When these agents are administered, it is important to prevent excessive lowering of the blood pressure.

Glasgow Coma Score

What is it and why is it important? Is the outcome of children any better than adults if they have the same GCS? Is there an age break for this? What is the significance of the fact that below age 7, there is no better pediatric outcome?

Raccoon eyes, periorbital ecchymoses, are one of the signs of a basilar skull fracture. Other clinical signs of this type of skull fracture are Battle's sign, retroauricular or mastoid ecchymosis, blood behind the tympanic membrane, and CSF otorrhea or rhinorrhea. Since the cribriform plate is disrupted in patients with basilar skull fractures, placement of tubes in the nose is to be avoided. Endotracheal and gastric tubes should be placed through the mouth. With conservative management, many patients with isolated basilar skull fractures do well. The most common morbidity is a persistent CSF leak.

Worsening pulmonary function in this setting may be due to the development of neurogenic pulmonary edema (NPE) [20], which can develop anytime from 2 h after the head injury to several days afterward. Although not certain, it is thought that a transient increase in sympathetic tone is responsible for the development of neurogenic pulmonary edema. This sympathetic discharge leads to increased PVR, accompanied by damage to the endothelium allowing leakage of fluid into the alveoli. The presentation includes hypoxemia, CXR findings of diffuse fluffy infiltrates but normal to low cardiac filling pressures. In most cases, neurogenic pulmonary edema resolves on its own. Pulmonary edema can significantly complicate the management of patients with raised ICP, however. Hypoxia must be avoided in all patients but the increase in cerebral blood flow that results from a lower PaO_2 can be very deleterious to those with raised ICP or limited intracranial compliance. The application of high PEEP to improve oxygenation will decrease cerebral venous drainage, again affecting ICP.

Glasgow Coma Score

The Glasgow Coma Scale was developed, surprisingly, in Glasgow, as a tool for quickly assessing the level of consciousness of patients with impaired consciousness or coma. The score can be done quickly and repeatedly as clinical conditions change. Various modifications have been made for use in children [21]. One limitation of the score is that it does not include an assessment of brainstem function. The GCS is useful for prognosticating pediatric head trauma. A child whose GSC is <5 has a relatively poor prognosis. While children with GCS 4–5 are likely to survive, approximately 50% of these children will have cognitive, academic or other neurologic deficits. Children with a GCS <3 have a 40–60% mortality and if such a child survives s/he will be very likely to have significant permanent neurologic deficits. Children who have a GCS of >6 have an 80–90% chance of recovery with minimal neurologic deficit.

Pancreatitis

A 3-year old is admitted to the ICU following blunt abdominal injury after hitting a wall and falling over her tricycle. She is in intense abdominal pain and is not intubated. She has a sentinel loop in her epigastrium on a flat plate X-ray of the abdomen (KUB). What is the significance of that? Her CT scan obtained via the ED shows a fractured pancreas. What do you think? Anything you would watch out for? What are the consequences of the release of pancreatic enzymes into the retro-peritoneal space? Does she need invasive cardiovascular monitoring for this problem? It hurts her to breathe. Is there anything you can do to help? She is developing atelectasis. What will you do to treat this problem? How will you support her intra-vascular volume? Why is this important? Under what circumstances should surgery be considered? Her serum calcium is now 6.4 mg%; is that important? Why did it happen? What symptoms would you look for? What could you do about it? What if her BUN is rising (let us say it is 24 mg% 16 h after admission)? Why is this important? What can you do about it? Why does this happen?

Activity	Best response	Score
Eye opening	Spontaneous	4
	To verbal stimuli	3
	To pain	2
	None	1
Verbal	Oriented	5
	Confused	4
	Inappropriate words	3
	Nonspecific sounds	2
	None	1
Motor	Follows commands	6
	Localizes pain	5
	Withdraws from pain	4
	Flexion to pain	3
	Extension to pain	2
	None	1

Pancreatitis

The most immediate threat to a child after blunt abdominal trauma is bleeding from injury to the spleen or liver. Other organs may also be injured. The pancreas and duodenum may be injured when a child suffers abdominal trauma from a high-speed deceleration or from child abuse. The hollow viscera may also be lacerated or torn from sites of attachment such as the ligament of Treitz. The evaluation of a child who has suffered blunt abdominal trauma must include a search for injuries to the GU system and the bony pelvis, the ribs, and the lumbar spine and sacrum. The child in this case suffered a relatively high-speed deceleration when she crashed against the handlebars of her bicycle. Her abdominal pain may be due to any of the injuries mentioned or a combination. CT scanning has become an essential part of the evaluation of trauma patients. Not only will this test reveal the presence of injuries to the liver or spleen, but it also can be used to visualize the kidneys and pancreas. The finding of a sentinel loop on KUB indicates the presence of an ileus. It is likely that there is inflammation in the epigastric area as a result of the trauma. If there was damage done to the pancreas in the event and pancreatic enzymes were released, a localized ileus is likely. Another KUB finding seen in acute pancreatic damage when the transverse and descending colon are affected is the so-called colon cutoff sign. The CT findings confirm the diagnosis of fractured pancreas. It is important that damage to the liver and spleen is ruled out by the CT.

Hemolytic Uremic Syndrome

A 4-year old with a 5-day history of diarrhea that seemed to be getting better has just been admitted to the ICU from the pediatrician's office with the following findings:

Pallor
Anuria
Tachycardia
Irritability
Ataxia
Tremors

His laboratory findings reveal a Hct of 24, BUN of 46, platelet count of 76,000, and a peripheral smear with evidence of microangiopathic hemolysis.

What do you think is going on? Whom would you consult? The renal service recommends dialysis. What is the patient's prognosis if dialysis continues for >2 weeks? Is there a risk for chronic nephropathy following 5 days of dialysis with apparent resolution?

The release of pancreatic enzymes can be quite harmful in these patients. The laboratory evaluation of this child should include serum calcium, amylase, lipase, and a CBC. The laboratory evaluation can help with prognostication. A poor prognosis is associated with serum calcium <7.5 mg/dL, a WBC count of 20,000, a PaO_2 of 60 mmHg, a BUN >20 mg/dL, and a base deficit >4 mEq/L. If the prognosis appears to be poor, management should be more aggressive [22–24]. It might be prudent to intubate the trachea and also institute invasive hemodynamic monitoring sooner rather than later. She will splint her breathing due to pain, and develop respiratory insufficiency. As the inflammation caused by the pancreatic enzymes released into the peritoneum increases, there will be greater and greater fluid transudation into the peritoneum, leading to intravascular volume depletion. The etiology of the hypocalcemia seen in these patients is due to saponifaction of fatty acids, sequestration of calcium in bones, and hypomagnesemia. Calcium is involved in cardiac conduction, neuromuscular transmission, and muscle contraction and all these are altered by hypocalcemia. Patients with hypocalcemia can exhibit cardiac arrthymias, a prolonged Q–T interval and seizures. They may experience tingling, numbness, and muscle weakness. Treatment is not only with IV calcium, as gluconate or chloride, but magnesium as well. If this child has an elevated BUN, it indicates prerenal azotemia, likely from fluid loss into the peritoneal space. The response should be to increase her intravascular volume. Pancreatic rest should be undertaken while she is watched and monitored carefully as described. A nasogastric tube should be placed and hyperalimentation should be started soon since these patients often must be kept NPO for several days or more than 1 week while the pancreas heals.

Hemolytic Uremic Syndrome

This patient has Hemolytic-Uremic Syndrome (HUS). He has had a typical prodrome of several days of diarrhea. In some cases, the diarrhea is bloody. HUS is characterized by microangiopathic hemolytic anemia, thrombocytopenia, and renal cortical injury. This condition occurs in children between 6 months and 4 years of age and it may occur sporadically or in epidemics in the USA. In other countries such as Argentina, HUS is endemic. The exact etiology is not known, although toxins have been implicated in many cases of HUS [25]. The syndrome is seen following colitis caused by certain E. coli or Shigella. Several viruses, such as EBV, influenza, and coxsackie, have also caused HUS. In most cases, it seems that the initial event in the development of HUS is injury to the vascular endothelium with subsequent platelet activation. Adhesion of platelets to the damaged endothelium leads to thrombocytopenia. Damage to RBCs during passage through damaged vascular beds results in the development of microangiopathic hemolytic anemia. The mechanism of renal damage also involves endothelial injury, specifically the endothelium of the glomerular capillaries. The laboratory evaluation of this patient should include, in addition to those tests noted above, a full set of electrolytes and evaluation of the coagulation system. Children with HUS may be dehydrated due to the

diarrhea. In addition there may be significant electrolyte abnormalities such as hyper- or hyponatremia, hyperkalemia, metabolic acidosis, and hypocalcemia. Seizures may be seen in affected children. There is no specific treatment for HUS other than careful supportive management of fluids and blood pressure and transfusion of blood products as the clinical condition dictates. Many children with HUS require dialysis but most children do recover and have normal renal function. Children who have had HUS should be followed for the development of hypertension or chronic renal failure. The best outcome is seen in children who have epidemic HUS with the typical prodrome. Familial cases or children who develop HUS at older ages do not have as favorable a prognosis.

Isopropyl Alcohol Poisoning

A 2-year old accidentally ingested about an ounce of isopropyl alcohol she happened to find laying around. Is this serious [1]? Why? Is isopropyl alcohol more toxic than ethanol? Methanol? Is it absorbed rapidly or slowly? She is admitted to the ICU, lethargic, confused, and stuporous. She appears to have intense abdominal pain, and is intermittently retching/vomiting. Is this bad? Her blood alcohol level is 110 mg%. One of the coworkers suggests ethanol therapy. Is this likely to be effective? Is there a role for ethanol therapy in any other alcohol poisoning? Is acute hemodialysis effective [2]? Should you just support and wait it out?

Isopropyl Alcohol Poisoning (1)

1. The toxic dose of isopropyl alcohol is approximately 1 mL/kg of the 70% solution in common use. An ounce ingestion (30 mL) in a 2-year old who probably weights between 10 and 15 kg will very likely lead to toxicity. Nearly one-fifth of an ingested dose is metabolized in the liver to acetone, another toxic CNS depressant. This child is exhibiting the usual signs of alcohol ingestion: CNS depression and GI disturbances. Occasionally, children develop hematemesis from gastritis and recurrent vomiting. With severe overdoses of alcohol, CNS depression is more significant and affected children will show hypotension, hypothermia, hypoventilation, and even respiratory arrest.

   Alcohol (ethanol, isopropyl alcohol, ethylene glycol) poisoning in pediatrics occurs either accidentally when a young child ingests the material or when an adolescent ingests it as an ethanol substitute or as a suicide attempt.

   Among the alcohols, ethylene glycol and methanol are the most toxic, followed by isopropyl alcohol (isopropanol) then ethanol in order of decreasing toxicity. All of the commonly ingested alcohols are absorbed from the GI tract very rapidly. The laboratory evaluation of patients in whom alcohol ingestion is known or suspected should include serum glucose and electrolytes, measurement of the alcohol level itself, and also a direct (i.e., by freezing point depression) measurement of the osmolality. Hypoglycemia is commonly seen in children who have ingested alcohol. With ingestion of alcohols other than isopropyl alcohol, there is often a significant anion gap. In children who have ingested ethylene glycol or methanol, an elevated anion-gap metabolic acidosis is a common lab finding. Ketosis, due to the presence of acetone, is seen in children who have ingested isopropyl alcohol. The finding of ketones in the blood without acidosis is suggestive of isopropyl alcohol ingestion. With any of the alcohols, however, an osmolar gap is seen, with the alcohols and their metabolites accounting for the increased actual osmolarity.

   Isopropyl alcohol is an irritant to the GI tract. Children who have ingested isopropyl alcohol exhibit abdominal pain, nausea and vomiting, and hematemesis secondary to gastritis.

   Treatment with activated charcoal is generally not effective because of this rapid absorption. Ethanol is a specific antidote for poisoning with either ethylene glycol or methanol. In cases of poisoning with methanol, toxicity is due to the formation of the metabolites formaldehyde and formic acid through the action of alcohol dehydrogenase on methanol. In the case of poisoning by ethylene glycol, the toxic metabolites formed by the action of alcohol dehydrogenase are glycoaldehyde and glycolic acid. In either situation, ingestion of methanol or ethylene glycol, administration of ethanol will slow the production of toxic metabolites by competing for the enzyme alcohol dehydrogenase, thereby decreasing the formation of the metabolites. With isopropyl alcohol poisoning, the toxicity is due to the isopropyl alcohol itself or acetone. The enzyme alcohol

dehydrogenase is not involved in the formation of acetone from isopropyl alcohol, so administration of ethanol to this child would only worsen the situation.

Hemodialysis is quite effective in removing isopropyl alcohol from the blood, but in most cases its use is unnecessary. Supportive treatment is recommended for most children with isopropyl alcohol poisoning, even when the blood alcohol level is as high as 200 mg%, a level associated with coma. In children who have hypotension is addition to CNS depression or in whom the blood alcohol level is >300 mg%, hemodialysis is indicated.

	Ethanol	Methanol	Isopropyl alcohol	Ethylene glycol
Toxicity	+	+++	++	+++
Metabolic acidosis	+	+++	−	+++
Osmolar gap	+	+	+	+
Anion gap	−	+	−	−
Ketosis	−	−	+	−
Rx	Support	Ethanol	Support	Ethanol
Clinical	Gastritis	Retinal edema	Gastritis	Renal failure

Annotated References

1. Marcadante KJ (2006) Respiratory failure. The acutely injured child. In: Kliegman RM, Marcdante KJ, Jenson HB, Behrman RE (eds) Nelson essentials of pediatrics, 5th edn. Elsevier Saunders, Philadelphia, pp 184–187.
   This chapter reviews acute respiratory failure from any cause in children including epidemiology, clinical and laboratory evaluation, management, and complications.

2. Marraro GA (2005) Protective lung strategies during artificial ventilation in children. Paediatr Anaesth 106:1813–1819
   This paper reviews various recruitment and ventilation strategies for patients with ARDS and included CT scans of adults during various respiratory maneuvers. Also discussed are the concepts of barotrauma and volutrauma.

3. Shock-Marcadante KJ (2006) The acutely injured child. In: Kliegman RM, Marcdante KJ, Jenson HB, Behrman RE (eds) Nelson essentials of pediatrics, 5th edn. Elseivier Saunders, Philadelphia, pp 187–195
   This chapter reviews the following categories of shock: hypovolemic, distributive, cardiogenic, distributive, and obstructive shock. General treatment principles and specific interventions for the various types of shock are discussed.

4. Holzman, R (2008) Trauma and casualty management. In: Holzman R, Mancuso TJ, Polaner DM (eds) A practical approach to pediatric anesthesia, 1st edn. Wolters Kluwer/Lippincott Williams and Wilkins, Philadelphia, p 637
   This chapter reviews general principles in the care of pediatric trauma victims as well as management of specific types of traumatic injuries including head injury,

spinal cord injury, and abdominal injuries. Also discussed is the organization of trauma centers for mass casualty situations.

5. Corrigan JJ, Boineau FG (2001) Hemolytic-uremic syndrome. Pediatr Rev 22(11):365–369
This paper reviews the epidemiology and management of HUS in children and also the immediate and longer term prognosis for recovery from this condition.

References

1. Riordan M, Rylance G, Berry K (2002) Poisoning in children 5: rare and dangerous poisons. Arch Dis Child 87:407–410
2. Trullas JC, Aguilo S, Castro P, Nogue S (2004) Life-threatening isopropyl alcohol intoxication: is hemodialysis really necessary? Vet Hum Toxicol 46:282–284
3. Ware LB, Matthay MA (2000) The acute respiratory distress syndrome. N Engl J Med 342:1334–1349
4. Bernard GR (2005) Acute respiratory distress syndrome: a historical perspective. Am J Respir Crit Care Med 172:798–806
5. Flori HR, Glidden DV, Rutherford GW, Matthay MA (2005) Pediatric acute lung injury: prospective evaluation of risk factors associated with mortality. Am J Respir Crit Care Med 171:995–1001
6. Pfenninger J (1996) Acute respiratory distress syndrome (ARDS) in neonates and children. Paediatr Anaesth 6:173–181
7. Hotchkiss RS, Karl IE (2003) The pathophysiology and treatment of sepsis. N Engl J Med 348:138–150
8. Seam N (2008) Corticosteroids for septic shock. N Engl J Med 358:2068–2069, author reply 70–1
9. Bendel S, Karlsson S, Pettila V et al (2008) Free cortisol in sepsis and septic shock. Anesth Analg 106:1813–1819
10. Marraro GA (2005) Protective lung strategies during artificial ventilation in children. Paediatr Anaesth 15:630–637
11. Carre JE, Singer M (2008) Cellular energetic metabolism in sepsis: the need for a systems approach. Biochim Biophys Acta 1777:763–771
12. Karasu A, Sabanci PA, Izgi N et al (2008) Traumatic epidural hematomas of the posterior cranial fossa. Surg Neurol 69:247–251, dicussion 51–52
13. Trenchs V, Curcoy AI, Morales M et al (2008) Retinal haemorrhages in- head trauma resulting from falls: differential diagnosis with non-accidental trauma in patients younger than 2 years of age. Childs Nerv Syst 24:815–820
14. Hayashi T, Kameyama M, Imaizumi S et al (2007) Acute epidural hematoma of the posterior fossa–cases of acute clinical deterioration. Am J Emerg Med 25:989–995
15. Orliaguet GA, Meyer PG, Baugnon T (2008) Management of critically ill children with traumatic brain injury. Paediatr Anaesth 18:455–461
16. Jussen D, Papaioannou C, Heimann A et al (2008) Effects of hypertonic/hyperoncotic treatment and surgical evacuation after acute subdural hematoma in rats. Crit Care Med 36:543–549
17. Taplu A, Gokmen N, Erbayraktar S et al (2003) Effects of pressure- and volume-controlled inverse ratio ventilation on haemodynamic variables, intracranial pressure and cerebral perfusion pressure in rabbits: a model of subarachnoid haemorrhage under isoflurane anaesthesia. Eur J Anaesthesiol 20:690–696

18. Wang HC, Chang WN, Chang HW et al (2008) Factors predictive of outcome in posttraumatic seizures. J Trauma 64:883–888
19. Frend V, Chetty M (2007) Dosing and therapeutic monitoring of phenytoin in young adults after neurotrauma: are current practices relevant? Clin Neuropharmacol 30:362–369
20. Sedy J, Zicha J, Kunes J et al (2008) Mechanisms of neurogenic pulmonary edema development. Physiol Res 57:499–506
21. Holzman R (2008) Trauma and casualty management. In: Holzman R, Mancuso TJ, Polaner DM (eds) A practical approach to pediatric anesthesia, 1st edn. Wolters Kluwer/Lippincott Williams and Wilkins, Philadelphia, p 637
22. Jackson WD (2001) Pancreatitis: etiology, diagnosis, and management. Curr Opin Pediatr 13:447–451
23. Pitchumoni CS, Patel NM, Shah P (2005) Factors influencing mortality in acute pancreatitis: can we alter them? J Clin Gastroenterol 39:798–814
24. Alvarez Calatayud G, Bermejo F, Morales JL et al (2003) Acute pancreatitis in childhood. Rev Esp Enferm Dig 95:40–44, 5–8
25. Zheng XL, Sadler JE (2008) Pathogenesis of thrombotic microangiopathies. Annu Rev Pathol 3:249–277

Index

Printed by Printforce, the Netherlands